Alternative Methodologies for the Safety Evaluation of Chemicals in the Cosmetic Industry

Nicola Loprieno
Science Faculty
University of Pisa
Pisa, Italy

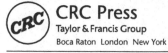
CRC Press
Taylor & Francis Group
Boca Raton London New York

CRC Press is an imprint of the
Taylor & Francis Group, an **informa** business

CRC Press
Taylor & Francis Group
6000 Broken Sound Parkway NW, Suite 300
Boca Raton, FL 33487-2742

Reissued 2019 by CRC Press

A Library of Congress record exists under LC control number:

Publisher's Note
The publisher has gone to great lengths to ensure the quality of this reprint but points out that some imperfections in the original copies may be apparent.

Disclaimer
The publisher has made every effort to trace copyright holders and welcomes correspondence from those they have been unable to contact.

ISBN 13: 978-0-367-24662-4 (hbk)
ISBN 13: 978-0-367-24663-1 (pbk)
ISBN 13: 978-0-429-28376-5 (ebk)

Visit the Taylor & Francis Web site at http://www.taylorandfrancis.com and the
CRC Press Web site at http://www.crcpress.com

PREFACE

As I read through the text of this book, I was struck by the fact that it forms an ideal transition between the beginning of the use of *in vitro* sciences as applied to toxicology and the beginning of the discipline of *in vitro* toxicology. The first papers and symposium programs that began to share the science of *in vitro* sciences as applied to toxicology are found in the mid-1970s and the first congress held at the end of the 1970s. Now some 20 years later, Professor Loprieno presents us with a magnificent categorization and presentation of information available for the evaluation of safety using *in vitro* techniques.

The cosmetic industry, throughout the world, has been a highly self-regulated industry providing quality products with a remarkable absence of toxicity. Societal pressures generating within the scientific community as well as the well-known social activism of the animal protectionists have led to the development of an incredible number of assays that can be used not only for the cosmetic industry but for product development and safety evaluation across all industry.

Directives 86/609/EEC and 93/35/EEC issued by the Council of Ministers of the European Economic Community, raise the need for quality *in vitro* methods to a new level. The latter directive, at its strike date of 1998, will force new practices for safety evaluation of personal care products throughout the world.

With this as the backdrop for Professor Loprieno's book, he has provided a remarkably comprehensive and complete look at the entire field. He thus provides the foundation for the next phase of significant growth for this discipline.

In his introductory comments, Professor Loprieno provides an excellent history of the approach of the European Communities. Because of his intimate knowledge of this area, the reader is provided an understanding of the developments that resulted in the legislation and thus has a better foundation on which to judge future developments.

The quantity and quality of information provided in the pages of this book are truly remarkable. The tables, the outlines, the lists, and the bibliography are magnificently comprehensive and complete. The book is being kept smaller in size than would be required for this amount of information by the use of outline form and tables that provide detailed information. This is a very scholarly work in a format that makes it extremely useful, not only for the present but as we move into more advanced and significant developments that will occur during the next decade.

Because of Professor Loprieno's long-standing personal involvement in many of these areas, one gets a global perspective of the field. Not only do the presentations provide a basic primer for the newly interested, but they provide exciting details for the serious student. One of the delightful aspects of reading through this book is the tremendous number of important quotes presented in the text from the entire field. As I read the text, I knew I was being treated to the author's thoughts and judgments regarding individual methods, how various aspects of the field developed and the important crossroads.

An additional understanding results from the presentation. Professor Loprieno points out that this is just the beginning. There are many methods we will need to develop that will be more sophisticated and more specific.

Each method that is presented is consistent in its format, training the reader to easily find the specific information the reader wants.

The concluding chapters of the book present the developing Galileo Data Bank, an important newly developed resource. Although the role of any database being developed is not yet fully clear, the Galileo Data Bank provides important and accessible data. It is an appropriate conclusion to this book as we move from the beginning of the field to more fully defining the discipline.

Professor Loprieno has written an important work that is exceedingly comprehensive, detailed, and remarkably accurate. This volume is a major contribution to the field.

Alan M. Goldberg, Ph.D.
Baltimore, Maryland
December 1994

ACKNOWLEDGMENTS

The author wishes to thank Dr. Gregorio Loprieno, M.D., Ph.D., for his collaboration and support during the development of this book, as well as for the selection and processing of the toxicity data of the Galileo Data Bank; Dr. Antonio Cecchi for typing and revising the English translation of the book; and, finally, Ms. Patrizia Lugo for her valuable suggestions in arranging and distributing information contained herein.

Also, the author is particularly in debt to Mr. Dimitry Angelis and Mr. Michael Van Beek, members of the EU-Commission, for their continuous stimulation in his interest in understanding the correlation between the scientific principles of the safety evaluation and the European Regulation in the field of cosmetics.

Considerable input to the development of the present book was represented by several technical reports prepared by the author to the EU-Commission, of which he is in debt to Mr. W. De Klerck, head of the EU-Unit 4 (Quality and Distribution of products).

ABOUT THE AUTHOR

Nicola Loprieno is, since 1975, a full professor of genetics at the Science Faculty of the University of Pisa, Italy, from which he graduated.

His research interest always has been in the field of chemical and radiation mutagenesis; he has worked in laboratories in the United Kingdom, Switzerland, and Sweden. His studies are reported in more than 200 scientific papers published in international papers and books.

He has been president of the Italian Association of Genetics, the European Environmental Mutagen Society, and the Italian Society for Environmental Mutagenesis.

He has participated as an expert in working groups of the International Agency for Research on Cancer (IARC) in Lyon, France, the World Health Organization (WHO) in Geneva, Switzerland and the Organization for Economic Cooperation and Development (OECD) in Paris, France.

At present, he is a member of both the Advisory Committee for Cosmetology in Brussels, Belgium and the Scientific Committee of the European Centre for Validation of Alternative Methodologies (ECVAM) in Ispra, Italy.

Pharmacology and Toxicology: Basic and Clinical Aspects

Mannfred A. Hollinger, Series Editor
University of California, Davis

Published Titles

Alternative Methodologies for the Safety Evaluation of Chemicals in the Cosmetic Industry, Nicola Loprieno

Angiotensin II Receptors, Volume I: Molecular Biology, Biochemistry, Pharmacology, and Clinical Perspectives, Robert R. Ruffolo, Jr.

Angiotensin II Receptors, Volume II: Medicinal Chemistry, Robert R. Ruffolo, Jr.

Basis of Toxicity Testing, Donald J. Ecobichon

Beneficial and Toxic Effects of Aspirin, Susan E. Feinman

Biological Approaches to Rational Drug Design, David B. Weiner and William V. Williams

Biopharmaceutics of Ocular Drug Delivery, Peter Edman

Chemical and Structural Approaches to Rational Drug Design, David B. Weiner and William V. Williams

Direct Allosteric Control of Glutamate Receptors, M. Palfreyman, I. Reynolds, and P. Skolnick

Genomic and Non-Genomic Effects of Aldosterone, Martin Wehling

Handbook of Pharmacokinetic and Pharmacodynamic Correlation, Hartmut Derendorf

Human Drug Metabolism from Molecular Biology to Man, Elizabeth Jeffreys

Human Growth Hormone Pharmacology: Basic and Clinical Aspects, Kathleen T. Shiverick and Arlan Rosenbloom

In Vitro *Methods of Toxicology*, Ronald R. Watson

Inflammatory Cells and Mediators in Bronchial Asthma, Devendra K. Agrawal and Robert G. Townley

Peroxisome Proliferators: Unique Inducers of Drug-Metabolizing Enzymes, David E. Moody

Pharmacology of the Skin, Hasan Mukhtar

Placental Toxicology, B. V. Rama Sastry

Platelet Activating Factor Receptor: Signal Mechanisms and Molecular Biology, Shivendra D. Shukla

Preclinical and Clinical Modulation of Anticancer Drugs, Kenneth D. Tew, Peter Houghton, and Janet Houghton

Stealth Liposomes, Danilo Lasic and Frank Marti

TAXOL®: Science and Applications, Matthew Suffness

Pharmacology and Toxicology: Basic and Clinical Aspects

Mannfred A. Hollinger, Series Editor
University of California, Davis

Forthcoming Titles

Alcohol Consumption, Cancer and Birth Defects: Mechanisms Involved in Increased Risk Associated with Drinking, Anthony J. Garro

Animal Models of Mucosal Inflammation, Timothy S. Gaginella

Antibody Therapeutics, William J. Harris and John R. Adair

Brain Mechanisms and Psychotropic Drugs, A. Baskys and G. Remington

Chemoattractant Ligands and Their Receptors, Richard Horuk

CNS Injuries: Cellular Responses and Pharmacological Strategies, Martin Berry and Ann Logan

Drug Delivery Systems, V. V. Ranade

Handbook of Mammalian Models in Biomedical Research, David B. Jack

Handbook of Methods in Gastrointestinal Pharmacology, Timothy S. Gaginella

Handbook of Pharmacology of Aging, 2nd Edition, Jay Roberts

Handbook of Theoretical Models in Biomedical Research, David B. Jack

Immunopharmaceuticals, Edward S. Kimball

Muscarinic Receptor Subtypes in Smooth Muscle, Richard M. Eglen

Neural Control of Airways, Peter J. Barnes

Pharmacological Effects of Ethanol on the Nervous System, Richard A. Deitrich

Pharmacological Regulation of Gene Expression in the CNS, Kalpana Merchant

Pharmacology in Exercise and Sport, Satu M. Somani

Pharmacology of Intestinal Secretion, Timothy S. Gaginella

Phospholipase A2 in Clinical Inflammation: Endogenous Regulation and Pathophysiological Actions, Keith B. Glaser and Peter Vadas

Placental Pharmacology, B. V. Rama Sastry

Receptor Characterization and Regulation, Devendra K. Agrawal

Receptor Dynamics in Neural Development, Christopher A. Shaw

Ryanodine Receptors, Vincenzo Sorrentino

Serotonin and Gastrointestinal Function, Timothy S. Gaginella and James J. Galligan

Targeted Delivery of Imaging Agents, Vladimir P. Torchilin

Therapeutic Modulation of Cytokines, M.W. Bodner and Brian Henderson

FOREWORD

This book introduces goals and approaches used in the field of European administrative regulation* for the control of chemical substances in the cosmetic sector in order to protect consumers' health by preventing unexpected consequent toxic effects. The book then critically inspects the various methodologies proposed by the toxicological scientific research as alternatives to the present use of animals.

The perspectives pointed out in the conclusions were reached while keeping in mind the operational strategies necessary for putting into practice the principles indicated in Council Directive 86/609/EEC, as well as in Council Directive 93/35/EEC, which amends for the sixth time the law regulating the production of cosmetic products in the European Communities (Council Directive 76/768/EEC) approved on July 14, 1993.

The guidelines of some *in vitro* toxicology tests based on extensive experimental studies published in the current scientific literature are also presented, according to the format already developed for similar tests approved for the *in vitro* genotoxicity test by the Commission of the European Communities or by the Organization for Economic Cooperation and Development. Examples of batteries including different methods applied to the safety evaluation of cosmetics are presented, after having listed and discussed the programs in development for the validation of alternative methodologies.

The basis for an *in vitro* toxicology database (the Galileo Data Bank) also is presented with the list of chemicals tested by means of different methodologies and examples of results obtained for groups of chemicals and formulations.

---

* The principal administrative bodies referred to in this work are the Council of Ministers and the Commission of the European Communities. There are three Communities — Economic (Common Market), Coal and Steel, and Atomic Energy (Euratom). Both the Council and the Commission issue Directives and Decisions on behalf of the collective Communities, which comprise 15 full members (see Chapter 1) and 60 affiliated nations.

TABLE OF CONTENTS

Chapter 1
INTRODUCTION 1
  1.1 Legislative Basis 1
  1.2 Cosmetic Ingredients 5

Chapter 2
THE ROLE OF TOXICOLOGY 9

Chapter 3
ANIMAL TOXICITY STUDIES 13
  3.1 Acute Toxicity Studies 13
  3.2 Dermal Irritation Studies 13
      3.2.1 Skin Irritation 14
      3.2.2 Skin Sensitization 14
      3.2.3 Photoallergic Reactions 14
      3.2.4 Phototoxicity 14
  3.3 Ocular Toxicity Studies 15
  3.4 Subacute, Subchronic, and Chronic Studies 15
  3.5 Carcinogenicity Studies 16
  3.6 Teratogenicity and Reproduction Toxicity Studies 16
  3.7 Toxicokinetic Studies 17
  3.8 Skin Absorption 17
  3.9 Mutagenicity Studies 17
  3.10 Animals Needed for Safety Evaluation of a Cosmetic Ingredient 19
  3.11 *In Vivo* Toxicity Testing Guidelines 20

Chapter 4
ALTERNATIVE METHODOLOGIES TO ANIMAL TESTING 25
  4.1 Acute Toxicity 27
  4.2 Dermal Irritation 29
      4.2.1 Physiochemical Analysis of the Properties of Chemicals Being
            Tested 30
      4.2.2 Precipitation (Turbidity) Test Systems 30
      4.2.3 Cell Culture Methods 30
      4.2.4 Tissue Culture Method Utilizing Epidermal Slices or Skin Explants 30
  4.3 Eye Irritation (Mucous Membrane) 31
  4.4 Structure-Activity Relationship Studies 37
      4.4.1 Chemical Descriptors 38
      4.4.2 Toxicological Data 38
      4.4.3 QSAR Techniques 39
  4.5 Teratogenicity 41
      4.5.1 Cell Cultures 41
      4.5.2 Organ Cultures 41
      4.5.3 Whole Embryo Cultures 41
  4.6 Genotoxicity and Carcinogenicity 42

Chapter 5
GUIDELINES FOR *IN VITRO* TOXICITY ASSAYS 45

Chapter 6
FUTURE DEVELOPMENTS 183
   6.1   Alternative Methodologies: State of the Art 183
   6.2   Methodologies Standardization 184
   6.3   Methodology Specificity 186
   6.4   Methodology Predictivity 186
   6.5   Alternative Methods: Perspectives 187
        6.5.1   Standardization of Specific Methodologies for the Predictive
                Evaluation of Potential Toxic Effects of Chemical Substances 188
        6.5.2   Implementation of a Database for the Sector of Cosmetic
                Ingredients 188
        6.5.3   Organization of a Database of Currently Available Results for the
                Evaluation of Safety of Cosmetic Ingredients Obtained or Being
                Developed with Alternative Methodologies 190
        6.5.4   Validation Studies on Alternative Methodologies 190

Chapter 7
IN VITRO TOXICITY DATABASE 207
   7.1   Introduction 207
   7.2   The Structure of the Galileo Data Bank 207
        7.2.1   Chemicals and Formulations 207
        7.2.2   Methods in GDB 209
        7.2.3   Biosystems in GDB 209
        7.2.4   Results in GDB 209
   7.3   Use of GDB 209
        7.3.1   Toxicological Profiles of Individual Chemicals 212
        7.3.2   Cytotoxic Activity of a Series of Chemicals on Different
                Biosystems Treated with the Same *In Vitro* Methods 212
        7.3.3   Comparison Between *In Vitro* and *In Vivo* Results 213
        7.3.4   Predictivity of *In Vitro* Methods vs. *In Vivo* Toxic Endpoints 213
   7.4   Cosmetic Ingredients 215

References 241

Appendix A: Acronyms 249

Appendix B: Cell Lines Reported in the Methods 252

Index 255

Chapter 1

INTRODUCTION

1.1 LEGISLATIVE BASIS

Council Directive 76/768/EEC of July 27, 1976,[1] regulates the production, manufacturing, and marketing of cosmetic products in the Member States (France, Germany, Belgium, The Netherlands, Denmark, Greece, Italy, United Kingdom, Ireland, Spain, Portugal, and Luxembourg) of the European Communities (EC), which includes the European Economic Community (EEC).* Council Directive 76/768/EEC was amended five times before the June 14, 1993, approval of Council Directive 93/35/EEC (the Sixth Amendment), which modified a set of articles pertaining to definitions, safety evaluation criteria, inventory, dossier, labeling, and related concerns.[2]

Article 2 of Council Directive 76/768/EEC, as modified by the Sixth Amendment, states that: "A cosmetic product put on the market within the Community must not cause damage to human health when applied under normal or reasonably foreseeable conditions of use, taking into account, in particular, the product's presentation, its labeling, any instructions for its use and disposal, as well as any other indication or information provided by the manufacturer or his authorized agent or by any other person responsible for placing the product on the Community market."

This Directive relates only to cosmetic products, not to pharmaceutical and medicinal products. Its main goal is the protection of consumers' health,[3] and it triggered several mechanisms to fulfill this requirement:

- a list of chemicals that must not be contained in finished products (Annex II).
- a list of substances that cosmetic products must not contain except those subjected to restrictions and conditions laid down in Annex III.
- lists of authorized substances that could include antioxidants, hair dyes, preservatives, coloring agents, and ultraviolet filters (Annexes IV, VI, VII).

Moreover, the EC Council of Ministers has stated that in order to update these lists, the EC Commission will make use of the scientific opinions expressed by a special committee of experts, the Scientific Committee on Cosmetology (SCC).[4] The SCC was established by the Commission on December 19, 1977, as stated by Commission Decision 78/45/EEC;[3] it was asked to assist the Commission in examining the complex scientific and technical problems involved in formulating and amending the rules that regulate the marketing of cosmetic products.

The SCC comprises 21 members who are qualified scientists in the fields of medicine, toxicology, biology, chemistry, and other similar disciplines.[5]

The SCC is consulted by the Commission regarding any scientific or technical problem arising in the field of cosmetic products, particularly those involving the safety of substances used in the preparation of cosmetic products and the composition and conditions of use of such products.

The SCC also has been asked to make it possible to perform the safety evaluation of cosmetic ingredients by:

1. analyzing the studies presented to the Commission and developed by the cosmetic industries regarding cosmetic ingredients that could represent a hazard to consumers;
2. evaluating the most recent scientific literature on different toxicological aspects relevant for safety evaluation of cosmetic ingredients;

1

---

* After January 1, 1995, three more Member States have joined the European Union: Sweden, Finland, and Austria.

3. requiring additional safety testing to examine any new potential hazard connected with a particular ingredient, thus making reassessment of its safety possible;
4. recommending a series of guidelines to be considered by the cosmetic industries when developing adequate studies to be used in safety evaluation of cosmetic ingredients;
5. updating the aforementioned guidelines in accordance with the scientific development of safety studies, and defining the safety levels of cosmetic ingredients in practical use.

The SCC defined the general guidelines[6] for the safety evaluation of cosmetic ingredients in the EC in 1982 and updated them in 1990 (Table 1.1).[3] These guidelines apply mainly to new cosmetic ingredients, but also can be adopted for other ingredients about which concerns about safety-in-use have been brought to notice, bearing in mind the relevant toxicity data already in existence.

In order to include a cosmetic ingredient in one of the Annexes to Directive 76/768/EEC (Annex III, IV, VI, and VII), COLIPA (the European Association of Cosmetic Industries) presents to the Commission a body of toxicological information obtained from studies developed on the cosmetic ingredient at issue. Such information relates to potential biological hazards of a cosmetic ingredient and to its safety evaluation based on a series of toxicological studies. In many cases, other relevant toxicological information is derived from experimental studies developed by research institutes and published in international scientific journals.

The safety evaluation of cosmetic ingredients presently applied by the SCC consists of the analysis of all studies available concerning the toxicological potential of the chemical sub-

TABLE 1.1
SCC Guidelines for the Safety Evaluation of Cosmetic Ingredients (SPC/803/-5/90)

When requested, the manufacturer shall provide the Commission with the information set out below:[a]

1. Acute toxicity (oral or by inhalation in the case of volatile substances)
2. Dermal absorption;
3. Dermal irritation;
4. Mucous membrane irritation;
5. Skin sensitization;
6. Subchronic toxicity (oral or by inhalation in the case of volatile substances);
7. Mutagenicity (bacterial test for gene mutations and *in vitro* mammalian cell culture test for chromosome aberrations);
8. Phototoxicity and Photomutagenicity (in the case of UV light-absorbing substances);
9. Human data (if available).

When considerable oral intake can be expected or when data on dermal absorption indicate a considerable penetration of the ingredients through the skin, taking into account the toxicological profile of the substance and its chemical structure, the following further information may be necessary:

10. Toxicokinetics;
11. Teratogenicity, reproduction toxicity, carcinogenicity, and additional genotoxicity.

There may be instances when it does not appear to be necessary, or it is not technically possible, to provide information; in such cases scientific justification needs to be given.

According to Article 7 of Council Directive 86/609/EEC, "regarding the protection of animals used for experimental and other scientific purposes," an animal study shall not be performed if another scientifically satisfactory method of obtaining the result sought, not entailing the use of an animal, is reasonably and practically available.

[a]   When applying for inclusion in positive lists (Annexes IV, VI, and VII of Directive 76/768/EEC[1]), manufacturers must present a dossier containing the information reported here.

TABLE 1.2
Directive 76/768/EEC, Article 4ᵃ

1. Without prejudice to their general obligations deriving from Article 2, Member States shall prohibit the marketing of cosmetic products containing:
   a. substances listed in Annex II;
   b. substances listed in the first part of Annex III, beyond the limits and outside the conditions laid down;
   c. colouring agents other than those listed in Annex IV, Part 1 with the exception of cosmetic products containing colouring agents intended solely to colour hair:
   d. colouring agents listed in Annex IV, Part 1, used outside the conditions laid down, with the exception of cosmetic products containing colouring agents intended solely to colour hair;
   e. preservatives other than those listed in Annex VI, Part 1;
   f. preservatives listed in Annex VI, Part 1, beyond the limits and outside the conditions laid down, unless other concentrations are used for specific purposes apparent from the presentation of the product;
   g. UV filters other than those listed in Part 1 of Annex VII;
   h. UV filters listed in Part 1 of Annex VII, beyond the limits and outside the conditions laid down therein.
   i. ingredients or combinations of ingredients tested on animals after 1 January 1998.

ᵃ Modified by the Sixth Amendment (Council Directive 93/35/EEC).[2]

stances under consideration. This analysis allows evaluation of the safety levels for consumers potentially exposed to chemicals such as ingredients of finished cosmetic products.

As in the case of other fields of application of chemical substances, such as food additives, drugs, industrial chemicals, and pesticides, the basis for cosmetic ingredient safety evaluation by the SCC has been the evaluation of toxicological studies presented by industries or published in the current scientific literature. At present, toxicological studies make use of animal tests, as well as other methods which have been developed according to guidelines defined by the Commission of the European Communities,[7,8] or the Organization for Economic Cooperation and Development (OECD), and approved by the international scientific community.[9]

Among several amendments, Article 4 of Council Directive 76/768/EEC as modified by the Sixth Amendment establishes that after January 1, 1998, cosmetic ingredients or their combinations tested on animals will not be allowed on the market (Table 1.2).

The amendment to Article 4 with subparagraph (i) is based also on the new wording of the Sixth Amendment, which states that: "Assessment of the safety of use of the ingredients employed in cosmetics and of the final product should take into account the requirement of Directive 86/609/EEC;[10] which concerns the protection of animals used for experimental and other scientific purposes."

Clearly, the legislature has intended to ban the testing on animals of cosmetic ingredients or combinations of ingredients in relation to the problem of the toxicity or safety evaluation of these specific chemicals or their combinations, but only provided that some alternative methodologies are available.

The Sixth Amendment, however, states: "If there has been insufficient progress in developing satisfactory methods to replace animal testing, and in particular in those cases where alternative methods of testing, despite all reasonable endeavors, have not been scientifically validated, the Commission shall, by January 1, 1997, submit draft measures to postpone the date of implementation of this provision." This requirement is not in conflict with Article 7 of Council Directive 86/609/EEC (Protection of Animals)[10] stating that, "An experiment shall not be performed, if another scientifically satisfactory method of obtaining the result sought, not entailing the use of an animal, is reasonably and practically available."

If it is not possible to adopt alternative methodologies as a substitute for all animal toxicity testing procedures in the safety evaluation of cosmetic ingredients, the Commission, having consulted the SCC, will submit a request to postpone the date of the implementation of such a ban.

A series of other improvements in the safeguarding of public health has been introduced for the regulation of cosmetics in the EC by the approval of the Sixth Amendment,[2] which specifies the following:

(A) The compilation by the Commission of the European Communities, no later than December 14, 1994, of an inventory of ingredients employed in products, in particular on the basis of information supplied by the industry concerned (Article 5a.1). The same article states that "Cosmetic Ingredient" shall mean any chemical substance or preparation of synthetic or natural origin, except for perfume and aromatic compositions, used in the composition of cosmetic products. The inventory shall contain information on:

(i) the identity of each ingredient, in particular its chemical name, the CTFA name, the European Pharmacopoeia name, the international nonproprietary names recommended by the World Health Organisation, the EINECS, IUPAC, CAS, and Color Index Numbers, and the common name;

(ii) the usual functions of the ingredient in the final product;

(iii) where appropriate, restrictions and conditions of use, and warnings that must be printed on the label. This inventory shall be updated periodically. It is indicative and shall not constitute a list of substances authorized for use in cosmetic products.

(B1) The manufacturer or his agent, or the person to whose order a cosmetic product is manufactured, or the person responsible for placing an imported cosmetic product on the Community market shall, for control purposes, keep the following information readily accessible to the competent authorities of the Member State concerned at the address specified on the label in accordance with Article 6(1)(a):

(a) The qualitative and quantitative composition of the product; in the case of perfume compositions and perfumes, the name and code number of the composition and the identity of the supplier.

(b) The physicochemical and microbiological specifications of the raw materials and the finished product, and the purity and microbiological control criteria of the cosmetic product.

(c) The method of manufacture complying with the good manufacturing practice laid down by Community law or, failing that, laid down by the law of the Member State concerned; the person responsible for manufacture or first importation into the Community must possess an appropriate level of professional qualification or experience in accordance with the legislation and practice of the Member State which is the place of manufacture or first importation.

(d) Assessment of the safety for human health of the finished product. To that end, the manufacturer shall take into consideration the general toxicological profile of the ingredient, its chemical structure, and the level of exposure. Should the same product be manufactured at several places within Community territory, the manufacturer may choose a single place of manufacture where that information will be kept available. In this connection, and when so requested for monitoring purposes, he shall be obliged to indicate the place so chosen to the monitoring authority/authorities concerned.

(e) The name and address of the qualified person or persons responsible for the assessment referred to in (d). That person must hold a diploma as defined in Article I of Directive 89/48/EEC in the field of pharmacy, toxicology, dermatology, medicine, or a similar discipline.[2]

(f) Existing data on undesirable effects on human health resulting from use of the cosmetic product.

(g) Proof of the effect claimed for the cosmetic product, where justified by the nature of the effect or product.

(B2) The assessment of the safety for human health referred to in Paragraph B1(d) shall be carried out in accordance with the principles of Good Laboratory Practice laid down in Council Directive 87/18/EEC of 18 December 1986 on the harmonization of laws, regulations and administrative provisions relating to the application of the principles of good laboratory practice and the verification of their application for tests on chemical substances.[2]

(B3) The information referred to in Paragraph B1 must be available in the national language or languages of the Member State concerned, or in a language readily understood by the competent authorities.

The requirement of Product Information (P.I.), laid down by the Authorities as from the text cited, is clearly related to the requirement that all information that could be needed "for control purposes" concerning the technical characteristics and safety of every cosmetic product placed on the market be promptly available. Thus the P.I. is set out so that information is easily accessible for overall assessment of the safety of the cosmetic product on the basis of all relevant knowledge.

1.2 COSMETIC INGREDIENTS

Ingredients are defined as any substances used in cosmetic products. Examples of ingredients are provided by those chemicals mentioned in Annexes III, IV, VI, and VII of Council Directive 76/768/EEC.[1]

Although many thousands of different cosmetic products are marketed within the EU countries, they are formulated from a much smaller number of ingredients. The European Inventory, as requested by the Sixth Amendment and adopted on June 28, 1995, contains between 7,000 and 8,000 individual substances. The presence of potentially harmful chemicals among cosmetic ingredients is limited to a small number of substances. Most raw materials employed in cosmetic products are recognized as harmless, based on their widespread human use by consumers over many decades and in sectors other than the cosmetic one (e.g., food additives and drugs).

Since 1976, different types of cosmetic ingredients have been reviewed by Council Directive 76/768/EEC, because of some concern deriving from their toxicological properties. Annex II of Council Directive 76/768/EEC[1] reports a list of substances that must not form part of the composition of cosmetic products: it includes 412 individual cosmetic ingredients or groups of related chemicals. The decision to exclude most of these 412 cosmetic ingredients from use in finished cosmetic products was made by the Commission when approving Council Directive 76/768/EEC of July 27, 1976.[1]

Since 1978, the list of forbidden substances in cosmetic products (Annex II of Council Directive 76/768/EEC[1]) has been increased by more than 50 chemicals. These chemicals, which had been used in cosmetic products for many years, were identified by the SCC as presenting a possible risk of cancer or other toxicity risk for the consumers.

As specified previously, the Commission has approved a series of technical directives regulating the use of different types of cosmetic ingredients, namely:

1. substances listed in the first part of Annex III of Council Directive 76/768/EEC subjected to the restrictions and conditions established (Article 4);[1]
2. coloring agents listed in the first part of Annex IV of Council Directive 76/768/EEC (Article 4);[1]
3. preservatives listed in the first part of Annex VI of Council Directive 76/768/EEC (Article 4);[1]
4. UV filters listed in the first part of Annex VII of Council Directive 76/768/EEC (Article 4).[1]

Due to their intrinsic toxicity, all these cosmetic ingredients can represent different types of risk for consumers.

There are 157 coloring agents that can contain cosmetic products under Council Directive 76/768/EEC:[1] for some of them, use is limited to a maximum of 5 ppm in the finished products.

According to their potential toxic effects, they are classified as:

*   Coloring agents allowed in all cosmetic products;
*   Coloring agents allowed in all cosmetic products except those intended to be applied in the vicinity of the eye: in particular eye make-up and eye make-up removers;
*   Coloring agents allowed exclusively in cosmetic products intended not to come into contact with the mucous membranes;
*   Coloring agents allowed exclusively in cosmetic products intended to come into contact with the skin only briefly.
*   Coloring agents which include nitro dyes, azo compounds, tryphenylmethane, xanthene, quinoline, anthraquinone, indigo, etc.

Preservatives are substances with very different chemical structures which are included in cosmetic finished products to preserve the cosmetic preparation from pathogenic microorganisms which could affect the health of consumers, or to prevent conversion of some ingredients to harmful substances caused by many types of microorganisms, during the use of a cosmetic product.

It has been proved that some of the preservatives used by the cosmetic industry belong to the class of moderately toxic substances. Because of the small concentration levels involved, a single intake of even a large amount of a cosmetic preparation will not lead to an acute toxic effect; in the case of preservatives penetrating the skin, daily use of a cosmetic preparation leads to long-term bodily absorption. Precisely because preservatives are included in several types of cosmetic finished products, when evaluating potential health risks to consumers' health, the possible absorption of certain amounts of active preservative ingredients by the human body must be taken into account.

The SCC has estimated that consumer exposure to several types of cosmetic products of various uses (hygiene, eye, nonrinse-off, and rinse-off products) may reach a total of 27.1 g/d

(SPC/1247/93 en).[11] The resulting consumer exposure to a preservative is a function of its permitted concentration in the finished products, which ranges from 0.1 to 2.0%. According to Council Directive 76/768/EEC[1] (Annex VI — Part 1), 46 preservatives can be permitted in the cosmetic finished products, and another 9 are allowed temporarily (Annex VI — Part 2).

Sunscreen preparations are available in a wide selection of protective strengths. The various preparations range from oils to liquid and cream emulsions, gels, spray foams, and even hair sunscreens.[12] Sunscreen agents present in sunscreen preparations can absorb UVA and UVB radiation, thus protecting the skin from erythema.

It is acknowledged widely that the use of sunscreens could protect consumers from certain types of skin cancer; however, no data on this subject are available at present.[13,14] When absorbing UV radiation, sunscreen ingredients undergo a change in chemical structure and may induce several types of toxicological effects on humans, including photomutagenic, photoallergic, phototoxic, and photocarcinogenic effects.

There are many substances and combinations of substances described in the literature as tanning agents. A few of these substances have been marketed in cosmetic preparations. Annex VII of Council Directive 76/768/EEC[1] contains seven different sunscreens that can be contained in cosmetic products; Annex VII, part 2, contains 13 sunscreens that are temporarily allowed to be contained in cosmetic products. In addition to the three categories of cosmetic ingredients, during the last 10 years the SCC has been involved in evaluating a fourth group of chemicals that are the basis for hair coloring finished cosmetic products.

Hair dyes can be divided into three types, depending on whether they color hair temporarily, semipermanently, or permanently. Dyes, dye intermediates, and other ingredients involved vary according to the type of hair product. A commercial formulation may contain several types of individual cosmetic ingredients, including nitrocompounds, aromatic compounds, amino compounds, oxidizing agents, and surface active agents.

In the past, a few of these chemical compounds were demonstrated to be carcinogenic and mutagenic to animals, and they were included in Annex II of Council Directive 76/768/ EEC.[1,15] Because of their possible chemical and metabolic interconversion of the amino group or the metabolic reduction of the nitro group present in the molecules of many hair dye ingredients, all these chemicals are termed amine-generated chemicals, among which possible derivations potentially harmful to consumers' health have been identified.

The Commission has accepted a series of opinions expressed by the SCC on a group of approximately 50 hair dyes.

In addition to cosmetic ingredients that are part of the positive lists, other chemicals used in the cosmetic sector could present a risk to the health of consumers. Depending on the qualitative relevance of the risk these chemicals might present, the Commission may submit them to the SCC analysis. Therefore, it is possible to distinguish two different categories of cosmetic ingredients in relation to current EC regulation, namely:

1. Cosmetic ingredients subject to regulatory requirements, such as those new substances to be included in Annexes III, IV, and VII of Council Directive 76/768/EEC;[1]
2. Cosmetic ingredients, of widespread use and present in the European Inventory, for which there is a need for P.I. to be reported in the Dossier in order to assure the safety of the finished products in which they are contained (see Sixth Amendment, part B1[d]).

The application of alternative methodologies, and in general of the new criteria to be derived by implementing the Sixth Amendment in the safety evaluation of cosmetic ingredients, should take into consideration the different meaning of the potential for harmful effects in relation to the two types of cosmetic ingredients mentioned above.

Chapter 2

THE ROLE OF TOXICOLOGY

The role of chemicals in industrial countries has increased considerably during the second half of this century. All types of industrial production in the present world economy make use of chemicals, obtained either from natural resources (plants, animals, microorganisms) or through synthetic processes.

The impact of chemicals upon our lives has resulted in an ever-increasing need to identify, assess, and evaluate the toxicity database of many chemical agents, especially those for which a direct human exposure is documented or predicted.

It is relatively easy to demonstrate that humans of every age are exposed to a myriad of air-, water-, and foodborne toxicants with varying properties. Public and official concerns about human contamination are focused on a vast array of chemicals, including industrial solvents, volatile organic compounds, agrochemicals, household products (e.g., detergents, cleaners, and paints), cosmetic products (e.g., shampoos, hair dyes, and sunscreens), and a plethora of prescription and nonprescription drug preparations.

Therefore, toxicity data related to chemical agents have become the basic information for regulating human exposure, by means of controlling a possible limitation of both their use and introduction on the market.

Toxicity data related to chemical agents consist of quantitative and/or qualitative results, obtained by a complex series of toxicity studies. These data represent one possible and acceptable way of estimating what the impact of a given chemical could be on the quality of human life, or whether there could be impairment of one or more typical normal biological processes representative of human life, such as the survival of cellular components of human tissue, the normal development of human organs, or the reproductive functions.[16]

Scientific literature contains thousands of reports dealing with adverse effects produced by chemicals on different organisms including man, such as acute and immediate (as well as delayed) adverse toxic effects, malformations, birth defects, neurological diseases, and cancers.

The primary purpose of a toxicity study on a chemical is to obtain biological information relevant for the estimation of the potential toxic adverse effects of the chemical that could result from a given human exposure. The main feature of a toxicity study is therefore represented by its ability to reproduce biological processes similar to those specific to human life, and to identify the possible adverse effects produced by chemicals.

Toxicity data to be used in the risk assessment of individual cases of human exposure to chemicals have thus far been obtained almost exclusively from animal studies. The scientific research during the last 50 years has been able to develop an experimentally well defined animal experiment for each of the adverse effects to be considered for risk assessment (Table 2.1).

During the 1970s and 1980s, several national agencies and international organizations, such as the OECD and the EEC, followed the criteria provided for them by internationally recognized scientists, and set up a series of guidelines on how to develop a toxicity study so that its result may be used for the regulation of a given chemical.

In the EC, for example, Directives 87/302/EEC and 92/69/EEC[7,8] — both amending Council Directive 67/548/EEC on the approximation of laws, regulations and administrative provisions relating to the classification, packaging, and labeling of dangerous substances — describe the test methods for the determination of toxicological properties listed in Annexes VII and VIII of Directive 79/831/EEC,[17] which "are based on those recognized and recommended by competent international bodies (in particular by OECD)." These two Directives

TABLE 2.1
Major Types of Animal Toxicity Tests

1. Acute Oral (dermal, inhalation) Toxicity
2. Acute Dermal Irritation-Corrosivity
3. Acute Eye Irritation-Corrosivity
4. Skin Sensitization
5. Subacute Oral (dermal,[a] inhalation[b]) Toxicity
6. Subchronic Oral[c] (dermal, inhalation) Toxicity
7. Teratology
8. Multigeneration Reproduction Toxicity
9. Toxicokinetics
10. Carcinogenicity
11. Chronic Toxicity
12. Genetic Toxicity[d]
13. Acute Delayed Neurotoxicity
14. Implantation Toxicity
15. Skin Painting Chronic Toxicity

[a] 14 to 28 d
[b] 21 to 28 d
[c] 90 d
[d] Only a few animal studies, the majority being represented by *in vitro* tests.

include 26 methods out of 36 that make use of animals; the 10 *in vitro* tests are all related to the evaluation of mutagenic properties of chemicals.

Moreover, Commission Directive 91/325/EEC[18] defines the criteria for the classification of dangerous chemical substances. These are classified based on their toxicological properties, identified through of animal toxicological tests, such as those described by the previous mentioned two directives (87/302/EEC and 92/69/EEC).[7,8] Council Directive 86/609/EEC[10] also has been considered. It concerns the protection of animals used for experimental and other scientific purposes. It refers to the use of animals in experiments that are undertaken for the development, manufacture, quality, effectiveness, and safety testing of drugs, foodstuff, and other substances or products (Article 3). The same Directive states, however, in its Article 23 that "the Commission and Member States should encourage research into the development and validation of alternative techniques which could provide the same level of information as that obtained in experiments using animals, but which involve fewer animals or which could entail less painful procedures, and shall take such other steps as they consider appropriate to encourage in this field."

Toxicology as a science has advanced in the second half of this century as the use of chemicals in pesticides, pharmaceuticals, and cosmetics has increased. The public has realized the value of toxicological testing, after a series of disasters including the Minamata disease (methylmercury poisoning in Japan), the thalidomide tragedy, the development of cancer in females exposed to diethylstilbestrol (DES) *in utero,* and the Seveso accident with the diffusion of the carcinogenic dioxin TCDD in the environment of a region in Italy.

There are two approaches to toxicology, one mechanistic, the other descriptive: both approaches affect the design of an experiment and the choice of biological endpoints to be measured.

The mechanistic toxicology is focused on the biochemical process by which a toxic effect is produced, such as, for example, the identification of a metabolic product derived in the liver of the animal exposed to a chemical and its ability to give rise to a liver tumor.

The descriptive toxicology relies on different analytical techniques, such as pathology, statistics, physiology, and pharmacology. This approach is concerned mainly with the final

TABLE 2.2
Toxicity Testing on Animals

Acute, Subacute, and Chronic Toxicty Testing: Determine the effect
of a chemical on health and mortality during various lengths
of exposure

Hypersensitivity Tests: Assess the tendency of a chemical to elicit
rashes and other allergic responses

Reproductive Toxicity Testing: Assess the effect of a chemical
on fertility and fecundity

Phototoxicity Tests: Determine the extent to which a chemical
is activated by sunlight, thereby enhancing its toxicity

Developmental Toxicity Tests: Evaluate the capacity of a chemical
to cause abnormalities in an embryo, fetus, or newborn

Toxicokinetic Studies: Explore the absorption, distribution metabolism,
storage and excretion of a chemical

Ocular — and Skin — Irritation Tests: Measure the ability
of a chemical to inflame or irritate the skin or eyes

Behavioral Tests: Monitor the effect of a chemical on cognitive
function during development and in the adult

observed adverse effect — for example, a tumor — and does not necessarily require an understanding of the mechanisms by which toxic effects have occurred.

Descriptive toxicology, for instance, indicates that a chemical substance is able to produce cancer in an animal, whereas mechanistic toxicology provides an approach to extrapolation from one species to another based on known similarities and differences in physiology. The closer to humans a test animal is biologically, or the greater the number of species in which the effect is detected, the more likely the cancer will be found to occur in humans as well.

Most of the toxicity test methods currently available are descriptive and involve the use of animals. However, there is increasing progress in scientific research that allows the identification of the elementary biological mechanisms by which a toxic effect is produced. This continuous and further understanding of the basis of toxicological effects will promote the development of reliable and scientifically valid *in vitro* toxicity tests in the future. These tests also could be used in extrapolating results. It is obvious, however, that whole-animal toxicity testing will probably continue to be needed in the following cases: when searching for effects in previously unknown target organs; in evaluating effects that represent an interaction of multiple-organ systems; in monitoring metabolism and pharmacokinetics; in evaluating healing or diminished responsiveness to the toxic substance; and in risk-assessment decisions. Animal use in toxicity testing seems, at present, unlikely to be entirely discarded in the foreseeable future.

Chapter 3

ANIMAL TOXICITY STUDIES

The primary purpose of any toxicological study is to obtain biological (biochemical, physiological, morphological) information indicative of toxicity that is reproducible, reliable, and dose-related, and which can be interpreted and/or extended to the assessment of health risks to humans. Detailed protocols have been established regarding how to conduct an animal toxicity test: they are designed so that high doses of agent are administered over varied periods of time by various routes to animals that are euthanized at predetermined time intervals to permit necroscopy, a biochemical and microscopic examination of the organs, and a comparison with results obtained from animals dying or becoming moribund during the treatment period.

3.1 ACUTE TOXICITY STUDIES

Acute toxicity studies are conducted on animals to ascertain the total adverse biological effects occuring during a finite period of time following the administration of single, frequently large, doses of an agent (or several doses repeated over a short interval of time). The effects observed in the animals usually are related directly to the amount of the chemical substance administered orally, dermally, or via inhalation.[18] The objectives of any acute toxicity test are to discover and report any adverse health effect that could be attributed to the chemical under evaluation.

Acute toxicity studies frequently are designed to express the potency of the toxicant in terms of the median lethal dose (LD_{50}), a value representing the estimated dose causing the deaths of 50% of the animals exposed under the defined conditions of the test. In the case of inhalation acute toxicity tests, the toxicant potency is presented as the median lethal concentration (LC_{50}), the estimated concentration in the environment to which the animals are exposed that will result in 50% mortality of the animal population exposed under the defined conditions of the test.

Commission Directive 93/21/EEC[17] classifies as "very toxic" a chemical agent that produces an LD_{50} at a dose ≤25 mg/kg in a rat population exposed by oral route, an LD_{50} at a dose ≤50 mg/kg in a rat or rabbit population exposed by a dermal route, or an LC_{50} at a dose ≤0.5 mg/l in a rat population exposed by inhalation for 4 h to an aerosol or particulate, or at a dose of ≤0.5 in a rat population exposed for 4 h to a gas or a vapor.

The same Directive classifies as "toxic" a chemical agent that produces in treated rats an LD_{50} respectively between 25 and 200 mg/kg (oral route), an LD_{50} between 50 and 400 mg/kg (dermal route), an LC_{50} between 0.25 and 2 mg/l/4h (inhalation exposure). A chemical agent is classified as harmful if the LD_{50} is between 200 and 2000 mg/kg (oral route), an LD_{50} between 400 and 2000 mg/kg) (dermal route), or if the LC_{50} is between 1 and 20 mg/l/4h.

Directive 92/69/EEC states that for oral and inhalation acute toxicity tests, and for the dermal acute toxicity (with healthy intact skin) at least ten rodents (five females and five males) are to be exposed at each dose level (at least three). However, a new approach to acute toxicity testing based on a fixed dose procedure that reduces the number of animals[19] has been proposed by the British Toxicology Society,[19] and adopted by EU-Commission Directive 92/69/EEC[8].

3.2 DERMAL IRRITATION STUDIES

For the regulation of many products and chemical agents, including cosmetic ingredients, that may come into direct contact with the skin, studies are performed on the skin of suitable animal species. Dermal irritation studies include at present direct irritation and sensitization tests; a cutaneous phototoxicity test and a cutaneous photosensitization test are also usually requested for UV-absorbing chemicals.

3.2.1 SKIN IRRITATION

In order to evaluate the ability of a chemical substance to cause skin irritation, the measurement of the edema (the accumulation of excess fluid in the subcutaneous fluid) and of the erythema (redness of the skin caused by engorgement of the capillaries) generally is performed on treated rats, or, more recently, on treated rabbits or guinea pigs, which have relatively sensitive skins. The test material will be applied to one abraded site and one intact site on the back of the abdomen. Since the material is to remain in place for 24 h after application, retraining boxes are used to prevent the animals from grooming themselves.

The predictive value of this methodology always has been debated, since different results have been obtained when animal data were compared with those obtained from human volunteers. The dermal application of some 40 cosmetic ingredients resulted in a degree of decreasing responsiveness in the following order: rabbit, guinea pig, albino rat, human, and swine.[20] Usually the rabbit produces false positive responses, and often mild or moderate irritant agents are not identified correctly by this methodology.

At least three healthy adult animals are used, according to Commission Directive 92/69/ EEC;[8] additional animals may be required to clarify equivocal responses.

3.2.2 SKIN SENSITIZATION

A dermal reaction exists whereby exposure to chemicals elicits little reaction, but following a second dermal exposure, an effect is seen that occurs earlier, is severe, and persists longer; subsequent exposures to the same chemical agent, even though weeks or years apart, result in a full-blown, allergy-like, delayed reaction to that chemical. It often occurs that this reaction can be elicited by a much lower concentration of the agent and on areas of the skin other than those involved in the initial contact. The allergic reaction observed in this study depends on the production of complexes between the chemical and certain proteins against which the animal develops antibodies; subsequent exposure to the same chemical (or to a closely related chemical) stimulates the immunity system to react and produce an allergic response.

The test animal used for this study is the guinea pig: 20 animals are used in the treatment group, and at least 10 are used in the control group.

3.2.3 PHOTOALLERGIC REACTIONS

A variety of chemicals (including thiazides, phenothiazine, hexachlorophene, and several natural compounds), cause an allergy-like reaction manifested in the form of an immediate urticaria, a persistent eczema, or a delayed popular eruction when dermally applied or ingested by an individual who is subsequently exposed to sunlight. All chemicals eliciting this type of reaction contain ring systems in their structures that are capable of absorbing UV light from sunlight. The light-induced activation of the chemical results in covalent binding of this reactive intermediate with cellular and plasma proteins to produce antigens that will stimulate antibody formation. The reactions that are observed as a result of the chemically treated skin's exposure to sunlight are of the antibody type or due to a cell-mediate immune response. The test animal used for this study is the guinea pig or the rabbit. A guideline on how to conduct such a study is being discussed by the OECD.

3.2.4 PHOTOTOXICITY

Phototoxicity is a very common reaction observed in human skin exposed to UV-light immediately after a chemical exposure: the supposed mechanism to explain this reaction involves again the formation of a chemical intermediate derived from the reaction of the chemical with the UV-light, which elicits a direct, local (dermal) cellular toxicity, consisting in a delayed erythema and hyperpigmentation, followed by desquamation of skin.

A guideline for developing this type of study is being discussed by the OECD.

The conclusion of a recent workshop organized by ECVAM on "*In Vitro* Phototoxicity Testing" is proposing a sequential approach to testing for photosensitization with a testing strategy based on *in vitro* phototoxicity tests followed, when negative results are produced, by human testing. If *in vitro* testing indicates a phototoxic potential, then animal testing may be necessary to determine a No Observed Effect Level (NOEL) for testing in humans.[21]

3.3 OCULAR TOXICITY STUDIES

A contact with chemicals as a consequence of an accident, or a normal contact with chemicals present in cosmetic products employed for human skin care, may produce ocular damages. The method to evaluate qualitative alterations produced in the eyes of exposed animals and to transform them into quantitative measurements is known as the Draize test. According to this method, the substance to be tested is applied in a single dose to one eye in each of several experimental animals (the species recommended is the adult albino rabbit); the untreated eye is used to provide control information. The degree of irritation is evaluated and graded at specific intervals, and it is further described to provide a complete evaluation of the effects. The duration of observations should be sufficient to evaluate fully either reversibility or irreversibility of the effects observed. In addition to the observations of the cornea, iris, and conjunctiva, any other lesions that are noted should be recorded and reported.

The test animal used for this study is the rabbit. At least three animals are used in this method. Additional animals may be required to clarify equivocal responses.

The Draize test has become a target for animal welfare groups and concerned scientists who claim that it is unnecessary and inhumane; they suggest that it causes unnecessary pain to animals, and is subjective and prone to such interlaboratory variation in results as to be completely unreliable.

As in all cases of animal studies, even for the ocular irritation test applied to rabbits, there are serious limitations in transferring the results to humans.

Furthermore, there are serious structural and physiological differences which make the rabbit eye an unsatisfactory model for the human eye, including the presence of a third eyelid in the rabbit lacking in humans; the reduced efficiency of the rabbit's tearing mechanism, when compared to man's; the differences in the pH of aqueous humor in human eyes (pH 7.2) and in those of the rabbit (pH 8.2); and the structure and thickness of the cornea.

3.4 SUBACUTE, SUBCHRONIC, AND CHRONIC STUDIES

Humans often are exposed repeatedly to a substance; this does not necessarily cause the same effects as an acute, one-time exposure.

The effects of chronic toxicity differ from those of acute toxicity when the test substance or its metabolites accumulate in the organism up to a toxic level, or when it causes irreversible effects that accumulate with each administration.

The simulation of a repeated human exposure to a chemical requires the development of two distinct types of studies; the short-term (subacute or subchronic, 21 or 90 d) and the long-term (chronic, 1 or 2 years) studies.

The subacute, subchronic, and chronic studies are designed to:

1. Assess possible cumulative effects of the repeated exposure as body burdens of the chemical and/or biotransformation products are acquired with time.
2. Examine the biological nature of the toxic effects caused by different dosages.
3. Determine the nature of macroscopic and microscopic organ or tissue damage as it develops, in relation to the different dosages.
4. Identify the approximate dosage at which altered physiological, biochemical, and morphological changes observed at higher dosages do not occur (No Observed Adverse Effect Level: NOAEL). This experimental value, which could be evaluated in the treated animals, is used to calculate the safety margin to be recommended for human exposure.

For a subacute oral toxicity study, which lasts 28 d, at least 10 animals (5 female and 5 male) are used at each dose level (usually 3 and a control group). For this study, the preferred species is the rat.

For a subchronic oral toxicity study, which lasts 90 d, at least 20 animals (10 female and 10 male) are used at each dose level (in general, 3 and a control group). For this study too, the preferred animal is the rat; in some cases, chemicals are tested also on a nonrodent species, such as the dog.

For a chronic oral toxicity study, which lasts the whole life span of the species selected, generally rats are used. Animals are usually treated 7 d per week; at least 40 animals (20 female and 20 male) are used at each dose level, normally 3 and a control group.

3.5 CARCINOGENICITY STUDIES

Carcinogenicity studies are largely based on animal investigation. Detecting human carcinogens by means of epidemiological investigations presents a special problem because a latency period of 20 years or more may occur. Animal testing, particularly on rodents, is useful because the latency period for tumor formation is much shorter (1 or 2 years for rodents); this allows potential human carcinogens to be detected during testing and before they are marketed. It is also much easier to control the animal environment than the human environment, and therefore to investigate causal relationships.

Carcinogenicity testing requires more animals than other tests. When tests are performed on rodents, at least 100 animals (50 female and 50 male) are used for each of the 3 doses and for a control concurrent group. Normally two species of rodents are used: the mouse and the rat.

Extensive examinations are made on multiple samples of 30 or more tissues and organs for each animal included in the study, thus providing normally 500,000 data to be analyzed for statistical reasons. An agent is defined as "carcinogenic" when it increases the frequency of tumors found in control animals, causes an earlier appearance of tumors, induces new types of tumors not found in control animals, or causes a multiplicity of neoplasms in different body sites.

3.6 TERATOGENICITY AND REPRODUCTION TOXICITY STUDIES

Teratogenicity studies allow the identification of those agents that induce structural malformations, metabolic or physiological dysfunctions, and behavioral alterations in the offspring, either at birth or in a defined postnatal period.

Reproductive toxicology is the study of the occurrence, causes, manifestations, and sequelae of adverse effects of exogenous agents on reproduction, which includes loss of libido, sterility, abortion, fetal death, perinatal death, and delayed toxicity.

The animals commonly used in the teratogenicity studies are the rat, the mouse, the hamster, and the rabbit. At least 20 rats, mice or hamsters, or 12 pregnant rabbits, are required at each dose level (three dose levels and a control): all female animals (treated and control) are sacrificed before the expected date of delivery.

In the reproduction toxicity studies, one generation or two generations of animals are investigated: the parent animals are treated for all their sexual cycles, during the mating period and thereafter (only the females during pregnancy and for the duration of the nursing period). In the case of two-generation study, the treatment is continued to F1 offspring during their growth into adulthood, mating and production of an F2 generation, until the F2 generation is weaned. The rat or the mouse are the preferred species: each treated and control group should contain a sufficient number of animals to yield about 20 pregnant females. At least three treated groups and a control group are used.

3.7 TOXICOKINETIC STUDIES

Toxicokinetic studies provide information on the mechanism of absorption, the substance distribution among the various body compartments, and metabolism and alimentation as well. They facilitate the interpretation of results from other tests, and their extrapolation of a foreign substance often will explain its toxicity or lack thereof (mechanistic approach).

Absorption of a substance by the body can occur through a variety of routes. If exposure takes place by inhalation, absorption can occur in the lungs, and in the gastrointestinal tract. If exposure occurs by mouth, absorption will occur as the substance passes through the gastrointestinal tract. With dermal exposure, the substance will be absorbed through the skin.

Toxicokinetic studies may be conducted in one or more appropriate animal species, and should take into account the species used or intended to be used in other toxicological studies on the same test substance.

For absorption and excretion studies, there should be initially four animals in each dose group. Both sexes may need to be studied; if there are sex differences in response, then four animals of each sex are to be tested.

When tissue distribution is studied, the initial group size should take into account both the number of animals to be sacrificed at each time point and the number of time points to be examined. When metabolism is being studied, the group size should be related to the needs of the study. In the case of single-dose administration, at least two dose levels are used: one with no toxic effects, and one that allows changes in toxicokinetic parameters or at which toxic effects occur.

3.8 SKIN ABSORPTION

The extent and rate of percutaneous absorption is of chief interest in the course of defining the need for specific toxicity studies of cosmetic ingredients.

Minipigs seem to be the most suitable animal for studying the percutaneous absorption of cosmetic ingredients; in some instances pig skin could be used by *in vitro* technology, although differences between *in vivo* and *in vitro* are observed depending on the part of the body from which the skin is obtained.

It has been suggested that penetration studies on cosmetic ingredients should be conducted on humans, by employing radiolabeled compounds. However, there are ethical considerations today that make it almost impossible to justify the use of radiolabeled compounds on humans.

3.9 MUTAGENICITY STUDIES

Chemical agents of different structure and use are able to react directly with the cellular DNA molecules, which represent the basis of genetic information for the development and functioning of a living organism, including man. The types of chemical consequences of the interaction between a genotoxic chemical and the DNA molecule and their biological significances have been analyzed in microorganisms, cell lines, insects, plants, and mammals, and can be described in molecular terms. Chemical agents also are able to react with the nuclear structures present in all cells of living organisms, known as chromosomes, where genes form the basis of structural organization of the individual genetic program. The consequences of the attack by chemicals on the chromosomal structure produce the well-known phenomena of chromosomal abnormalities (gaps, breaks, interchanges, minutes, rings, dicentrics, polycentrics, nondisjunctions, etc.) that have been recognized to be present in populations exposed to a genotoxic agent.

In the last 25 years, scientific research has demonstrated that these molecular changes induced in the DNA molecules, or these chromosomal abnormalities induced by chemicals (therefore called genotoxic chemicals), are occurring almost in the same way in cells of all living organisms. In mammals, including man, all these alterations represent the causes of severe genetic diseases, as they are transmitted to the progeny of an affected individual (mutations). Thus for this sector of mutagenicity/genotoxicity studies, the mechanistic approach is operating well, because it is possible to document that a given chemical is producing damages to DNA or chromosome structure. In this case, the extrapolation of the intrinsic reactions between the DNA or the chromosomes and the chemicals from testing organisms to mammals, including humans, is fully possible and complete.

There are several whole-animal tests for evaluating the mutagenic potential of a chemical agent, such as the *in vivo* mammalian bone-marrow cytogenetic test, the micronucleus test, the rodent dominant lethal test, the *in vivo* mammalian germ-cell cytogenetics, the mouse spot test, and the mouse heritable translocation test. A specific sector of scientific research, however, has demonstrated that several nonanimal *in vitro* tests are fully alternative to the use of mammals, and international agencies such as EPA, WHO, OECD, and EEC have long since approved adequate guidelines for performing *in vitro* mutagenicity studies, due also to the extensive international collaborative research that has validated these methodologies through an intensive interlaboratory cooperative work.

In the EC legislation, *in vitro* mutagenicity studies are accepted for the initial screening of the mutagenic chemicals, as well as for additional information (as it is reported in Commission Directive 87/302/EEC[7]); the initial assessment of the mutagenic activity consists of assays for gene (point) mutation in bacteria and for cytogenetic damage in mammalian cells (*in vitro*); suitable methods for these "base set" studies were described in Commission Directive 92/69/EEC.[8] Supplementary studies that are suitable for the verification and/or extension of results obtained in the base set are described in Directive 87/302/EEC.[7]

All EC-approved *in vitro* guidelines refer to:

1. Commission Directive 92/69/EEC:[8]
   - *In vitro* mammalian cytogenetic test (chromosome aberrations);
   - *Escherichia coli* — reverse mutation assay (gene mutations);
   - *Salmonella typhimurium* — reverse mutation assay (gene mutations).
2. Commission Directive 87/302/EEC:[7]
   - Gene mutation — *Saccharomyces cerevisiae* (gene mutations);
   - Mitotic recombination — *Saccharomyces cerevisiae* (mitotic recombination);
   - *In vitro* mammalian gene mutation test (gene mutations);

- DNA damage and repair — unscheduled DNA synthesis (UDS), mammalian cells *in vitro* (DNA damage);
- Sister chromatid exchange (SCE) assay *in vitro* (chromosome damages);
- *In vitro* mammalian cell transformation test (genetical changes).

It has been demonstrated extensively that the initial biological reaction of the development of a tumor is a change in certain types of genes (oncogenes or tumor suppressor genes) represented by different types of mechanisms, such as DNA base-pairs change (both qualitative and quantitative) and DNA repair process (chromosomal abnormalities, mitotic recombinations, and gene conversion). These reactions are the same ones that produce mutations or genotoxic effects, as described above. Therefore, genotoxicity tests have been employed during the last 20 years for screening carcinogenic agents. For each one of the above-mentioned *in vitro* mutagenicity tests, as well for whole mammals *in vivo* mutagenicity tests, specific parameters have been evaluated, such as:

Sensitivity: Number of carcinogens found mutagenic among a number of carcinogens tested.
Specificity: Number of noncarcinogens found nonmutagenic among a number of non-carcinogens tested.
Accuracy: Number of correct test results among the number of chemicals tested.
Predictivity: Number of carcinogens found positive (mutagenic) among the number of positive results obtained.
Prevalence: Number of carcinogens among the number of chemicals tested.

The percent value of each one of these parameters varies according to the mutagenicity test, or a combination of different mutagenicity tests, considered. By these same criteria, the batteries of tests to be employed in the prescreening of carcinogenic chemicals have also been defined.

Loprieno et al.[22] have documented that the accuracy of correct identification by means of genotoxicity assays of carcinogenic and noncarcinogenic chemicals increases from 68.6% with the use of the Salmonella test alone to 71.6% if the Salmonella test is combined with the Chromosome Aberration *in vitro* test, and to 92.5% if these two *in vitro* tests are combined with an *in vivo* test, such as the rodent bone marrow micronucleus test. The correspondent values for positive predictivity are 63.9, 82.7, and 95.6%, respectively.

At the end of the 1970s, more than 100 methods were described in the literature for assessing the mutagenic or genotoxic potential of a series of chemical substances. After several international cooperative research trials[23,24] that included more than 50 laboratories in the world and different classes of chemicals, a few methods have been accepted by the international scientific community as valid for assessing the mutagenic potential of chemicals. Protocols have been defined through several discussions at OECD and EEC levels, and their updating is continuous.

3.10 ANIMALS NEEDED FOR SAFETY EVALUATION OF A COSMETIC INGREDIENT

The number of animals employed in hazard evaluation has been estimated by following the guidelines for safety evaluation of cosmetic ingredients in the EC, as recommended by the SCC, with the basic information needed in the case of those cosmetic ingredients included in the positive lists, such as the coloring agents, preservatives, hair dyes, and sunscreens, also keeping in mind the protocols reported in Commission Directives 87/302/EEC[7] and 92/69/EEC.[8] Table 3.1 shows that approximately 200 animals are needed to present a base dossier for these types of chemical ingredients.

TABLE 3.1
Number of Animals Employed in the Safety Evaluation Scheme
(Basic Set) Recommended by the Scientific Committee on
Cosmetology of the European Commission

Type of Study	Species	Number
Acute Toxicity (oral) 3 doses + control	Rat	40
Dermal Absorption	Rat/Mouse	10
Dermal Irritation	Rabbit	3
Mucous Membrane Irritation	Rabbit	3
Skin Sensitization	Guinea pig	30
Subchronic Toxicity (oral) 90 d; 3 doses + control	Rat	80
Subtotals		
	Rat	130
	Rabbit	6
	Guinea pig	30
Total		**166**

In the case of additional information regarding other toxicological endpoints such as carcinogenicity, teratogenicity, toxicokinetics, and chronic toxicity, it is possible to estimate that for fewer than ten new cosmetic ingredients put on the market each year in the EC, some 1000 animals would be needed to complete the basic information for the safety evaluation of one new cosmetic ingredient. This means a total consumption of no more than 5000 animals for new ingredients (2000 for basic studies and 3000 for additional studies on three of ten new cosmetic ingredients).

If one considers that COLIPA submits to the Commission no more than one or two new dossiers per year, the total number of animals requested to fulfill the recommendation of the SCC may be estimated not to exceed 1,000 per year! In the cosmetic sector at least, this number is rather distant from the 2 million medical experiments performed on living animals in 1990 as indicated by FRAME.[25]

In Great Britain, the 1992 *Statistics of Scientific Procedures on Living Animals*[26] reported that 3082 animals (954 rats, 1922 guinea pigs, and 206 rabbits) had been employed in scientific procedures for safety evaluation of cosmetic and toiletries products. This number represents 0.1% of all animals used in the safety evaluation in that country during 1992.

In the EC, the SCC has released during 1993 a final opinion on 43 cosmetic ingredients, namely 8 sunscreens, 5 preservatives, and 30 hair dyes. The toxicological dossier of each of those cosmetic ingredients includes a body of toxicological studies considered to represent an adequate set of information relating to the potential hazard to consumers' health. The toxicological studies present in the dossier were essentially conducted in Europe, with the exception of the majority of the long-term carcinogenicity studies, which were developed in the United States under the National Toxicology Program sponsored by the U.S. government. It could be assumed that the period of time for developing these studies is 10 years.

By analyzing data presented to the SCC, it is reasonable to assume that approximately 39,000 laboratory animals were needed to develop those studies, and namely 5 species: rats (21,000), mice (14,500), guinea pigs (2,600), rabbits (700), and hamsters (100). This is only a rough estimate of the impact of the cosmetic ingredient evaluation system based on animal models, with an average of approximately 900 laboratory animals per cosmetic ingredient, based on a 10-year evaluation.

The highest number of laboratory animals reported by the Commission for the safety evaluation of cosmetics and toiletry products refers mainly to studies such as quality control, finished products, etc., rather than to the safety evaluation of cosmetic ingredients as those regulated by EU-Council Directive 76/768/EEC.[1]

3.11 *IN VIVO* TOXICITY TESTING GUIDELINES

Commission Directives 87/302/EEC[7] and 92/69/EEC[8] defined guidelines for the determination of toxicological properties in the Member States of the EC. Animal tests and studies shall be conducted by taking into account humane principles and international development in the field of animal welfare.

Particular attention should be given to Council Directive 86/609/EEC[10] on the approximation of laws, regulations, and administrative provisions of the Member States regarding the protection of animals used for experimental and for other scientific purposes.

According to Article 7 of this Directive, experiments making use of animals shall not be performed if another scientifically satisfactory method of obtaining the result sought, not entailing the use of an animal, is reasonably and practically available. Moreover, all experiments shall be designed to avoid distress and unnecessary pain and suffering to experimental animals.

Guidelines established by Commission Directives 87/302/EEC[7] and 92/69/EEC[8] refer to the following animal tests:

1.	Acute Toxicity (Oral)	Directive 92/69/EEC[8]
2.	Acute Toxicity (Oral) (Fixed Dose Method)	Directive 92/69/EEC[8]
3.	Acute Toxicity (Inhalation)	Directive 92/69/EEC[8]
4.	Acute Toxicity (Dermal)	Directive 92/69/EEC[8]
5.	Acute Toxicity (Skin Irritation)	Directive 92/69/EEC[8]
6.	Acute Toxicity (Eye Irritation)	Directive 92/69/EEC[8]
7.	Skin Sensitization	Directive 92/69/EEC[8]
8.	Repeated dose (28 d) Toxicity (Oral)	Directive 92/69/EEC[8]
9.	Repeated dose (28 d) Toxicity (Inhalation)	Directive 92/69/EEC[8]
10.	Repeated dose (28 d) Toxicity (Dermal)	Directive 92/69/EEC[8]
11.	Mutagenicity (*in vivo* mammalian bone-marrow cytogenetic test, chromosomal analysis)	Directive 92/69/EEC[8]
12.	Mutagenicity (Micronucleus Test)	Directive 92/69/EEC[8]
13.	Subchronic Oral Toxicity Test (90-d repeated oral dose study making use of rodent species)	Directive 87/302/EEC[7]
14.	Subchronic Oral Toxicity Test (90-d repeated oral dose study making use of nonrodent species)	Directive 87/302/EEC[7]
15.	Subchronic Dermal Toxicity Study (90-d repeated dermal dose study making use of rodent species)	Directive 87/302/EEC[7]
16.	Subchronic Inhalation Toxicity Study (90-d repeated inhalation dose study making use of rodent species)	Directive 87/302/EEC[7]
17.	Teratogenicity Study — Rodent and Nonrodent	Directive 87/302/EEC[7]
18.	Chronic Toxicity Test	Directive 87/302/EEC[7]
19.	Carcinogenicity	Directive 87/302/EEC[7]
20.	Combined Chronic Toxicity/Carcinogenicity Test	Directive 87/302/EEC[7]
21.	One-Generation Reproduction Toxicity Test	Directive 87/302/EEC[7]
22.	Two-Generation Reproduction Test	Directive 87/302/EEC[7]
23.	Toxicokinetics	Directive 87/302/EEC[7]
24.	Rodent Dominant Lethal Test	Directive 87/302/EEC[7]
25.	*In vivo* Mammalian Germ-Cell Cytogenetics	Directive 87/302/EEC[7]
26.	Mouse Spot Test	Directive 87/302/EEC[7]
27.	Mouse Heritable Translocation	Directive 87/302/EEC[7]

With the approval of Council Directive 86/609/EEC (Protection of the Animals),[10] several modifications of the procedures to be followed in conducting certain types of toxicity studies were brought to the attention of scientists.

For instance, to determine acute oral toxicity an alternative method (the "Fixed Dose Procedure") not utilizing death as a specific endpoint was introduced.[19] It makes use of fewer animals and results in less pain and distress than the classical determination of acute oral toxicity. The fixed dose method is conducted in two stages: in a preliminary study, the effect of various dose administered orally by gavage to single animals of one sex are investigated sequentially; in the main study, the substance is administered orally by gavage to groups of five male and five female animals at one of the preset dose levels (5, 50, 500, or 2,000 mg/kg);

The number of animals used is reduced to a scientifically acceptable minimum: only five animals of the same sex are tested for methods 1 and 4; only ten animals (and only five for the negative control group) are used for the determination of skin sensitization by means of the guinea pig maximization test (method 7). The number of animals needed for the positive control when using mutagenicity *in vivo* also is lowered (methods 11 and 12);

Pain and distress of animals during the tests are minimized; animals showing severe and enduring signs of distress and pain may need to be euthanized; dosing test substances in a way known to cause marked pain and distress due to corrosive or irritating properties need not be conducted (methods 1, 2, and 3);

Testing with insignificant high doses is avoided by introducing limit tests, not only in the acute toxicity tests (methods 1, 2, and 3) but also in the *in vivo* tests for mutagenicity (methods 11 and 12);

A strategy of testing for irritation allows not performing of test or its reduction to a single animal study, when sufficient evidence can be avoided;

The possibility of using *in vitro* tests or other criteria for defining irritation properties of a chemical was recognized. Scientific evidence of irritation properties can be based on the physicochemical properties of the substance, or on the results of well validated *in vitro* tests;

Before deciding to perform a skin irritation study (method 5) or an acute toxicity eye irritation study (method 6), careful consideration needs to be given to all information available on a substance to minimize testing of substances under conditions likely to produce severe reactions.

The following information can be useful when considering whether a complete test, a one-animal study, or no further testing is appropriate:

1. Physicochemical properties and chemical reactivity. Strongly acidic or alkaline substances (whose pH was demonstrated to be 2 or lower, or equal or greater than 11.5, for example) may not require testing for primary dermal irritation if corrosive properties can be expected. Alkaline or acidic reserve also should be taken into account;
2. If convincing evidence of severe effects in well-validated *in vitro* tests is available, a complete test may not be required;
3. Results from acute toxicity studies. If an acute toxicity test by the dermal route was conducted with the substance at the limit dose level (2,000 mg/kg body weight) and no skin irritation was observed, further testing for skin irritation may be unnecessary. In addition, testing of materials that have been shown to be highly toxic by the dermal route is unnecessary;
4. Results from skin irritation studies. Materials that have demonstrated definite corrosive or severe skin irritation in a dermal irritation study should not be tested further for eye irritation, because they might produce severe effects to the eye.

Guidelines for testing chemical substances for their toxicological hazard definition were developed and approved at the OECD level.[9]

The following guidelines have recently been amended and published:

1.	Acute Oral Toxicity	OECD No. 401
2.	Acute Dermal Toxicity	OECD No. 402
3.	Acute Inhalation Toxicity	OECD No. 403
4.	Acute Dermal Irritation/Corrosion	OECD No. 404
5.	Acute Eye Irritation/Corrosion	OECD No. 405
6.	Skin Sensitization	OECD No. 406
7.	Repeated Dose Oral Toxicity, Rodent: 28- or 14-d Study	OECD No. 407
8.	Subchronic Oral Toxicity, Rodent: 90-d Study	OECD No. 408
9.	Subchronic Oral Toxicity, Non-Rodent: 90-d Study	OECD No. 409
10.	Repeated Dose Dermal Toxicity: 21/28-d Study	OECD No. 410
11.	Subchronic Dermal Toxicity: 90-d Study	OECD No. 411
12.	Repeated Dose Inhalation Toxicity: 28- or 14-d Study	OECD No. 412
13.	Subchronic Inhalation Toxicity: 90-d Study	OECD No. 413
14.	Teratogenicity	OECD No. 414
15.	One-Generation Reproduction Toxicity Study	OECD No. 415
16.	Two-Generation Reproduction Toxicity Study	OECD No. 416
17.	Toxicokinetics	OECD No. 417
18.	Acute Delayed Neurotoxicity of Organophosphorous Substances	OECD No. 418
19.	Subchronic Delayed Neurotoxicity of Organophosphorous Substances: 90-d Study	OECD No. 419
20.	Acute Oral Toxicity — Fixed Dose Method	OECD No. 420
21.	Carcinogenicity Studies	OECD No. 451
22.	Chronic Toxicity Studies	OECD No. 452
23.	Combined Chronic Toxicity/Carcinogenicity Studies	OECD No. 453
24.	Genetic Toxicology: Micronucleus Test	OECD No. 474
25.	Genetic Toxicology: *In vivo* Mammalian Bone Marrow Cytogenetic Test — Chromosomal Analysis	OECD No. 475
26.	Genetic Toxicology: Rodent Dominant Lethal Test	OECD No. 478
27.	Genetic Toxicology: Mammalian Germ-Cell Cytogenetic Assay	OECD No. 483
28.	Genetic Toxicology: Mouse Spot Test	OECD No. 484
29.	Genetic Toxicology: Mouse Heritable Assay	OECD No. 485
30.	Genetic Toxicology: Unscheduled DNA Synthesis (UDS) Test with Mammalian Liver Cells *In vivo* (May 1994)	(to be approved)

These guidelines were the basis for detailing the corresponding guidelines approved by the EC's regulatory authorities as well as by Japan and the United States.

Chapter 4

ALTERNATIVE METHODOLOGIES TO ANIMAL TESTING

It seems suitable to include here a series of quotations from the last 5 to 10 years referring to the subject of alternative methods, especially to introduce controversial attitudes existing on the problem of a possible introduction of *in vitro* methodologies of any kind, within the framework of safety evaluation for chemical substances in general, and for cosmetic ingredients in particular.

Although animal models are of limited value in predicting toxic hazard for man, there is as yet little evidence that it will be possible in the foreseeable future to dispense entirely with live animal testing. The immediate prospect for a significant reduction in the scale of live animal experimentation stems from a reappraisal of current animal procedures, better experimental design and analysis, better use of available data on the toxicity of previously investigated compounds, and refinement of the questions being asked in toxicological investigations. Current methods in toxicity testing have evolved over several decades. Each chemical or series to be studied should be regarded as a novel, often unique, problem requiring a specifically designed program of investigations. Total abolition of the need for animal experimentation is a long-term goal because, with few exceptions, alternative approaches and methodologies are not yet developed to the point where they conceivably could be considered as adequate total replacements. More effort should be put into the development and validation of alternative techniques.[27]

Although most laws do not explicitly require animal testing, requirements of safety implicitly require that the best available means for determining safety be used. Thus, alternatives are not likely to be used widely until they can be shown to be at least as valid and reliable as the tests being replaced. Meeting these criteria is probably not overly difficult with some alternatives that involve reduction or refinement, but it may be harder to replace whole-animal testing totally with *in vitro* methods.[28]

In recent times, alternative methods in biomedical research and safety evaluation of chemicals and compounds have come increasingly to the fire. This development represents the confluence of several factors:

- accelerating developments in basic biologic methodology and understanding, especially *in vitro*,
- increasing realization of the wastefulness of such tests as the classic LD_{50} and Draize, once useful but now considered archaic, and
- increasing insistence from the public and animal rights groups that new understandings and methodologies be pressed into service of reducing animal use and alleviating animal suffering.[29]

The purpose of hazard evaluations of cosmetics, household products, and pharmaceutics is to protect human and animal life from levels of exposure to chemical agents that could have deleterious effects. It provides the basic knowledge for treatment should such exposure occur. In the area of testing cosmetic and household products, the media and animal rights activists have confused the issues of testing and biological research.[30]

Before any new *in vitro* test can become a regular, routine source of toxicological data, it will have to be validated. That means it must be shown to be reliable (to give consistent results in different laboratories and at different times in the same laboratory) and meaningful (to provide information that contributes to chemical safety evaluation). To promote acceptance, toxicologists must also begin to compile databases for *in vitro* tests so that better predictions can be drawn from the results.

The *in vitro* methodologies for evaluating the toxicological potential of chemical substances which have been reported in the literature have not yet been sufficiently validated for use in areas other than screening for mutagenicity/genotoxicity and for prescreening for severe irritation.
Moreover, the *in vitro* methodologies so far available have not yet been adequately validated in other areas to be included in regulatory guidelines at this time.
Alternative means different types of procedures which eliminate, reduce, or refine the use of animals in toxicity testing.[31]

Scientists have been and are searching for alternative methods to the use of animals in biomedical and behavioral research for a variety of reasons, including an interest in the welfare of animals, a concern for the increasing costs of purchasing and caring for animals and because in some areas alternative methods may be more efficient and effective research tools. In current usage, the term "alternative methods" includes replacement for mammals, reduction in the use of animals, and refinements in experimental protocols that lessen the pain of the animals involved.
The search for alternatives to the use of animals in research and testing remains a valid goal of researchers, but the chance that alternatives will completely replace animals in the foreseeable future is nil.[32]

Short-term tests provide a great deal of information relevant to the evaluation of the safety of chemicals, particularly the mechanisms of action, but are not yet developed to the stage where they can replace long-term animal tests as a basis for safety judgment.

- The prospects for developing *in vitro* tests for acute, local effects are encouraging.
- A relatively single set of *in vitro* cytotoxicity tests will identify most substances likely to cause acute systemic toxicity. However, the full potential of such assays will require a better understanding of the proportion of chemicals exerting an effect through general cytotoxic action compared with those affecting "organizational aspects" of the whole organism.
- Chronic effects are unlikely to be detected using currently available *in vitro* procedures.[33]

More research with *in vitro* methods should be carried out on molecular and cellular mechanisms of toxicity, including the identification of specific tissue, organ and system targets and responses.
The contributions already being made to toxicology as a result of the exploitation of *in vitro* methods should be more readily recognised by all toxicologists, and welcomed as the basis of a more scientific approach to toxicity testing.[34]

The field of *in vitro* toxicity testing is a rapidly evolving scientific endeavour. Initially, the scientific approaches to toxicity testing were focussed mainly on applying existing technologies from other fields of biomedical research to the problem at hand. In more recent years we have seen a shifting of emphasis to second-generation methods that are designed to address the *in vitro* toxicity testing problem from a more mechanistic approach. In coming years the new approaches will move through the cycle of research, development, validation, and ultimately acceptance by both the scientific and regulatory communities. In the past (for example, with the Ames Assay) this cycle has taken 10 to 15 years to come full term.[35]

In the following sections, methodologies under consideration or proposed for safety evaluation will be examined for each sector of toxicology.

4.1 ACUTE TOXICITY

It must be asked whether model systems using bacteria, cell cultures or tissues could contribute to the assessment of acute toxicity of chemical substances. This idea is based on the assumption that adverse effects on structure and function of a single cell could predict toxicity in the whole animal.[36]

This statement may well represent the problem of how to overcome the present classification of chemical substances on the basis of a single value of LD_{50}, which indicates mainly the death of the animal and which depends on the reaction between a chemical and specific receptors or regulatory systems functioning only in the whole animal, in relation also to the pharmacokinetic and metabolic fate of the chemical in whole organism.

Thanks to improved cell culture techniques, experimental models have been developed to assess important biological characteristics such as:

- membrane permeability;
- active and passive transport of ions and other compounds through the membrane;
- cellular respiration and energy metabolism;
- integrity of the cytoskeleton;
- growth inhibition and cell viability;
- inhibition of cell cycle controlling factors;
- measurements of macromolecular synthesis (DNA, RNA, proteins);
- changes in cell morphology;
- release of specific proteins;
- release or uptake of dyes or radioactive markers;
- ATP levels.

It already has been recognized by scientists that cell culture methods can provide preinformation (in the form of screening tests), and are useful in establishing dosages for the whole-animal experiment, thus reducing the number of animals used in testing. Information obtained by means of these different cell methods can certainly be used for building up information on specific groups of chemical substances. This information can be used for evaluating related chemicals, or for establishing a ranking order of toxicity. It also allows the selection of the least toxic compound in a series of chemically related substances.

Moreover, most of these endpoints are quantitative and can be used to elaborate dose-response curves, thus allowing the determination of the lowest effective dose (LED), a parameter useful for a further comparison with other chemicals, or for characterizing the intrinsic cellular toxicity of a chemical or of a mixture of chemicals (formulations).

On behalf of international organizations, such as the Scientific Committee on Problems of the Environment (SCOPE), the International Council of Scientific Unions (ICSU), the International Program on Chemical Safety (IPCS) of the WHO, the United Nations Environmental Program (UNEP) and the International Labor Organization (ILO), a recent working group has examined the problem of alternative methods for evaluating toxicity. It has indicated the present limitations of use for such methods:[33]

1. Basic cytotoxicity tests do not evaluate the capacity of highly specialized cells to carry out their organ-specific functions.
2. Some kind of toxicity involves the interactive influence of different types of cells. Toxic responses involving hormonal and nervous adjustment and immunological responses, for example, are typical of those involving organizational features characteristic of the whole organisms. This sort of response requires *in vivo* testing.
3. Many chemicals require previous biotransformation before they can exert a toxic effect on cells. In such cases, tests with hepatocytes or other metabolically competent cells could be used to supplement tests on less competent cells. However, it should be noted that hepatocyte cultures undergo differentiation and, as a consequence, may modify their capacity to metabolize xenobiotic chemicals.
4. *In vitro* concentrations of substances may be difficult to relate to concentrations in intact animals because of distribution phenomena (e.g., blood-brain barrier).
5. Most tissue culture systems involve such short incubation and observation times that they may be predictive only for acute *in vivo* effects. It is doubtful whether such tests can be used in predicting chronic toxicity.

The present scientific literature indicates the following methods as examples of those used to study the toxicity of chemicals:

- Cell Proliferation Assay[37]
- Neutral Red Uptake (NRU)[37-40]
  The following cell lines are used:
  - Rabbit tracheal epithelium;
  - Rat hepatocytes;
  - Human epidermal keratinocytes;
  - SIRC cell line;
  - Balb/c 3T3-L1 cell line;
  - Keratinocytes, clonetics;
  - Human fetal dermal fibroblasts cell line.

- Tetrazolium Salt (MTT assay)[37,40]
  The following cell lines are used:
  - Rabbit tracheal epithelium;
  - Keratinocytes, clonetics;
  - Human fetal dermal fibroblasts cell line.

- LDH Release[37]
  The following cell lines are used:
  - Rabbit tracheal epithelium;
  - HEp-2 cell line.

- Colony Formation Assay[40,41]
  The following cell lines are used:
  - Rabbit cornea cells;
  - FRSK cell line;
  - ARLJ301-3 cell line;
  - Balb 3T3 cell line;
  - SIRC cell line.

- Agar Overlay Test (AOT)[39]

- Total Protein Content (Lowry method)[39]
- Total Protein Content (Bio-rad assay)[39,40]
  The following cell lines are used:
  - Keratinocytes clonetics;
  - Human fetal dermal fibroblasts cell line;
  - HEp-2 cell line;
  - Balb/c 3T3 cell line.

- Total Protein Content (Kenacid blue method KB)[39]
- Tetrahymena Motility Assay[40]
- Neutral Red Release[39]

According to a review prepared by Paganuzzi-Stammati et al.,[42] the most commonly used endpoints as markers of toxic effects in cell cultures are the following:

- Synthesis or Release of Specific Molecules: Collagen mat, heme, hemoglobin, albumin, urea, lipoprotein, a-aminolevulinicacid, bile salts, metallothionein, glycosamino-glycans, proline and hydroxyproline, energy-dependent choline accumulation, histamine release, and c-AMP.
- Synthesis, Activity or Release of Specific Enzymes: β-glucuronidase, lactate-dehydrogenase, oubain-insensitive ATPase, 4,6-P-dehydrogenase, ASAL, glycogenphosphorylase, glutamic-oxalacetic transaminase, glutamic-pyruvic transaminase, acetylcholinesterase, and renin.
- Interactions of Compound with Cells: Phagocytosis, cytoplasmatic inclusions, intracellular accumulation, siderosome formation, uptake and/or binding of compound to cytosol and lipoproteins, mitogenic response.
- Alterations of Metabolic Pathways: Methaemoglobin reduction, 5-methyltetra-hydropholate accumulation, glucose-transport, hormone-stimulated gluconeogenesis, lipid peroxidation, fat accumulation, and glucosamine and galactose incorporation.
- Cell Surface Activities: Adhesiveness, Con-A agglutination, antibody-mediated rosette formation, complement deposition on treated cell membrane, chemotactic migration, antagonism with Histidine-H1 receptor, GABA-mediated postsynaptic inhibition, spike frequency, membrane polarization, fiber retraction and outgrow, and electrophysiological alteration.

In conclusion, at this stage of research, many methods not using whole animals have been employed in the testing of toxicity of chemical compounds and have been proposed as replacement for the LD_{50}: these methods range from the use of animal cells and tissue cultures to plant cells, bacteria, and invertebrates such as Paramecium and Tetrahymena. Attempts already have been made to validate some of the most currently used or promising methodologies with a small series of chemicals.

There is not available, however, a database containing the results of toxicity testing with nonanimal assays, which could allow a validation at a higher level, taking into account different sets of data and data from animal toxicity studies.

4.2 DERMAL IRRITATION

The Fund for the Replacement of Animals in Medical Experiments (FRAME) Toxicity Committee, after working for two years (1988–90), presented its conclusions on the problem of alternative methods to the dermal irritation studies using animals.[34]

Alternatives, according to this committee, can be classified into four groups as follows:

4.2.1 PHYSIOCHEMICAL ANALYSIS OF THE PROPERTIES OF CHEMICALS BEING TESTED

Usually, this relates to partition coefficient for predicting percutaneous absorption, and possibly, chemical structure. Validated quantitative structure-activity relationship (QSAR) data also can be used at this stage.

4.2.2 PRECIPITATION (TURBIDITY) TEST SYSTEMS

Such systems are exemplified by SKINTEX™, a technique that has been developed commercially, consisting of an artificial keratin barrier matrix and a reagent of dermal proteinaceous constituents, including collagen, globulin, glycosaminoglycans, and mucopolysaccharides. There are reservations over the limited mechanistic base of SKINTEX™.

4.2.3 CELL CULTURE METHODS

In vitro approaches have concentrated almost exclusively on assessing the primary toxic response to chemical insult. This approach has been applied to tissue-specific, differentiated cell types, such as mast cells, macrophages, polymorphonuclear cells, and keratinocytes, in which functional endpoints such as degranulation phagocytosis, migration and keratinozation or stratification have been measured. The approach has also, however, been applied to a wide range of cell types from other tissues of origin, with measurement of more general biochemical processes, such as cell viability, membrane integrity and enzyme leakage, DNA or protein synthesis, and cell replication, to name but a few.

4.2.4 TISSUE CULTURE METHOD UTILIZING EPIDERMAL SLICES OR SKIN EXPLANTS

Techniques have been developed that use intact skin isolated from both animals and man. The short-term maintenance of living preparation of freshly prepared skin over nutrient media, has been studied as a means of assessing skin irritant potential. While viable skin *in vitro* is avascular and will not retain aspects of the *in vivo* inflammatory response, it does permit measurements of a wide range of general biochemical indices of tissue toxicity, similar to those measured with cells in culture, as well as histological examination for morphological changes.

According to Deleo,[43] the development of systems for skin irritations is not as advanced; a number of the test systems that appear promising have been adapted to be used in the evaluation of skin-irritant chemicals by incorporating a relevant cell type in one specific evaluation methodology. Examples of these test systems are reported in Table 4.1.

The European Chemical Industry Ecology and Toxicology Center (ECETOC) presented a monograph in July 1990 dealing with the problem of describing various aspects of the assessment of skin irritation/corrosive potential of substances and preparations including the use of alternative testing procedures.[44]

TABLE 4.1
Test Systems to be Used for Skin Irritation Studies

In Vitro System	Endpoint
Human fibroblast and keratinocytes	Neutral red incorporation
Human keratinocytes	[³H] Uridine incorporation cellular protein
Skin organ culture (human, guinea pig, rabbit)	[¹⁴C] Leucine incorporation cellular vacuole formation
Cell-free (macromolecular mixture: SKINTEX™)	Physical/chemical reaction
Human keratinocytes	Cell growth inhibition and enzyme and ion leakage
3T3 fibroblasts (XB-2 keratinocytes)	Neutral red uptake, MTT clearage, hexosaminidase leakage, colony area, cell number, keratin staining
Keratome skin in diffusion chamber	Amino acids uptake, enzyme release
Fibroblast culture with keratin/agar overlay	Histochemistry, [³H] thymidine uptake, chromium release

According to the working group, "It has not been possible to identify a single *in vitro* or *in vivo* method which will adequately assess the skin irritation potential for all materials and all exposure situations."

The working group has discussed several "new *in vivo* experimental methods" to substitute for the Draize Primary Skin Irritation Test, which include:

- use of alternative species;
- methods to reduce the subjective nature of observation;
- alternative to patch test techniques;
- other indicators of irritant response.

The committee has classified a series of alternative *in vitro* approaches that use cell lines, skin tissues and nonbiological approaches. Some of them are presented in Table 4.2.

Usually all *in vitro* cytotoxicity methodologies available were adapted to cutaneous irritation studies. The basis for an adequate evaluation of these methodologies is, once again, the availability of an extensive toxicology database to allow a comparison between groups of chemicals whose irritation potential has been studied on whole animals or humans. What, moreover, is lacking is an *in vivo* skin irritation database to allow the comparison of the value of varying methodologies when applied to the same chemical substance.

4.3 EYE IRRITATION (MUCOUS MEMBRANE)

In a recent critical review of the *in vitro* alternative methods to the animal eye irritation it has been suggested that a battery of tests will be required to replace or reduce the use of the rabbit eye irritation test.

The available test protocols suggested as alternative methods are reported in Table 4.3.

The most critical considerations on these methods include the following aspects:

- lack of standardization;
- noncommercial availability of the tests;
- the nonbiological nature of some of them;
- the nature of the endpoint considered in the assay that does not correspond to the *in vivo* problems;
- the subjectivity of the evaluation of the results;
- the qualitative nature of the results, which does not inform about the extent of damage;

A recent evaluation of alternatives to the Draize eye test made available by the *in vitro* Toxicology Task Force of the U.S. Pharmaceutical Manufacturers Association (1990)[45] has concluded that "no single *in vitro* test system or battery of tests is currently capable of replacing the Draize eye test for ocular toxicity." However, the individual tests differ in their level of scientific merit:

- Tests promising for their relevance in *in vivo* ocular toxicity
  - Enucleated Superfused Rabbit Eye System;
  - Corneal Cup Model/Leukocyte Chemotactic Factors;
  - Corneal Opacity Test.

- Tests of questionable relevance to ocular toxicity but which provide estimates of nonspecific cytotoxic potential
  - Balb/c 3T3 Cells/Morphological Assay (HTD);
  - BHK Cells/Growth Inhibition;

TABLE 4.2

Different Alternative *In Vitro* Approaches to Substitute for the Draize Test

	Test System	Testing Procedures and Evaluation	Result
A.	**Cell Cultures**		
1.	3T3 Swiss mouse fibroblast	Cytotoxicity: Effects on cell proliferation, cell metabolism, cell membrane integrity	18 chemicals tested: 27% false positive
2.	XB-2 cell line	Keratinocyte differentiation: impairment of stratification and keratinization	
3.	C3H-10 T^1/$_2$ cells	Prelabeling with ^{3}H Arachidonic acid: total release of label into media	3 surfactants tested: correct classification
4.	Mouse embryo fibroblast cell line		
5.	Human keratinocytes		
6.	Differentiating keratinocytes (from rat sublingual epithelium)	Evaluation of total protein content, Acid phosphatase release, prolinase activity	1 chemical tested: suitable for testing
7.	Human keratinocytes	Grown on 3T3 mouse fibroblast; evaluation of lactate dehydrogenase, N-acetyl-ß-glucosaminidase and K+ concentration	Few chemicals tested: correlation with skin toxicity
8.	Guinea pig kidney fibroblast	Capacity to inhibit DNA-synthesis	Several chemicals tested: ranking
9.	Rat peritoneal mast cells	Cytolytic release of radioactively-labeled ^{51}Cr-chromate cytoplasmatic protein, release of histamine	Sodium laurate the most potent
10.	HEp-2 cells	Cell growth assay, Total protein content = IC$_{50}$ values	A series of n-alkylbenzoates: good correlation with IC$_{50}$ and skin toxicity
11.	Permanent cell line BALB/c 3T3 (mouse fibroblast)	Neutral red uptake, Uridine uptake inhibition assay	14 chemicals tested: good correlation
12.	KB cells (oral epidermal carcinoma)	Uridine uptake inhibition assay = UI$_{50}$	11 chemicals tested: r = 0.92 with 10 chemicals and skin irritation other chemicals tested

13.	3T3-L1 cells (mouse embryo)	Total cell protein, Neutral red uptake, morphological effects (ID_{50}; HTD)	30 chemicals tested: close correlation between the 3 methods. No *in vivo* data comparison
14.	Human endothelial cell cultures from umbilical cords	Production and release of prostanoids	2 chemicals tested: POSITIVE results
15.	Mouse connective tissue cells and mouse liver cells	Cytotoxicity evaluation by total purine and pyrimidine = GI_{50}, total protein content = ID_{50} and Acid Phosphatase (ACP) and LDH release	16 anesthetics: good correlation with rabbits, *in vivo*; 10 different chemicals: $r = 0.8$
16.	HEp-2 cells		
17.	KB cells	Uridine uptake inhibition assay = UI_{50}	5 chemicals tested: bad correlation
B.	**Skin Cultures**		
1.	Hairless mice	Measurement of enzyme activity (GOT, MDH, LDH, and glucose)	Different chemicals: correlation depending on chemical class
2.	Mouse skin	^{3}H-Thymidine and ^{14}C-Leucine incorporation (DNA and proteins); release of LDH, GOT, GPT, MDH	1 chemical tested: good correlation between *in vivo* and *in vitro* changes
3.	Mouse skin	Skin culture for 20 h: release of LDH	5 chemicals tested: good correlation between *in vivo* and *in vitro* data
4.	Full thickness, clipped skin of young rabbits	Energy status, tissue respiration and release of AST, MDH, LDH	6 chemicals tested: good correlation
5.	Hairless mouse and human skin	Histochemical changes, Oxygen uptake in mouse skin. Measurement of 5H groups, K^+ permeability and test chemical permeability in human skin	9 chemicals tested: no correlation with *in vivo* data
6.	Human skin epithelium	Cytotoxicity (LID and MID)	
7.	Embryotic chick spleen explants		18 chemicals tested: different results with the 2 cultures. Good correlation with patch-test

TABLE 4.2 (Continued)
Different Alternative *In Vitro* Approaches to Substitute for the Draize Test

	Test System	Testing Procedures and Evaluation	Result
8.	Calf and human skin discs	Thickness measurements	Series of alkyl sulfates: good correlation
9.	Rat skin slices	Leakage of AcP, LDH, and N-AG	3 chemicals tested: no correlation
10.	Human and rabbit skin keratome slices	Histological and histochemical determinations	7 chemicals tested: some correlation
11.	Epidermal slices of rat skin	Lysis of stratum corneum	63 chemicals tested: classification
12.	Epidermal slices of rat and human skin	Lysis of stratum corneum	59 chemicals tested: good correlation between human skin and animal data
13.	Rat epidermal slices	Lysis of stratum corneum	63 chemicals tested: classification
14.	Pig-Epidermis test	Swelling behavior of the isolated epidermis	Some surfactants tested: r = 0.84
15.	Epidermal permeability on isolated human epidermis	Radioactive chemicals tested	4 chemicals tested: good correlation with skin irritation
C.	**Nonbiological**		
1.	Zein-test	Solubilization of maize protein	16 chemicals tested: good correlation with *in vivo* data
2.	Hydrophobicity	Measured by HPLC and TLC	Some chemicals tested: inverted correlation
3.	Collagen swelling	—	Some chemicals tested: good correlation
4.	Hemolytic test (rabbit erythrocytes)	50% emolysis (EC$_{50}$)	16 chemicals tested: no correlation
5.	SKINTEX™ (Dermal Irritation Assay)	Mixture of chemicals	42 different chemicals tested: 94% equivalence
6.	Lysis of rabbit polymorphonuclear leukocyte (PMNL) granules	Lysis of granules with a spectrophotometer	Different chemicals tested: some POSITIVE correlation

7.	Alkali/acid reserve	Calculation of pH	34 chemicals tested: good correlation
8.	*In vivo* electrical resistance measurement (ERM) in rat skin	—	12 different chemicals tested: good correlation
9.	Structure activity relationship (TOPKAT)	QSARs studies	526 compounds tested: 90–95% of correct prediction

From ECETOC, Monograph No. 15, 1990, modified.

Table 4.3

Examples of Alternatives to Ocular Irritation Tests	
Methods	**Effects**
Neutral Red Assay Agarose Diffusion Method	Cell Viability and Membrane Integrity
Total Protein Content	Cell Growth Evaluation
Sylicon Microphysiometer	Metabolism Impairment
Fluorescein Leakage Test	Epithelium Damage
Chorioallantoic Membrane (CAM/HET–CAM)	Inflammation
Bovine Corneal Opacity	Cell and Tissue Physiology
Eyetex™	Protein Structure Modification

- BHK Cells/Colony Formation Efficiency;
- BHK Cells/Cell Detachment;
- SIRC Cells/Colony Forming Assay;
- Balb/c 3T3 Cells/Total Protein;
- BCL-D1 Cells/Total Protein;
- LS Cells/Dual Dye Staining;
- RCE-SIRC-P815-YAC-1/Cl Release;
- L929 Cells/Cell Viability;
- Bovine Red Blood Cell/Hemolysis;
- Rabbit Corneal Cell Cultures/Plasminogen Activator;
- LS Cells/ATP Assay;
- Balb/c 3T3 Cells/Uridine Uptake Inhibition Assay;
- Balb/c 3T3 Cells/Neutral Red Uptake;
- HeLa Cells/Metabolic Inhibition Test (MIT-24);
- Bovine Eye Cup/Histamine (Hm) and Leukotriene C4 (LT-C4) Release.

- Scientifically inadequate tests
  - Epidermal Slice/Electrical Conductivity (irrelevant to eye);
  - Rabbit Ileum/Contraction Inhibition (irrelevant to eye; pharmacological model);
  - Chorioallantoic Membrane (CAM) (irrelevant to eye; *in vitro* test; poor correlation);
  - Rat Peritoneal Cells/Histamine or Serotonin Release (irrelevant to eye);
  - Rat Vaginal Explant/Prostglandin Release (irrelevant to eye);
  - Rabbit Corneal Epithelial Cells/Wound Healing (potentially relevant to repair studies, but not injury);
  - Protein Matrix Assay (physiochemical reaction irrelevant to eye);
  - Computer Based/Structure-Activity Relationship (SAR) (output limited to database input; inadequate for novel structures/mixtures);
  - Tetrahymena/Motility (irrelevant to eye; questionable relevance to mammals).

There is widespread opinion that there is a need to continue in developing new methods for eye irritation evaluation based on fundamental research, with the objectives of improving some of the more interesting methodologies and developing additional methods in the area of recovery and repair of ocular damage.

There is also a need to develop both the scientific basis for mixture toxicology (e.g., formulations of finished cosmetic products); and for new methods and approaches to handle mixtures, solids, and water-insoluble materials, as only water-soluble compounds have generally been tested so far. There is also a need for quantitative structure-activity approaches. Although empirical approaches to the development of structure-activity relationships have been initiated, there has been scarce development of quantitative structure-activity relationships based on mechanistic understanding.[46]

It should be mentioned that a mixed procedure including animals and *in vitro* cell culture has been proposed.[47]

4.4 STRUCTURE-ACTIVITY RELATIONSHIP STUDIES

For many years, several attempts were made to relate all kinds of biological activity to chemical and molecular structures of compounds, on a qualitative as well as on a quantitative basis. This correlation refers to the previously defined acronyms SAR and QSAR.

A QSAR applies various techniques to define a relationship between a biological activity of a series of chemicals, and one or more parameters, called the "chemical descriptors", that are able to describe the chemical and molecular structure of substances. Among all biological activities, toxicity plays an active role in our present problem. Toxicity, as any other biological activity, is the result of the interaction between "sites" present in the molecular structure of a chemical compound and specific receptors present in the cell, as, for instance, the DNA molecule.

In QSAR studies, the molecular structure of a series of chemical compounds can be expressed by means of different substituent chemical groups in the molecule, by structural fragments of molecules, or by physical and chemical properties referred to a chemical molecule.

The system represented by QSAR is developed originally by comparing a series of toxicological effects displayed by a rather high and complex series of chemicals, with their specific parameters, represented by "chemical descriptors"; then, results are employed for predicting similar toxicological properties displayed by unknown chemicals, namely those for which no biological studies have yet been developed.

Validity of prediction ability of any QSAR system depends on the scientific value of the system itself, namely, on the quality of original biological data of those chemical substances identified unique for the construction of the QSAR system.

Any QSAR system is based on three different components:

1. the chemical descriptor;
2. the biological data, namely the toxicological data referred to given toxic endpoints;
3. the system to construct the correlation.

4.4.1 CHEMICAL DESCRIPTORS FOR QSAR

*   Physicochemical descriptors
    *   Melting point
    *   Boiling point
    *   Vapor pressure
    *   Dissociation constant (pKa)
    *   Activation energy
    *   Reaction rate constant (K)
    *   Partition coefficient (P)
    *   Coefficient from reverse-phase chromatography (Rm)
    *   Solubility in water (S)
    *   Parachor
    *   Hammet constant (δ)
    *   Taft polar substituent constant (d)
    *   Ionization potential
    *   Dielectric constant
    *   Dipole moments
    *   H bonding (HB)
    *   Quantum chemical data (atomic charge, bound energy, bound indices, resonance, energy, electron donating character, electron accepting character, electrostatic potential, distribution and Dewar numbers, π-bond reactivity, electron polarizability).

*   Steric descriptors
    *   Molecular volume
    *   Molecular surface area
    *   Molar refractivity (MR)
    *   Substructure shape
    *   Taft steric substituent constant (Es)
    *   Verloop STERlMa constants (L; B1-B5)

*   Structural descriptors
    *   Atom and bond fragment
    *   Substructures
    *   Substructure environment
    *   Number of atoms in a given structural element
    *   Number of rings (in polycyclic compounds)
    *   Molecular connectivity (extent of branching)

For each of these descriptors, or at least for those that have been selected to construct the QSAR system, the relationship should be defined with the toxicological endpoint to be taken into consideration, on the basis of results obtained from experimental studies.

4.4.2 TOXICOLOGICAL DATA AND QSAR

Toxicological data represent a crucial point in all QSAR systems developed so far. Usually, those interested in these studies do not perform, in their laboratories, the toxicological database. They are not toxicologists and therefore the main sources of their biological data are represented by the scientific literature. Not all scientific papers adequately describe experiments performed and results obtained, and some scientific journals are less stringent in publishing submitted papers than others. Therefore, for those who are less experienced in the field, all the literature data are listed together and used for the study of relationships in the QSAR system they are interested in. By doing so, the toxicological value of the data used is rather low, since the collection of biological data includes some very reliable ones (similar data obtained in different laboratories with the same expertise) and others of poor reproducibility.

Another difficulty related to toxicological data is represented by the fact that their qualitative and quantitative determination is not always precise, depending on the toxicological endpoint. For example, LD_{50} values represent a final endpoint that depends on several receptors in tissues and organs present in the whole animal: their reactions are not always in quantity the same. There are several criteria for toxicological data acceptability in QSARs; one may be that one presented by ECETOC's expert group: "Sufficient toxicological data, ideally generated via standard protocols and evaluated according to comparable criteria, must be available if a valid QSAR has to be developed. The important variables should be identical or comparable throughout any set of data used, but this requirement cannot always be met (it is never met). Where such variables differ within the data set, they should be evaluated critically for their effect on the QSAR, as much differences may greatly affect the outcome of biological assay."[48]

In our experience, when we decided to build up a database of mutagenicity data (*Salmonella typhimurium* gene mutations, chromosome aberrations in mammalian cells grown *in vitro*, and micronucleus in bone narrow cells of rodents) for more than 3000 chemicals[22] we decided to reevaluate all available biological data, in order to apply the same comparable criteria.

4.4.3 QSAR TECHNIQUES

Here is a list of some techniques used by different authors:

- Simple graphical plots or equations
- Regression analysis
- Pattern recognition

Examples of QSAR studies in the field of toxicology are the following:

- Oral LD_{50}, mouse/rat
- Inhibition of tissue-culture growth
- Teratogenicity
- Irritation of respiratory tract in mouse
- Skin absorption
- Receptor binding.

All these studies have been developed using a selected group of chemical substances. We must underline that when we tried to study the correlation between the growth inhibition of tissue culture and the LD_{50}, the correlation found was poor.[65] The same happened when a selected group of 567 chemicals from a total of 3600 chemicals was used to define the QSAR system for the prediction of LD_{50}: slightly more than 80% of the predicted values were within a factor of 10 higher or lower than the measured values.

The conclusion on the validity of QSAR studies to predict different toxicity endpoints of unknown chemicals is that the QSARs applied in toxicology are still the subject of considerable research, while the possibility to apply QSAR techniques to practical problems is still limited.

Where a specific toxic effect is of interest or concern in choosing chemicals for product development, certain QSARs may be useful for ranking the candidate chemicals. QSARs also may be useful for choosing from a series of chemicals those that should have priority for toxicity studies, and for deciding which toxic endpoint should be studied.

SAR or QSAR models should be used as alternatives to animal bioassays in the context of other information for the chemicals of concern. Thus, just as bioassays and *in vivo* methods have their limitations, so do SAR models.

These also include the sometimes limited database on which an SAR model is based, the temptation to extrapolate beyond the confines of the model, and the noise inherent in the bioassays on which models are based. Within these constraints, SAR models have a considerable potential in reducing the number of animals used in toxicity testing.

Particular interest was aroused by the application of QSARs in the field of carcinogenic predictivity of those chemicals analyzed for their mutagenicity. Valid results were obtained with the method that employs descriptors derived from the atomic structure of molecules, with binding connections included; they belong to the number-of-atom type, number and type of binding, molecular weight of compounds, number of rings (fragment descriptors), or partition coefficients, or geometrical descriptors (molecular volume, main axes, and molecular main axes ratio).

These methods, which have been adjusted through a series of databases, can be employed for the evaluation of new compounds of unknown activity if their structure is inserted for analysis. The latter is compared with the other descriptors of molecules that already have been inserted and that constitute the reference set (training set). In case of overlap, the probability that the new compound may be active is calculated on the basis of the probabilities that the overlap of descriptor parts may or may not be relevant to the reference set activity. Many among these methods use databases that are not alike (i.e., nonanalogous compounds) and do not belong to the qualitative type: in other words, they cannot predict an expected power (i.e., reversion/nanomolecules), unless the compound being examined belongs to a particular class of activity or whether it does not.

Among these methods, we should quote the Free Wilson, the ADAPT (Automated Data Analysis using Pattern-recognition Techniques), CASE, and Enslein's methodology.[49,50]

Within the scope of a wide classification of mutagenic/nonmutagenic compound, CASE was able to correctly classify 88% of the database compounds with TA98 strain of *Salmonella typhimurium* (Ames' Assay) and 84% of those with TA100 strain. Even a QSAR type assay could be performed, as data were inserted in semiquantitative form.

The Enslein method has been applied to mutagenesis and carcinogenesis, by taking into consideration the database obtained from the International Agency for Research on Cancer (IARC) monographs; 343 compounds were used, together with 120 noncarcinogenic and 223 carcinogenic ones.

The databases were chemically rather different, as they contained a variety of chemical compound classes; 79 descriptors were employed (e.g., molecular refractivity, etc.). The discriminating equation classified correctly between 87%, and between 78 and 80% of noncarcinogens.

Ashby has described a set of "structural alerts" that he considers to be associated strongly with carcinogenic potential in rodents and mutagenic activity in the Ames test.[51]

The further increase of databases in the field of genotoxicity and carcinogenicity of chemical compounds will be a good source for further studies of QSAR type in toxicology. This success of QSARs for genotoxicity and carcinogenicity data is also the result of the development of knowledge in these particular sectors of research, in which the mechanistic approach is based on sound scientific knowledge.

4.5 TERATOGENICITY

In whole animals the teratogenic effect is represented by any kind of malformations (morphological and functional) occurring in the embryo; the target, however, is not only the embryo, but also the fetus, the placenta, and the mother. This situation complicates the development of a unique *in vitro* test for teratogens: the knowledge of the mechanism by which a class of chemicals produces teratogenic effects may influence the choice of the *in vitro* test system.

Examples of possible tests are represented by:

- Cell Cultures
  - cell lines
  - primary cell culture
- Organ Cultures
  - nonmammalian
  - mammalian
- Whole Embryo Cultures

4.5.1 CELL CULTURES

These are represented by different established (differentiated) cell lines, such as:

- mouse ovarian tumor cells;
- human embryonic palatal mesenchymal cells;
- neuroblastoma cells.

The endpoints evaluated consist of: cytotoxic effects; cell proliferation; cell attachment; cell communication; cell differentiation.

Among the primary cell cultures available for the study of teratogenic compounds, those employed have been represented by (1) the embryonic limb mesenchymal cells; and (2) mild brain neural cells from rat embryos. Cell growth and toxicity and cell differentiation have been used as endpoints (it has been reported that by using these methodologies, 93% of chemicals tested were identified correctly as teratogens, and 89% of the nonteratogens were identified correctly).

4.5.2 ORGAN CULTURES

The organ culture system used most extensively to study teratogens *in vitro* is the "limb bud culture system," which undergoes extensive morphological and biochemical differentiation that can be evaluated; it allows the study of morphogenesis, cartilage formation, and muscle formation. Other systems are represented by human digits, palatal shelves, lenses, and different sex organs: by these methods, teratogenic effects on organogenesis have been studied.

4.5.3 WHOLE EMBRYO CULTURES

Some consideration has been given to the use of nonvertebrate and nonmammalians embryos, such as hydra system, chick embryos, fish embryos, and frog embryos.

Among the mammalian embryos, rat or mouse postimplantation embryos have been used, on which 17 morphological stages of embryonic development have been identified. The applicability of the whole-embryo technique as a routine method is limited because it is expensive, too sensitive to disturbances, often of unknown origin, and prone to abnormal development even under normal conditions. Furthermore, a maximum period of culture is too short if compared with the entire period of organogenesis. Testing of compounds that are insoluble or soluble in toxic solvents is difficult, and false positives are common with surface-active compounds.[52]

There are many other excellent examples in the use of *in vitro* methods to study teratogenic mechanisms. At present, none of the *in vitro* assays has been sufficiently evaluated, or been sufficiently predictive, as to gain wide acceptance as an all-purpose screen for developmental toxicants. Rapid *in vitro* screens could be, however, used to rank in order the teratogenic potential of chemical families so that the ones with the least toxicity could be developed further.[53]

Two assays for testing *in vitro* teratogens have been used by the National Toxicology Program (NTP) in the U.S.:

1. The MOT assay measures the attachment of ascitic mouse ovarian tumor cells (MOT cells) to a lectin (concanavalin A-) coated surface. Cellular adhesiveness is a generic property of embryonic cells; therefore, it is assumed that inhibition of adhesiveness by a chemical indicates teratogenic potential. The test chemical is added to a suspension of MOT cells which have been exposed to radiolabeled thymidine, and a plastic sheet coated with concanavalin A is placed in the culture vessel. Over a period of hours, the MOT cells normally adhere to the lectin-coated surface. Inhibition of this phenomenon by teratogens can be assessed by counting the radioactivity associated with the plastic sheets and by comparison with control values.
2. The HEMP assay measures the growth and proliferation of Human Embryonic Palatal Mesenchyme (HEMP) cells in the presence of test agents. Growth and division of cells is a fundamental process in developing tissues, and inhibition of this would be indicative of developmental toxicity. The HEMP cells are plated at a low density in tissue culture dishes. After 24 h, the test agent is added, and the cultures are maintained for an additional 72 h without a media change. At the end of this period, the number of cells present is counted using a Coulter counter.

More than 100 substances, including teratogens and nonteratogens, have been tested on MOT assay, in combination with a metabolic activation system (S-9); results have indicated an "accuracy" of 79% (corrected identified teratogens and nonteratogens).

Approximately 100 substances have been tested on HEMP assay, in the presence and absence of rat liver S-9 (metabolic activation system); results have indicated a predictive value of 64% (prediction *in vivo* teratogens).

The NTP has used these two combined methodologies (MOT/HEMP) in a battery, and reported 72% of agreement with the *in vivo* data.

4.6 GENOTOXICITY AND CARCINOGENICITY

As already stated, genotoxicity and/or mutagenicity produced by chemical agents can be evaluated by means of a series of *in vitro* methodologies, using mammalian and submammalian (microorganisms) cells; whole insects, such as *Drosophila melanogaster*, and plant cells also can be employed.

All different DNA and chromosome alterations described so far as responsible for human genetic diseases can be evaluated by testing chemicals for the following effects:

*   gene (molecular) mutations, such as DNA based;
*   changes, intercalations, transversion, transitions, etc.;
*   chromosome aberrations;

- chromosome number anomalies, such as nondisjunction, polyploidy, aneuploidy;
- sister chromatid exchanges (SCE);
- unscheduled DNA synthesis (UDS), or DNA damages;
- mitochondrial mutations.

Generally speaking, the primary evaluation of the potential for genotoxicity of chemical substances makes use of two basilar *in vitro* methodologies, such as the *Salmonella typhimurium* Ames' assay (gene mutation) and the *in vitro* mammalian chromosome aberration test (chromosome aberration). The results observed with these two systems can be verified in other *in vitro* assays, or, in a particular case of relevance for human exposure of chemicals being tested, when these two tests have produced positive results, specific animal tests may be used, with the aim of identifying the same potentiality in some *in vivo* tissues.

The database for these two methodologies applied to chemical substances accounts for more than 10,000 chemicals belonging to all possible chemical classes.

At the University of Pisa we have collected and reevaluated approximately 4,000 chemicals (identified by their CAS or EINECS numbers) tested with these two methodologies, and comparison has been made between these results and those obtained in animal genotoxicity or carcinogenicity studies.[22]

New *in vitro* methodologies have been developed and validated recently through an international cooperative research supported by the EC Commission. They allow the evaluation of the introduction of aneuploidy in mammalian cell grown *in vitro* or human lymphocytes.

A recent development refers to the use of Salmonella Ames' assay and the mammalian chromosome aberration assay in the testing of photomutagenic compounds which are relevant in the sector of cosmetic ingredients (sunscreen), according to the recommendation presented by the SCC.[54-56]

Genotoxicity and mutagenicity *in vitro* results normally are used to prescreen for carcinogenicity. As discussed before, the target for the toxic effects producing mutations and/or cancer is DNA. There are enough databases that correlate, at least for 80%, positive results obtained in *in vitro* genotoxicity tests with positive results obtained in the long-term carcinogenicity animal studies. The same holds true for noncarcinogens. Relevant information has been accumulated in the scientific literature that has permitted the identification of "structural alerts" present in the molecular structure of chemical substances that are responsible for mutagenic/carcinogenic properties of compounds.[51] By combining molecular data and *in vitro* genotoxicity data, it is possible today to rely on these simple conclusions and consider a chemical substance a candidate for producing tumors in whole-animal studies. This represents the most interesting achievement in the field of toxicity testing apart from the use of animals. Carcinogenicity studies require the higher number of animals and they involve the daily treatment of several hundred animals of two species for all their lives.

Chapter 5

GUIDELINES FOR *IN VITRO* TOXICITY ASSAYS

Guidelines for nonanimal toxicity testing procedures can be derived from the analysis of the scientific literature, where the protocols used for the individual study reported in the paper are described.

The test systems based on nonanimal models can be classified on the basis of both the biological component (i.e., epithelial cell culture, liver cell culture, yeast species, prokaryotic or eukaryotic organism, enucleated rabbit eyes, etc.) and on the basis of the endpoint measurement (i.e., cell toxicity, enzyme release, protein content, DNA fragmentation, etc.).

Frazier et al.[46] have described a series of protocols of *in vitro* toxicity testing procedures alternative to the Draize ocular irritation test. The list is reported in Table 5.1.

The *In Vitro* Techniques in Toxicology (*INVITTOX*) database was arranged by ERGATT/FRAME in Nottingham, England.[27] The production of protocols is the core activity of *INVITTOX*. The aim is to provide precise, up-to-date technical information on *in vitro* techniques. Each protocol is a self-contained document that includes detailed instructions on how to perform the technique. The rationale behind the technique is summarized, and the performance of the system in relation to others is assessed. The particular advantages and shortcomings of the system are discussed, and possible applications are indicated. A list of references relating to the technique is provided and, where possible, representative experimental data are included.

The protocols are written by *INVITTOX* staff in consultation with the scientists who have provided the information. These informants need not necessarily be the originators of the systems described, but they should use them regularly and should have been involved in their further development.

The information is sent to *INVITTOX* in any form convenient to the informant, usually as preprints or reprints containing a description of the method. *INVITTOX* staff extract relevant details and produce a draft protocol. Sometimes, when more than one source document is being used, discrepancies in the descriptions are noted. These, together with points on which more detail is needed, are sent as a list of questions to the informant. The answers, together with any other comments or changes that the informant might suggest, form the basis of a new revised draft. This process is repeated through as many drafts as are necessary, until both the informant and *INVITTOX* are satisfied, at which point the protocol is made available to registered users of *INVITTOX*. In this way, the informant retains full control of the content of the protocol, while being subjected to a minimum of effort.

All informants are asked whether they are willing to become contacts for the protocols concerned. In cases where this permission is given, the protocol will feature the contact name and address, so that any user encountering difficulties has direct access to an experienced user of the system.

INVITTOX protocols are not peer reviewed, although in many cases they are based on information derived from already published, refereed papers. The policy of *INVITTOX* is to accept all information that is offered, in the belief that the best judgment on a technique will come from people who have tried to use it. For this reason, a questionnaire is sent out with each protocol, in which users are asked to comment on the document and also on the method described. In particular, we are interested in hearing of any problems that have arisen and any modifications that have been introduced. Information from the questionnaires will at some point be incorporated into the protocols, so that the protocols will come to mirror the current consensus on the best way of performing a technique. Unfortunately, the return rate for questionnaires has been rather low. This could, of course, be due to the fact that *INVITTOX*

TABLE 5.1
List of Test Protocols

A. Morphology
    1. Enucleated Superfused Rabbit Eye System
    2. Balb/c 3T3 Cells/Morphological Assays (HTD)

B. Cell Toxicity
    1. Adhesion/Cell Proliferation
        a. BHK Cells/Growth Inhibition
        b. BHK Cells/Colony Formation Efficiency
        c. BHK Cells/Cell Detachment
        d. SIRC Cells/Colony Forming Assay
        e. Balb/c 3T3 Cells/Total Protein
        f. BCL-DI Cells/Total Protein
    2. Membrane Integrity
        a. LS Cells/Dual Dye Staining
        b. Thymocytes/Dual Fluorescent Dye Staining
        c. LS Cells/Dual Dye Staining
        d. RCE-SIRC-P815-YAC-I/Cr Release
        e. L929 Cells/Cell Viability
        f. Bovine Red Blood Cell Hemolysis
    3. Cell Metabolism
        a. Rabbit Corneal Cell Cultures/Plasminogen Activator
        b. LS Cells/ATP Assay
        c. Balb/c 3T3 Cells/Uridine Uptake Inhibition Assay
        d. Balb/c 3T3 Cells/Neutral Red Uptake
        e. HeLa Cells/Metabolic Inhibition Test (MIT-24)

C. Cell and Tissue Physiology
    1. Epidermal Slice/Electrical Conductivity
    2. Rabbit Ileum/Contraction Inhibition
    3. Bovine Cornea/Corneal Opacity
    4. Proptosed Mouse Eye/Permeability Test

D. Inflammation/Immunity
    1. Chorioallantoic Membrane (CAM)
        a. CAM
        b. HET-CAM
    2. Bovine Corneal Cup Model/Leukocyte Chemotactic Factors
    3. Rat Peritoneal Cells/Histamine Release
    4. Rat Peritoneal Mast Cells/Serotonin Release
    5. Rat Vaginal Explant/Prostaglandin Release
    6. Bovine Eye Cup/Histamine (Hm) and Leukotriene C4 (LT-C4) Release

E. Recovery/Repair
    1. Rabbit Corneal Epithelial Cells/Wound Healing

F. Other
    1. EYTEX Assay
    2. Computer Based/Structure Activity Relationship (SAR)
    3. Tetrahymena/mobility

From Frazier, J. M., et al., *Evaluation of Alternatives to Acute Ocular Irritation Testing — Alternative Methods in Toxicology 4,* Mary Ann Liebert, New York, 1987. With permission.

protocols are in many cases serving as a collection of information on available techniques, and that the techniques themselves are not yet being used. Future plans at *INVITTOX* include contacting all recipients of selected protocols to solicit their comments.

A number of *INVITTOX* protocols already have been updated based on further information received from the original informant. In such cases, it is *INVITTOX* policy automatically to send out the updated version to everyone who has requested the protocol at any time in the past.

Table 5.2 presents a list of protocols on *in vitro* techniques to be used for toxicity testing and stored in the *INVITTOX* data bank.

The descriptions of the 50 *in vitro* methodologies (see list below) in this chapter have been elaborated with the collaboration of Dr. Maria Nieri, Dr. Elena Bosco, and Dr. Gregorio Loprieno, by considering the methods described by the individual authors reported in the document and adapting them to the format used by OECD and EEC for similar guidelines which have been included in the Galileo Data Bank (see page 209).

The guidelines (Exposure Concentrations, Culture Conditions, Metabolic Activation, Reference Substances, Evaluation and Interpretation of the Data, etc.) could be improved in the future when a series of parameters will be completed, in connection with similar attempts made in the past, for example by the Center for Alternatives to Animal Testing in 1984,[46] or on the basis of the ERGATT/FRAME Data Bank of *INVITTOX*.

Some guidelines are already adopted for testing chemicals for their genotoxic potential; they have been validated in the past and are used in different fields (industrial chemicals, pesticides, food additives, cosmetic ingredients, and drugs).

- Agar overlay test (AOT)
- Bovine corneal opacity and permeability (BCOP) assay
- Chorioallantoic membrane (CAM) test
- Cell metabolic cooperation assay
- Cell metabolic cooperation assay for analysis of gap junction intercellular communication (GJIC)
- Cell proliferation assay
- Chromium-51 release assay
- Co-culture clonal survival assay
- Colony formation assay
- Dual dye staining (acute cellular toxicity)
- Dye transfer assay for analysis of GJIC
- Enucleated eye test (EET)
- Epidermal slice technique for skin corrosive potential
- *Escherichia coli* — reverse mutation assay
- EYTEX™ assay
- Gene mutation test — *Saccharomyces cerevisiae*
- HET — CAM test
- *In vitro* acute hepatotoxicity test
- *In vitro* mammalian cell gene mutation test
- *In vitro* mammalian cell transformation test
- *In vitro* mammalian cytogenetic test
- *In vitro* measurement of inflammatory mediators
- *In vitro* percutaneous absorption assay
- *In vitro* photomutagenicity mammalian cytogenetic test
- *In vitro* Syster chromatid exchange assay (SCE)
- Inibition of tumor cell attachment

TABLE 5.2
INVITTOX Protocol List 6 (17.2.1993) of Alternative Methods

1. Bovine Isolated Cornea Test
2. Rabbit Isolated Terminal Ileum
3a. The Frame Modified Neutral Red Uptake Cytotoxicity Test
3b. The Frame Cytotoxicity Test (Kenacid Blue)
4. Model Cavity Method
5. Isolated Rat Glomeruli And Proximal Tubules
6. Human Lymphocyte Cytotoxicity Assay
7. The Isolation And Culture Of Rat Hepatic Cells
8. *Allium* Test
9. A Cytotoxicity Test Using Perfused Cell Cultures: The Use Of Membrane Permeability As A Measure Of Cytotoxicity In Perfused Cell Cultures
10. Reactive Metabolite Formation By Fortified Liver Microsomes
11. Whole Rat Brain Reaggregate Culture
12. Polymorphonuclear Leukocytes Locomotion
13. Hepatoma Cell Cultures As *In vitro* Models For Hepatotoxicity
14. Hel 30 Cytotoxicity Test
15. Hen's Egg Test (HET)
16. Cytotoxicity And Genotoxicity In Primary Cultures Of Human Hepatocytes
17. MTT Assay
18. Unscheduled DNA Synthesis in Hepatocyte Cultures Assessed By The Nuclei Procedure
19. Alkaline Unwinding Genotoxicity Test
20. Isolation Of Rat Hepatocytes
21. Bovine Spermatozoa Cytotoxicity Test
22. *Tetrahymena Thermophila* Ocular Irritancy Test
23. Rat Hepatocyte Flow Cytometric Cytotoxicity Test
24. Cytoskeletal Alterations As A Parameter For Assessment Of Toxicity
25. Laser Diffraction Measurement Of Tumor Spheroids
26. The Skin Test
27. Human Skin Fibroblast/Collagen Lattice Cytotoxicity Test
28. Human Esophageal Culture
29. Human Thyroid Culture
30. The Ames Test
31. Agarose Overlay Assay
32. Dust Toxicity in Rat Alveolar Macrophage Cultures
33. Yeast Growth Rate Cytotoxicity Test
34. Yeast Plasma Membrane H^+-Atapase Toxicity Test
35. Chinese Hamster Ovary Cell Na+/K+ -Atapase Test
36. Chinese Hamster Ovary (CHO) Cell Proliferation Test
37. Red Blood Cell Test System
38. L929 Cytotoxicity Test
39. V79 Cytotoxicity Test For Membrane Damage
40. SIRC Cytotoxicity Test
41. Rabbit Articular Chondrocyte Functional Toxicity Test
42. Liver Slice Hepatotoxicity Screening System
43. Colorimetric Cytotoxicity Assays For Anchorage Dependent Cells
44. Cell Culture Phototoxicity Test
45. The *Dunaliella Tertiolecta* Test: A Marine Test Assay Procedure
46. Balb/C 3T3 Cytotoxicity Test
47. HET-CAM Test
48. Lung Cell Assay
49. H-4-II-E Rat Hepatoma Cell Bioassay
50. HEp-2 Cytotoxicity Test For Implant Materials
51. Llc-Rk$_1$ Cell Screening Test For Nephrotoxicity
52. Quantitative Video Microscopy Of Intracellular Motion And Mitochondrial Specific Fluorescence
53. Automated *In vitro* Dermal Absorption (AIDA) Procedure
54. The FRAME Neutral Red Release Assay

TABLE 5.2 (Continued)
***INVITTOX* Protocol List 6 (17.2.1993)**

55. The Pollen Test System
56. Hen's Egg Test — Yolk-Sac Blood Vessel Assay
57. Human And Bovine Lens Epithelial Culture
58. UV Absorption As An Approximation For Cell Number
59. *In vitro* Fertilization Sperm Toxicity Test
60. Eye Lens Organ Culture
61. An *In vitro* Model For Studies Of Prostaglandin H Synthase (PHS)-Mediated Genotoxicity Of Xenobiotics
62. Screening System of Promoters Using *ras* Transfected BALB/c-3T3 Clone (BHAS 42)
63. α-Methyl Glucose Uptake In Isolated Proximal Tubular Cells
64. The Neutral Red Cytotoxicity Assay
65. Lucifer Yellow Intercellular Exchange Assay For Tumor Promoters
66. *In vitro* Prediction Of The Maximum Tolerated Dose

- LDH release
- Method for *in vitro* cytotoxicity testing
- Method for *in vitro* neurotoxicity test
- Methods of assessment of thyrotoxicity
- Micromass teratogen test
- Micronucleus test
- Microtubule disassembly
- Mitotic recombination test — *Saccharomyces cerevisiae*
- Neutral red release (NRR)
- Neutral red uptake (NRU)
- Photomutagenicity bacterial assay
- Protein Synthesis Inhibition
- QSAR applied to the Draize test — 1
- QSAR applied to the Draize test — 2 (multi-CASE methodology)
- QSAR applied to the Draize test — 3
- *Salmonella typhimurium* — reverse mutation assay
- Sex-linked recessive lethal test in *Drosophila melanogaster*
- Tetrahymena motility assay
- Tetrazolium salt assay (MTT)
- The pollen tube test
- Total protein content (Bio-rad assay)
- Total protein content (Kenacid blue method, KB)
- Total protein content (Lowry method)
- Unscheduled DNA synthesis

AGAR OVERLAY TEST (AOT)

1. METHOD

1.1 Introduction, 1.2 Definition, and 1.3 Reference Substances (to be defined)

1.4 Principle of the Test Method

The AOT is a cytotoxic assay used to identify a reduction of cell viability on established cell lines exposed to test chemicals. The endpoint is determined by a vital stain uptake that is revealed by an area of discolored cell and lysis in the monolayer. AOT allows to assay both liquid and solid test compounds and is recommended by the FDA to test Class III Soft Contact Lenses. Currently the test also is used in the United States in the screening of solid or semisolid cosmetics for irritative potential. The most interesting aspect of AOT is the possibility of using the chemicals undiluted, thus avoiding both the problem of solubility of the substances and toxicity of the solvents and affording the possibility of better mimicking the Draize eye irritation test or an accidental exposure in humans.

1.5 Quality Criteria (to be defined)

1.6 Description of the Test Method
1.6.1 Preparations
Established cell lines: L929, ATCC (CCL1), NCTC929, clone of strain L., are used.

1.6.2 Test Conditions
Number of Cultures
(to be defined)

Use of Negative and Positive Controls
Blank plate (no sample-placement on the overlay), or negative control plates (100 μl saline or solvent, adsorbed on filter paper) and adequate positive control plates (1 cm² rubber glove) are used.

Exposure Concentrations
(to be defined)

Culture Conditions
(to be defined)

Metabolic Activation
(most chemicals require metabolic activation)

1.6.3 Procedure
1.6.3.1 Preparation of Cultures
Cell Lines: cells from culture flasks are tripsinized and a cell suspension produced at 4×10^5 viable cells/ml in 1X medium; 4 ml/plate of cell suspension is dispensed onto an appropriate number of 60 mm tissue culture plates, then the cells are incubated at 37°C in a humidified 5% CO_2 incubator for 24 h. Then the medium is carefully removed from plates and the confluent cell monolayer is covered by 4 ml/plate of a mixture 2% agarose and 2X media, maintained at 42°C. After 15 min, 4 ml of Neutral Red vital stain (0.01% in medium) is added to the agar surface and the plates left in dimmed lighting at room temperature for at least 10 min: then the excess stain is discarded.

Culture Medium (1X): RPMI 1640 supplemented with glutamine 2 mM, 100 IU/ml penicillin, 100 μg/ml streptomycin and 10% FCS.

1.6.3.2 Treatment of the Cultures with the Test Substance
Cell Lines: 100 μl of the liquid chemicals or dilution thereof are absorbed on filter paper and deposited onto the agar surface (in the case of powder, 100 mg of chemical are distributed on the agar surface covering about 1 cm²). All plates are incubated in 5% CO_2 atmosphere

at 37°C for 22 to 24 h. At the end of treatment time the plates are examined for evidence of cytotoxicity.

1.6.3.3 Analysis

Cytotoxicity is determined according to the following criteria: the plates are examined macroscopically and microscopically (by inverted light microscope) for evidence of discoloration and lysis (% of lysed cells within the decoloration zone); the results are expressed in terms of Response Index (Zone Index-Lysis Index), the zone index being an estimate of the size of the zone of unstained cells beneath the sample, and the lysis index indicating the percentage lysis within that zone. The grading is as follows:

Zone Index

0 = no detectable zone around or under sample
1 = zone limited to area under sample
2 = zone no greater than 0.5 cm in extension from the sample
3 = zone no greater than 1 cm in extension from the sample
4 = zone greater than 1 cm in extension from sample but not involving entire plate
5 = zone involving entire plate

Lysis Index

0 = no observable lysis
1 = less than 20% cells lysed
2 = less than 40% cells lysed
3 = less than 60% cells lysed
4 = less than 80% cells lysed
5 = more than 80% cells lysed

The sample is not regarded as cytotoxic on the test system when lysis did not occur even if discoloration is seen. In this case discoloration could result from technical bias (e.g., diffusion, dye interferences).

2. DATA

3. REPORTING
3.1 Test Report

The test report shall, if possible, include the following information:

- test conditions: detailed description of treatment and sampling schedule, dose levels, toxicity data, negative and positive controls;
- dose/effect relationship when possible;
- statistical evaluation;
- discussion of the results;
- interpretation of the results.

3.2 Evaluation and Interpretation
(to be defined)

ALTERNATIVE TO ANIMAL TEST

This method may be used in the screening for potential eye irritant chemicals.

BIBLIOGRAPHY

Commission of the European Communities, Collaborative Study on the Evaluation of Alternative Methods to the Eye Irritation Test — Part 1, Doc. XI/632/91 V/E/1/131/91, Brussels, 1991, p. 13.

Commission of the European Communities, Collaborative Study on the Evaluation of Alternative Methods to the Eye Irritation Test — Part II, Doc. XI/632/91 V/E/1/131/91, Brussels 1991, p.152.

Gettings, S.D., J. J. Teal, D. M. Bagley, J. L. Demetrulias, L. C. Di Pasquale, K. L. Hintze, M. G. Rozen, S. L. Weise, M. Chudkowski, K. D. Marenus, W. J. W. Pape, M. Roddy, R. Schnetzinger, P. M. Silber, S. M. Glaza and P. J. Kurtz, The CTFA evaluation of alternatives program: An evaluation of *in vitro* alternatives to the Draize primary eye irritation test (Phase 1) Hydro-alcoholic formulations; (Part 2) Data analysis and biological significance, *In Vitro Toxicology*, Vol. 4, No. 4, p. 247, 1991.

INVITTOX, Protocol No. 31, November 1991.

Rougier, A., M. Cottin, O. De Silva, R. Roguet, P. Catroux, A. Toufic and K. G. Dossou, *In vitro* methods: Their relevance and complementarity in ocular safety assessment, *Lens and Eye Toxicity Research*, Vol. 9, No. 3–4, p. 229, 1992.

BOVINE CORNEAL OPACITY AND PERMEABILITY (BCOP) ASSAY

1. METHOD

1.1 Introduction, 1.2 Definition, and 1.3 Reference Substances (to be defined)

1.4 Principle of the Test Method

This assay allows investigation of two important components of eye irritation, opacity and permeability, in a 1-day experiment, using an ocular tissue. It represents a useful approach to predict the irritant potential of compounds in development and process intermediates (which include a wide variety of chemical classes with variable physical characteristics).

1.5 Quality Criteria (to be defined)

1.6 Description of the Test Method

1.6.1 Preparation

Equipment

Corneal holders are specially made of plastic with glass disks on the lateral sides. Corneas are inserted between two chambers (5 ml each) and firmly clamped in place with screws. Holes in each compartment allowed medium filling and exhausting of bubbles. The opacitometer was composed of a black plastic box containing compartments for both treated and control corneas, light sources, and photocells. The difference between photocell signals was measured electronically and displayed on a digital dial. Due to a saturation mechanism, particularly with low illumination, the response of photocells is generally not linear. However, the system is designed to give a linear response over a wide range of light transmission, and an arbitrary reference is used to calibrate the apparatus in the linear portion of the curve. This is achieved, with no cornea in the apparatus, by setting an opacity value of 100 with the aid of an opaque, homogeneous, sheet of cellulose placed in the "experimental" compartment. Such an internal standard has been defined in preliminary experiments as a value corresponding approximately to the opacity produced by a 5% solution of benzalkonium chloride. It has been verified that the apparatus gives linear responses for up to 2.5 times this value.

1.6.2 Test Conditions
Number of Cultures
　Four corneas per group (test chemical or vehicle treatment) are used.

Use of Negative and Positive Controls
　Negative control (vehicle) is used.

Exposure Concentrations
　(to be defined)

1.6.3 Procedure
1.6.3.1 Preparation of Cultures
　The bovine eyes are collected in a local abattoir and transported to the laboratory immersed in a salt solution (Hanks). They are generally used within 2 h of the killing of animals. All eyes are carefully examined, and those presenting defects, such as neovascularization, pigmentation, opacity, and scratches, were discarded. Selected corneas are dissected with a 2 to 3 mm rim of sclera attached for easier handling. The iris and lens are removed, and the corneas are rapidly mounted into holders. Both chambers are then filled with MEM supplemented with 1% fetal bovine serum (FBS), and corneas are incubated for 1 h in a water bath at 32°C. This operation allows the corneas to equilibrate with the external medium.

1.6.3.2 Treatment of the Cultures with the Test Substance
　Fresh MEM + 1% FBS is placed in the posterior compartment and the anterior compartment (epithelium side) receives the test compound or its vehicle.

1.6.3.3 Analysis
Opacity Measurement
　The apparatus measures differences in light transmission between treated and control corneas. Thus, on each experimental day, two corneas are exposed to the vehicle, and the one that remained more clear is used as a control for all test corneas. Usually corneas treated with MEM or with PEG-400 remains very clear in the short-term treatment and incubation periods used, although a slight opalescence in a control cornea is observed on a very few occasions.

Fluorescein Assay
　After opacity readings are completed, medium is removed from the holders. Fresh medium is added to the posterior compartment, and 1 ml of a 5 mg/ml Na-fluorescein solution in Dulbecco's phosphate-buffered saline (DPBS) is put in contact with the epithelium. Corneas are incubated horizontally for 90 min, then the amount of the dye that passes through the cornea in the posterior compartment is measured spectrophotometrically at 490 nm.

2. DATA

3. REPORTING
3.1 Test Report
　The test report shall, if possible, include the following information:

- test conditions: detailed description of treatment and sampling schedule, dose levels, toxicity data, negative and positive controls;

- dose/effect relationship when possible;
- statistical evaluation;
- discussion of the results;
- interpretation of the results.

3.2 Evaluation and Interpretation
(to be defined)

4. ALTERNATIVE TO ANIMAL TEST
This method may be used in the screening for potential eye irritant chemicals.

BIBLIOGRAPHY

Gautheron, P., M. Dukic, D. Alix and J.F. Sina, Bovine corneal opacity and permeability test: An *in vitro* assay of ocular irritancy, *Fundamental and Applied Toxicology*, Vol. 18, p. 442, 1992.

Gautheron, P., J. Giroux, M. Cottin, L. Audegond, A. Morilla, L. Mayordomo-Blanco, A. Tortajada, G. Haynes, J.A. Vericat, R. Pirovano, E. Gillio Tos, C. Hagemann, P. Vanparys, G. Deknudt, G. Jacobs, M. Prinsen, S. Kalweit and H. Spielmann, Interlaboratory assessment of the bovine corneal opacity and permeability (BCOP) assay, *Toxicology in Vitro*, Vol. 8, No. 3, p. 381, 1994.

Muir, C. K., Four simple methods to assess surfactant-induced bovine corneal opacity *in vitro*: Preliminary findings, *Toxicology Letters*, Vol. 22, p. 199, 1984.

CHORIOALLANTOIC MEMBRANE (CAM) TEST

1. METHOD

1.1 Introduction, 1.2 Definition, and 1.3 Reference Substances (to be defined)

1.4 Principle of the Test Method
The CAM of the chick embryo is a complete tissue including arteries, capillaries and vein: the vessels contain erythrocytes and leukocytes of the same maturity as those of the developing embryo and are likely to respond to chemical-induced inflammatory stimuli. For this, the CAM has been proposed as a possible means of predicting the irritant potential of chemicals for the conjunctival tissue of the rabbit, as observed in the Draize test. The assay is based on the evaluation of the macro/micro alterations of the membrane, after an appropriate treatment time.

1.5 Quality Criteria (to be defined)

1.6 Description of the Test Method
1.6.1 Preparations
Hen's egg chorioallantoic membrane is used.

1.6.2 Test Conditions
Number of Cultures
Six to 15 eggs for each experimental point are used.

Use of Negative and Positive Controls
(to be defined)

Exposure Concentrations

Generally, four dilutions of test compounds are used; the four concentrations cover the range from no response to minor responses to severe effects.

Culture Conditions

Eggs that appear abnormal or with damaged membranes are discarded.

Metabolic Activation

(most chemicals require metabolic activation)

1.6.3 Procedure

1.6.3.1 Preparation of Cultures

Hen's Egg: Fertile eggs, day 0, are incubated at 37°C. On day 3 of incubation, the shell is penetrated in two places. First, near the pointed end of the egg a small opening is ground in the shell and the shell membrane is exposed. With a shortened needle and syringe the shell membrane is penetrated and 1.5 to 2 ml of albumen is removed and discarded. The second opening is a rectangular window. The window is closed with transparent tape until the next step (Zwilling technique).

To reduce the possibility of contamination from shellborne bacteria, the fertile hen's egg is placed in a dessicator containing a vial of 0.25 ml formalin to which an excess of potassium permanganate is added. The dessicator is then sealed and the eggs are left in the resultant formaldehyde vapor for 1 h. The eggs are stored in a cool room (5 to 12°C) prior to incubation. Eggs are then coded, incubated (Marsh Roll-X automatic incubator, Robin Haigh Incubators, with a relative humidity of 56%) and processed as above.

1.6.3.2 Treatment of the Cultures with the Test Substance

Hen's Egg: On day 14, the tape is removed opening the window. A Teflon™ ring, 10 mm in internal diameter, is placed on the CAM. The ring serves as a marker of the test site and as container for the preparation to be tested. An aliquot of the test sample is placed in the ring, using an Eppendorf pipette. The window is closed again with tape and the egg returned to the incubator. Three days later, on day 17 of incubation, the tape is removed and the CAM examined.

After a treatment procedure like that reported above, the treated CAM is examined macroscopically at 4, 24, and 48 h (after treatment) and is then prepared for histological examination.

1.6.3.3 Analysis

The criteria used for macroscopic rating of lesions on the CAM are listed below:

* size;
* contours and surface (raised, flat, or depressed edges, raised smooth, granular or shaggy, transparent or opaque);
* color (white, yellow, red, brown, grey, or black);
* retraction of surrounding CAM;
* spokewheel pattern of vessels;
* overall grade of severity;
* necrosis (confirmed microscopically).

The evaluation is made on individual eggs, all bearing coded numbers arranged at random. The scored sites are subdivided as follows:

- necrotic lesion of 5 mm or more (3+);
- necrotic lesion between 3 and 5 mm (2+);
- fleshy lesion less than 3 mm (1+);
- membrane without recognizable lesion (0).

The percentage of positive eggs is determined by adding up the numbers of eggs with scores of 2+ and 3+, and dividing this number of positives by the total number of viable eggs in the series (50% positive).

Other Classification
Reactions are grouped according to three grades of effect:

- Slight: macroscopically there is very little change from normal, with some drying and wrinkling of the CAM, while histologically, virtually no response is observed.
- Moderate: the lesion is well defined, with persisting blood vessels and some hemorrhage within the lesion. Microscopically a proliferative lesion is seen with hyperplasia of the ectoderm and endoderm coupled with a mesodermal response. Frequently there is a loss of ectoderm continuity over the center of the lesion with underlying disorganized regeneration.
- Severe: the lesion is well defined, with "ghost blood vessels" within the lesion. Histologically, full-depth or virtually full-depth necrosis is observed.

2. DATA

3. REPORTING
3.1 Test Report
Animal strains must be mentioned.

3.2 Evaluation and Interpretation
(to be defined)

4. ALTERNATIVE TO ANIMAL TEST
It may be used in the screening for potential eye irritant chemicals.

BIBLIOGRAPHY

Bagley, D. M., L. H. Bruner, O. De Silva, M. Cottin, K. A. F. O'Brien, M. Uttley and A. P. Walker, An evaluation of five potential alternatives *in vitro* to the rabbit eye irritation test *in vivo*, *Toxicology In Vitro*, Vol. 6, No. 4, p. 275, 1992.

Gettings, S.D., J. J. Teal, D. M. Bagley, J. L. Demetrulias, L. C. Di Pasquale, K. L. Hintze, M. G. Rozen, S. L. Weise, M. Chudkowski, K. D. Marenus, W. J. W. Pape, M. Roddy, R. Schnetzinger, P. M. Silber, S. M. Glaza and P. J. Kurtz, The CTFA evaluation of alternatives program: An evaluation of *in vitro* alternatives to the Draize primary eye irritation test (Phase 1) Hydro-alcoholic formulations; (Part 2) Data analysis and biological significance. *In Vitro Toxicology*, Vol. 4, No. 4, p. 247, 1991.

Lawrence, R. S., M. H. Groom, D. M. Ackroyd and W. E. Parish, The chorioallantoic membrane in irritation testing, *Food and Chemical Toxicology*, Vol. 24, No. 6/7, p. 497, 1986.

Leighton, J., J. Nassauer and R. Tchao, The chick embryo in toxicology. An alternative to the rabbit eye, *Food and Chemical Toxicology*, Vol. 23, No. 2, p. 293, 1985.

Parish, W. E., Ability of *in vitro* (corneal injury — eye organ — and chorioallantoic membrane) tests to represent histopathological features of acute eye inflammation. *Food and Chemical Toxicology*, Vol. 23, No. 2, p. 215, 1985.

CELL METABOLIC COOPERATION ASSAY

1. METHOD

1.1 Introduction, 1.2 Definition, and 1.3 Reference Substances (to be defined)

1.4 Principle of the Test Method

Many mechanisms are belived to be applicable to chemical teratogenesis and to result in growth retardation, impaired function, physical malformation, or death. Because cell-cell communication through chemical messengers is a fundamental event required for the differentiation of embryonal cells, some authors proposed the inhibition of intercellular communication as a possible mechanism of teratogenesis. This endpoint is evaluated by means the of V79 cell metabolic cooperation assay: it is dependent on the transfer, by way of gap junctions, of the toxic phosphorilated metabolite of 6TG from wild-type 6TGs cells to 6TGr cells when the two types of cells are co-cultured. The 6TGr are unable to metabolize 6TG to a toxic substrate, and survive to form colonies when intercellular communication is inhibited and the transer of phosphorilated 6TB from adjacent 6TGs is blocked. Range of doses is determined by means of cytotoxicity and cloning efficiency assays. This assay has been proposed as screen assay for developmental toxicants though some possible limitations are evident (e.g., species-, organ-, and cell-specificity of inhibitors of intercellular communication, the lack of metabolic activation systems in V79 cells, and the use of a single endpoint to predict developmental toxicity).

1.5 Quality Criteria (to be defined)

1.6 Description of the Test Method
1.6.1 Preparations
Chemicals are dissolved in absolute ethanol, acetone, DMSO (1% of the medium volume) or serum-free culture medium (up to 10% of the medium in the dish): volume of medium in culture dishes is adjusted accordingly to maintain a total volume of 5 ml. Chinese hamster lung fibroblasts (V79 cell line) are used (6TGs cells): the 6TG^r cells are derived from X-ray-irradiated wild-type 6TGs cells.

1.6.2 Test Conditions
Number of Cultures
Twelve dishes per concentration are used in V79 metabolic cooperation assay; four dishes per concentration are used in cloning efficiency assay.

Use of Negative and Positive Controls
Each cloning assay and metabolic cooperation assay includes a solvent control (negative control) and 4 mg/ml of 12-O-tetradecanoylphorbol-13-acetate (TPA) as a positive control.

Exposure Concentrations
Test chemicals are initially evaluated in a preliminary cytotoxicity assay to determine the concentrations ranging from nontoxic to cytostatic effect. Two or three independent cloning efficiency assays are then performed to define a concentration range, of approximately one order of magnitude, that extends from nontoxic concentrations to slightly toxic concentrations. Ideally, the three lowest concentrations would result in 100% cloning efficiency, and the

highest concentration would cause a significant reduction in cloning efficiency. The purpose of identifying a concentration that is cytotoxic is to determine the maximum nontoxic concentration for final testing in the metabolic cooperation assay where five concentrations are used.

Culture Conditions
   (to be defined)

Metabolic Activation
   (most chemicals require metabolic activation)

1.6.3 Procedure

Cells are maintained in culture medium containing 3% FBS. The culture medium is modified Eagle's minimum essential medium (MEM) with Earle's salts containing a 50% increase in all vitamins and essential amino acids, and 1 mM-pyruvate. Cultures are incubated at 37°C in a 5% CO_2/air atmosphere. The cells are transferred by trypsinization two to three times a week, and used within 2 months of thawing. Stock cultures are cryopreserved in Eagle's MEM containing 5% serum and 5% DMSO.

Cytotoxicity Assay

Cells are plated at 4×10^5 6TGr cells per 60-mm plastic culture dish. After a 4-h attachment period, test chemicals are added to dishes at approximately one-half log dilutions ranging from 0.001 to 10,000 µg/ml, depending on estimated toxicity of the chemicals. Following a 3-d growth period, cells are evaluated microscopically to detemine cytostasis or cytotoxicity.

Cloning Efficiency Assay

One hundred 6TGr cells are seeded in each 60-mm dishes. After a 4-h attachment period, dishes are treated with the appropriate concentration of test chemical or vehicle alone. Following a 3-d growth period, culture medium containing test chemical is replaced with fresh culture medium, and the incubation continues. After a 6- to 7-d growth period, cultures are rinsed with phosphate-buffered saline and stained and fixed with 1% crystal violet (1 g dissolved in 10 ml ethanol and diluted to 100 ml with water). Colonies are counted and compared with untreated cultures.

1.6.3.1 Preparation of Cultures

V79 Metabolic Cooperation Assay: 100 6TGr cells are co-cultured with 4×10^5 6TGs cells in 5 ml of medium in 60-mm dishes.

1.6.3.2 Treatment of the Cultures with the Test Substance

Test chemicals are added 4 h after plating 6TGr and 6TGs cells, and 6TG is added 15 min later to a final concentration of 10 µg/ml. After 3 d, medium is replaced with fresh medium containing only 6TG but without the test chemical; 3 to 4 d later, cells are washed with PBS and fixed and stained with 1% crystal violet. A final cloning efficiency assay is performed concomitantly with the metabolic cooperation assay.

1.6.3.3 Analysis

For both the metabolic cooperation assay and the final cloning efficiency assay, Dunnett's test is used to compare the number of colonies in cultures treated with the test compounds with control cultures: the level of $p < 0.01$ is considered statistically significant. In the cloning efficiency assay, any concentration that significantly reduces colony number is considered cytotoxic.

The results of each chemical assay are reduced to a single summary score. The summary scores separate the chemicals into three categories:

- a positive (+) score, if chemicals inhibits metabolic cooperation at at least two noncytotoxic concentration;
- a negative (-) score, if chemicals do not significantly inhibit metabolic cooperations at any concentration;
- an equivocal (=) score, if chemicals inhibit intercellular communication at less than two noncytotoxic concentrations.

2. DATA

3. REPORTING
3.1 Test Report and 3.2 Evaluation and Interpretation
(to be defined)

4. ALTERNATIVE TO ANIMAL TEST
It may be used in the screening for potential teratogenic chemicals.

BIBLIOGRAPHY

Toraason, M., J.S. Bohrman, E. Krieg, R.D. Combes, S.E. Willington, W. Zajac and R. Lagenbach, Evaluation of the V79 cell metabolic cooperation assay as a screen *in vitro* for developmental toxicants, *Toxic. In Vitro*, Vol. 6, No. 2, pp. 165–174, 1992.

CELL METABOLIC COOPERATION ASSAY
FOR ANALYSIS OF GJIC

1. METHOD

1.1 Introduction, 1.2 Definition, and 1.3 Reference Substances (to be defined)

1.4 Principle of the Test Method
Gap junction intercellular communication (GJIC), one of several specialized connections that form among adjacent cells, may become aberrant in the carcinogenic process particularly when non-DNA reactive (epigenetic) carcinogens are involved. The alteration of cell communication has been suggested as an endpoint for the development of screening tests for potential promoters. Among these, the V79 cell metabolic cooperation assay it is dependent on the transfer, by means of gap junctions, of the toxic phosphorilated metabolite of 6TG from wild-type 6TG^s cells to 6TG^r cells when the two types of cells are co-cultured. The 6TG^r are unable to metabolize 6TG to a toxic substrate, and survive to form colonies when intercellular communication is inhibited and the transfer of phosphorilated 6TG from adjacent 6TG^s is blocked. Range of doses is determined by means of preliminary cytotoxicity assays. The usefulness of this assay is still uncertain: a possible limitation stems from the organ specificity of certain chemicals.

1.5 Quality Criteria (to be defined)

1.6 Description of the Test Method
1.6.1 Preparations
    Chemicals are dissolved in absolute ethanol, acetone (2% of the medium volume), or serum-free culture medium and distilled/deionized water (up to 20% of the medium in the dish). Volume of medium in culture dishes is adjusted accordingly to maintain a total volume of 5 ml. Chinese hamster lung fibroblasts (V79 cell line) are used (6TG^s cells); the 6TG^r cells are derived from X-ray-irradiated wild-type 6TG^s cells.

1.6.2 Test Conditions
Number of Cultures
    Twenty dishes per concentration are used in V79 metabolic cooperation assay; four dishes per concentration are used in preliminary assay.

Use of Negative and Positive Controls
    Each cytotoxicity and metabolic cooperation assay includes a solvent control (negative control) and 4 ng/ml of 12-O-tetradecanoylphorbol-13-acetate (TPA) as a positive control. Each cytotoxicity assay includes a medium control without solvent.

Exposure Concentrations
    Test chemicals are initially evaluated in a preliminary cytotoxicity assay to determine the concentration ranges required to produce little or no cytotoxicity. Then, five concentrations, ranging from nontoxic to marginally cytostatic are selected for the second toxicity determination (clonal assay). Five or six concentrations, producing 70 to 100% cell survival in the second assay, then are evaluated in a third cytotoxicity determination (identical to the second). Five or six chemical concentrations are selected, based on the concentrations that produce 70 to 100% cell survival in the third assay, and evaluated by the metabolic cooperation assay.

Culture Conditions
    (to be defined)

Metabolic Activation
    (most chemicals require metabolic activation)

1.6.3 Procedure
    Cells are maintained in culture medium containing 3% FBS (Flow). The culture medium is modified Eagle's minimum essential medium (MEM, Gibco) with Earle's salts containing a 50% increase in all vitamins and essential amino acids except glutamine, 100% increase in the nonessential amino acids and 1 mM-pyruvate. Cultures are incubated at 37°C in a 5% CO$_2$/air atmosphere. The cells are passaged by trypsinization (0.01% trypsin-Worthington Biochemicals-solution prepared in calcium-and magnesium-free PBS) two to three times a week, and used within 2 months of thawing. Stock cultures are cryopreserved in Eagle's MEM containing 5% serum and 5% DMSO. To eliminate cell clumping, all cultures are transferred on the day before use and then are reseeded at the appropriate density on the day the experiment is initiated.

Cytotoxicity Assay
    Cells are plated at 4×10^5 6TG^r cells per 60-mm plastic culture dish (Lux). After a 4-h attachment period, test chemicals are added to dishes at approximately 1 to 2 log dilutions

ranging from 0.001 to 10,000 µg/ml, depending on estimated solubility and/or toxicity of the chemicals. Following a 3-d growth period, cells are evaluated microscopically to detemine cytostasis or cytotoxicity.

Clonal Assay

One hundred 6TG^r cells are seeded in 60-mm dishes. After a 4-h attachment period, dishes are treated with the appropriate concentration of test chemical or vehicle alone. Following a 3-d growth period, culture medium containing test chemical is replaced with fresh culture medium, and the incubation continues. After a 6- to7-d growth period, cultures are rinsed with phosphate buffered saline and stained and fixed with 1% crystal violet (1g dissolved in 10 ml ethanol and diluted to 100 ml with deionized water). Colonies are counted and compared with untreated cultures.

1.6.3.1 Preparation of Cultures

V79 Metabolic Cooperation Assay: 6TG^s cells are co-cultured with 4×10^5 6TG^s cells in 5 ml of medium in 60-mm dishes.

1.6.3.2 Treatment of the Cultures with the Test Substance

Test chemicals are added 4 h after plating 6TG^r and 6TG^s cells, and 6TG^s is added 15 min later to a final concentration of 10 M. After 3 d, medium is replaced with fresh medium containing only 6TG but without the test chemical; 3 to 4 d later, cells are washed with PBS and fixed and stained with 1% crystal violet.

1.6.3.3 Analysis

Means and standard deviations of colonies per dish are calculated per hour for each experimental group. Values from treated cells in the metabolic cooperation assay are compared with values from cells treated only with solvent with Dunnett's test: data are analyzed relative to controls at the <0.01 confidence level.

A chemical is classified as positive if it inhibits metabolic cooperation at two sequential concentration levels and if the cloning efficiencies in the concurrent cytotoxicity assay are at least 70% of the solvent control. A chemical that does not statistically inhibit metabolic cooperation at any concentration is scored as negative. Chemicals are scored as equivocal if they statistically inhibit metabolic cooperation only at a single concentration level and/or if greater than 30% cytotoxicity relative to controls occurs at the statistically positive concentration levels.

2. DATA

3. REPORTING
3.1 Test Report and 3.2 Evaluation and Interpretation
(to be defined)

4. ALTERNATIVE TO ANIMAL TEST

This test method may be used in the screening for potential tumor promoter/carcinogenic chemicals.

BIBLIOGRAPHY

Bohrman, J. S., J. R. Burg, E. Elmore, D. K. Gulati, T. R. Barfknecht, R. W. Niemeier, B. L. Dames, M. Toraason and R. Langenbach, Interlaboratory studies with the Chinese hamster V79 cell metabolic co-operation assay to detect tumor-promoting agents, *Environmental and Molecular Mutagenesis*, Vol. 12, p. 33–51, 1988.

CELL PROLIFERATION ASSAY

1. METHOD

1.1 Introduction, 1.2 Definition, and 1.3 Reference Substances (to be defined)

1.4 Principle of the Test Method
The cell proliferation assay is an easy and rapid method to evaluate the effect of test chemicals on cell proliferation of primary cultures: this is performed using an image analysis method and has been suggested to be a sensitive marker to determine the acute toxicity of chemicals.

1.5 Quality Criteria (to be defined)

1.6 Description of the Test Method
1.6.1 Preparations
Test chemicals are prepared in distilled water or DMSO and then diluted in serum-free culture medium; final DMSO concentration does not exceed 1%.
Primary cultures (rabbit tracheal epithelium) are used.

1.6.2 Test Conditions
Number of Cultures
Twenty-five control culture dishes are used; triplicate cultures are tested for each experimental point.

Use of Negative and Positive Controls
A negative control is used.

Exposure Concentrations
Test chemicals are applied in only a single concentration.

Culture Conditions
(to be defined)

Metabolic Activation
(most chemicals require metabolic activation)

1.6.3 Procedure
1.6.3.1 Preparation of Cultures
Primary Cultures: Tracheas are removed from rabbits and the epithelium is separated from the underlying cartilage and cut into 2-mm explants. The explants are grown on collagen matrix and covered with minimum essential medium (MEM).

1.6.3.2 Treatment of the Cultures with the Test Substance
Primary Cultures: Chemicals are applied on day 2 of culture and inhibition of growth is determined on days 3, 4 and 6; the evolution of cultures is observed until day 6 (96 h of treatment) without any change of culture medium.

1.6.3.3 Analysis
Culture growth is evaluated by an image analysis system. Cultures are photographed daily. The photographs are then analyzed by a computer connected with a CCD camera IVC 500

(Sony), which measured the ratio of outgrowth surface area to explant surface area. A standard curve of outgrowth surface area to explant surface area ratio vs. the number of days of culture is drawn on the mean of 25 control culture dishes. Surface ratios of treated cultures are evaluated by the image analysis method and then expressed as a percentage of control culture values. Because intertrachea variability, cells from the same trachea are used to make all the tests with the same chemical. Up to 30 cultures are obtained from a single trachea; 13 measurements are made on each trachea.

2. DATA

3. REPORTING
3.1 Test Report
The test report shall, if possible, include the following information:

- test conditions: detailed description of treatment and sampling schedule, dose level applied, toxicity data, negative and positive control;
- cell cultures;
- animal species/strain;
- discussion of the results;
- interpretation of the results.

3.2 Evaluation and Interpretation
(to be defined)

4. ALTERNATIVE TO ANIMAL TEST
This test method may be used in the screening for potential toxic chemicals.

BIBLIOGRAPHY

Blanquart, X. X., S. Romet, A. Baeza, C. Guennou and F. Marano, Primary cultures of tracheal epithelial cells for the evaluation of respiratory toxicity, *Toxicology In Vitro,* Vol. 5, No 5/6, p. 499, 1991.

CHROMIUM-51 RELEASE ASSAY

1. METHOD

1.1 Introduction, 1.2 Definition, and 1.3 Reference Substances (to be defined)

1.4 Principle of the Test Method
The chromium-51 release assay is a cytotoxicity assay that is rapid and easy to perform. It employs continuous cell lines and primary cell cultures that are known to label readily using 51_{Cr}. The assay determines the ability of chemical compounds to effect cytolysis *in vitro* by measuring 51_{Cr} release.

1.5 Quality Criteria (to be defined)

1.6 Description of the Test Method
1.6.1 Preparations
A cell line (P815) is used.

1.6.2 Test Conditions
Number of Cultures

The assay is carried out in quadruplicate for each experimental point; controls are performed in octuplicate.

Use of Negative and Positive Controls

A "spontaneous release" control, consisting of medium plus cells, and "total 51_{Cr} release" control, consisting of cells and 15% saponin detergent, are used as background controls.

Exposure Concentrations
   (to be defined)

Culture Conditions
   (to be defined)

Metabolic Activation
   (most chemicals require metabolic activation)

1.6.3 Procedure
1.6.3.1 Preparation of Cultures
   (to be defined)

1.6.3.2 Treatment of the Cultures with the Test Substance

Cells are seeded and labeled using 51_{Cr}. After the incubation time with test compounds has been completed, plates are centrifuged and supernatants are collected and counted using a gamma counter.

1.6.3.3 Analysis

The toxic effect is expressed as a CR_{50} value, i.e., the concentration of test chemical resulting in 50% release of 51_{Cr} compared to controls. Appropriate replicate wells are averaged and the percent 51_{Cr}-release calculated as follows:

$$\%51Cr - \text{release} \frac{(\text{CPM experimental release} - \text{CPM spontaneous release})}{(\text{CPM total release} - \text{CPM spontaneous release})} \times 100$$

Dose-response curves are constructed and the concentration of test material resulting in 50% release of 51_{Cr} is determined by interpolation.

2. DATA

3 REPORTING
3.1 Test Report
The test report shall, if possible, include the following information:

- test conditions: detailed description of treatment and sampling schedule, dose levels, toxicity data, negative and positive controls;
- dose/effect relationship when possible;
- statistical evaluation;
- discussion of the results;
- interpretation of the results.

3.2 Evaluation and Interpretation
(to be defined)

4. ALTERNATIVE TO ANIMAL TEST
This method may be used in the screening for potential eye irritant chemicals.

BIBLIOGRAPHY

Gettings, S.D., J. J. Teal, D. M. Bagley, J. L. Demetrulias, L. C. Di Pasquale, K. L. Hintze, M. G. Rozen, S. L. Weise, M. Chudkowski, K. D. Marenus, W. J. W. Pape, M. Roddy, R. Schnetzinger, P. M. Silber, S. M. Glaza and P. J. Kurtz, The CTFA evaluation of alternatives program: An evaluation of *in vitro* alternatives to the Draize primary eye irritation test (Phase 1) Hydro-alcoholic formulations; (Part 2) Data analysis and biological significance, *In Vitro Toxicology*, Vol. 4, No. 4, p. 247, 1991.

Shadduck, J. A., J. Everitt and P. Bay, Use of *in vitro* cytotoxicity to rank ocular irritation of six surfactants, in *In Vitro Toxicology: A Progress Report from the Johns Hopkins Center for Alternatives to Animal Testing*, Vol. 3, A. M. Goldberg, Ed., Mary Ann Liebert, New York, 1985, p. 641–649.

CO-CULTURE CLONAL SURVIVAL ASSAY

1. METHOD

1.1 Introduction, 1.2 Definition, and 1.3 Reference Substances (to be defined)

1.4 Principle of the Test Method
The co-culture clonal survival assay is a test for the detection of reduction of cell viability induced by chemicals. It is founded on the co-culturing of wild-type cells and ouabain-resistant cells (OUAr); this assay measures the relative cloning efficiency of chemically treated cells in high-density cell cultures.

1.5 Quality Criteria (to be defined)

1.6 Description of the Test Method
1.6.1 Preparations
Established cell lines BALB/3T3 clone A31 are used.

1.6.2 Test Conditions
Number of Cultures
Three cultures for each experimental point repeated in separate experiments are used.

Use of Negative and Positive Controls
Negative control (untreated or solvent) and positive control (benzo[a]pyrene) are used.

Exposure Concentrations
Four concentrations of each test compound are used.

Culture Conditions
Appropriate culture medium and seeding density are used.

Metabolic Activation
(most chemicals require metabolic activation)

1.6.3 Procedure
1.6.3.1 Preparation of Cultures

1.6.3.2 Treatment of the Cultures with the Test Substance
OUAr and wild-type cells are seeded at appropriate density. After a growing time, they are treated (at first with the test chemical and then with ouabain), then allowed to grow for an additional period, fixed, and stained.

1.6.3.3 Analysis
The result is reported as RCE_{50} (or LD_{50}). This is the concentration that results in 50% RCE (relative cloning efficiency) of chemically treated cells relative to untreated cultures.

2. DATA

3. REPORTING
3.1 Test Report
The test report shall, if possible, include the following information:

- test conditions: detailed description of treatment and sampling schedule, dose levels, toxicity data, negative and positive controls;
- dose/effect relationship when possible;
- statistical evaluation;
- discussion of the results;
- interpretation of the results.

3.2 Evaluation and Interpretation (to be defined)

4. ALTERNATIVE TO ANIMAL TEST
This method may be used in the screening for potential toxic chemicals.

BIBLIOGRAPHY

Matthews, E. J., Chemical-induced transformation in BALB/c-3T3 cells: relationship between *in vitro* transformation and cytotoxicity, carcinogenesis and genotoxicity. In *Mutation and Environment. Part D: Carcinogenesis*, Mendelsohn, M. L. and R. J. Albertini, Eds., Wiley-Liss, New York, 1990, p. 229–238.

Matthews, E. J., Transformation of BALB/c-3T3 cells: II. Investigation of experimental parameters that influence detection of benzo[a]pyrene-induced transformation. *Environmental Health Perspectives Supplements*, Vol. 101, Suppl. 2, p. 293, 1993.

Matthews, E. J., J. W. Spalding and R. W. Tennant, Transformation of BALB/c-3T3 cells: V. Transformation responses of 168 chemicals compared with mutagenicity in *Salmonella* and carcinogenicity in rodent bioassays. *Environmental Health Perspectives Supplements*, Vol. 101, Suppl. 2, p. 347, 1993.

COLONY FORMATION ASSAY

1. METHOD

1.1 Introduction, 1.2 Definition, and 1.3 Reference Substances (to be defined)

1.4 Principle of the Test Method
The colony formation assay is a test for the detection of reduction of cell viability induced by chemicals. It consists in counting colonies containing a minimum number of cells, each

arising from a single surviving cell. Compared with other cytotoxicity assays, it has a high sensitivity because the exposure to the chemicals occurs in a condition of a low cell density. The colony formation assay, using both primary cell cultures and established cell lines, has a good correlation with the Draize rabbit eye irritation test *in vivo* and is an attractive method for the screening of chemicals.

1.5 Quality Criteria (to be defined)

1.6 Description of the Test Method
1.6.1 Preparations
Chemicals are dissolved in PBS, DMSO, ethanol, or 50% ethanol in PBS on a weight/weight basis (detergents, glycols, oils, and final concentrations of solvents of 0.5% produce no effects on cell survival) or are prepared weight/volume with volume/volume dilutions in sterile medium without serum or antibiotics (hydro-alcoholic formulations). Sample preparations are not subject to pH adjustment and are sterilized only with a filter.

Primary cultures (RC-1 cells; rat bone-marrow cells) and established cell lines ARLJ301-3; BALB 3T3; FRSK; SIRC, ATCC (CCL 60) V79 are used.

1.6.2 Test Conditions
Number of Cultures
Three or four cultures are used for each dose.

Use of Negative and Positive Controls
A negative control (if necessary, cultures of various age) is used.

Exposure Concentrations
(to be defined)

Culture Conditions
Appropriate culture medium, seeding density, dosing time and dosing-endpoint time are used. Monolayer or three-dimensional culture systems are utilized.

Metabolic Activation
(most chemicals require metabolic activation)

1.6.3 Procedure
1.6.3.1 Preparation of Cultures
Primary Cultures: RC-1 cells (rabbit cornea cells) are cultured in Eagle's MEM with 10% fetal calf serum (Biocell Co., Carson, CA) in a humidified incubator at 37°C in an atmosphere of 5% CO_2: 500 cells are each plated onto 60-mm dishes.

Both medullary and endosteal rat femoral-marrow cells are used to generate single-cell suspensions, which are incubated at 33°C in 5% CO_2 and a humidity greater than 90% for 2 to 6 h in Fischer's medium conditioned with 10% FBS and 10% equine serum, and supplemented with hydrocortisone hemisuccinate (463 µg/l), nonessential amino acids, fungizone, and antibiotics (complete medium). Nonadherent cells are cryopreserved and adherent cells are cultivated for three to four passages, lifted with collagenase, and seeded onto pretreated nylon filtration screens (8 mm × 45 mm; numbers 3 through 210/36, Tetko, NY) at a density of 10^6 to 10^7 cells/ml; 10^6 freshly prepared or cryopreserved hematopoietic cells are inoculated onto the template when three or four of every five mesh openings contain stromal cell processes (about 5 to 7 d).

Cell Lines

FRSK cells (fetal rat skin keratinocytes cell line) are cultured in Eagle's MEM with 10% fetal calf serum (Biocell Co., Carson, CA) in a humidified incubator at 37°C in an atmosphere of 5% CO_2: 200 cells are plated onto each 60 mm dishes.

ARLJ301-3 cells (rat liver cell line) are cultured in William's medium with 10% fetal calf serum (Biocell Co., Carson, CA) in a humidified incubator at 37°C in an atmosphere of 5% CO_2: 500 cells are each plated onto 60-mm dishes.

Balb 3T3 cells (mouse whole embryo cell line) are cultured in Eagle's minimum essential medium with 10% fetal calf serum (Biocell Co., Carson, CA) in a humidified incubator at 37°C in an atmosphere of 5% CO_2: 100 cells are each plated onto 60-mm dish.

Confluent culture of SIRC (rabbit corneal cell line) are trypsinized for 5 min to prepare single-cell suspensions for seeding assay dishes. Relatively few cells are seeded onto each culture dish. Ham's F12 medium is used, supplemented with 10% heat-treated (30 min, 56°C) fetal calf serum, 100 IU/ml penicillin and 100 µg/ml streptomycin.

1.6.3.2 Treatment of the Cultures with the Test Substance
Primary Cultures and Cell Lines

From18 to 24 h after inoculation, the cells are treated with chemicals and incubated for 6 d (BALB 3T3 and FRSK) or 7 d (ARLJ301-3 and RC-1 cells). On day 7 or 8 after plating, the cells are fixed by methanol and stained with 5% Giemsa solution.

Suspended nylon screen bone-marrow cultures of various ages (10 to 208 d) are fed for 21 to 24 h with medium containing several concentrations of test compounds. Cultures are washed and incubated for an additional 2 d in complete medium. Enzyme-liberated adherent-zone cells are analyzed with colony-forming unit culture (CFU-C) assay as follows: cells derived from the adherent zone are incubated at 37°C in 5% CO_2, in complete medium for 2 h; 10^5 viable cells are plated into 10 mm × 35 mm Lux dishes containing 0.6 g Noble agar in 100 ml DMEM with 75 mg DEAE dextran and 3 g L-asparagine and 250 ml decomplemented rat serum. Pokeweed mitogen spleen-cell-conditioned medium is used as a source of colony-stimulating activity. A CFU-C is a progenitor cell that will give raise to a colony consisting of 30 cells or more after 8 to 10 d of culture.

For SIRC, adherent cells are washed to remove growth media, then exposed to test chemicals in the culture dishes for 1 h. Exposed cells are washed to remove the test materials and growth media is replaced in the dishes. Treated cells are then incubated for 1 week to allow them to undergo replication and form distinct colonies, each colony arising from a single surviving cell. Colonies are fixed and stained with 0.1% crystal violet in denatured ethanol (SDA-3A).

1.6.3.3 Analysis

The colonies that have more than 30 to 50 cells are counted. Between 50 and 100 colonies per dish are formed in the control. The ID_{50} values (50% inhibition dose of colony formation) are calculated as the relative percentage of the controls. Numbers of CFU-C per 10^5 cells are counted.

2. DATA

3. REPORTING
3.1 Test Report

The test report shall, if possible, include the following information:

- test conditions: detailed description of treatment and sampling schedule, dose levels, toxicity data, negative and positive controls;

- dose/effect relationship when possible;
- statistical evaluation;
- discussion of the results;
- interpretation of the results.

3.2 Evaluation and Interpretation
(to be defined)

CFU-C is a more accurate index of haematotoxicity when used in conjunction with phenotypic measurements, evaluated by flow cytometry.

4. ALTERNATIVE TO ANIMAL TEST
This method may be used in the screening for potential eye irritant chemicals.

BIBLIOGRAPHY

Bondy, G.S., C.L. Armstrong, B.A. Dawson, C. Heroux-Metcalf, G.A. Neville and C.G. Rogers, Toxicity of structurally related anthraquinones and anthrones to mammalian cells *in vitro, Toxicology in Vitro,* Vol. 8, No. 3, p. 329, 1994.

Gettings, S.D., J. J. Teal, D. M. Bagley, J. L. Demetrulias, L. C. Di Pasquale, K. L. Hintze, M. G. Rozen, S. L. Weise, M. Chudkowski, K. D. Marenus, W. J. W. Pape, M. Roddy, R. Schnetzinger, P. M. Silber, S. M. Glaza and P. J. Kurtz, The CTFA evaluation of alternatives program: An evaluation of *in vitro* alternatives to the Draize primary eye irritation test (Phase 1) Hydro-alcoholic formulations; (Part 2) Data analysis and biological significance, *In Vitro Toxicology,* Vol. 4, No. 4, p. 247, 1991.

Matthews, E. J., Transformation of BALB/c-3T3 cells: II. Investigation of experimental parameters that influence detection of benzo[a]pyrene-induced transformation. *Environmental Health Perspectives Supplements,* Vol. 101, Suppl. 2, p. 293, 1993.

Matthews, E.J., J. W. Spalding and R. W. Tennant, Transformation of BALB/c-3T3 cells: V. Transformation responses of 168 chemicals compared with mutagenicity in Salmonella and carcinogenicity in rodent bioassays. *Environmental Health Perspectives Supplements,* Vol. 101, Suppl. 2, p. 347, 1993.

Naughton, B.A., B. Sibanda, D. Triglia and G. K. Naughton, Rat bone-marrow cell proliferation and differentiation as an index of the effects of xenobiotics *in vitro, Toxicology In Vitro,* Vol. 5, No. 5/6, p. 389, 1991.

North-Root, H., F. Yackovich, J. Demetrulias, M. Gacula, Jr., and J. E. Heinze, Evaluation of an *in vitro* cell toxicity test using rabbit corneal cells to predict the eye irritation potential of surfactants. *Toxicology Letters,* Vol. 14, p. 207, 1983.

Sasaki, K., N. Tanaka, M. Watanabe and M. Yamada, Comparison of cytotoxic effects of chemicals in four different cell types, *Toxicology In Vitro,* Vol. 5, No. 5/6, p. 403, 1991.

DUAL DYE STAINING (ACUTE CELLULAR LETHALITY)

1. METHOD

1.1 Introduction, 1.2 Definition, and 1.3 Reference Substances (to be defined)

1.4 Principle of the Test Method
Dual dye staining is a cytotoxicity assay for the measurement of cell-membrane integrity by using fluorescein diacetate and ethidium bromide. The cells are exposed to a buffer solution containing the two dyes. Cells are freely permeable to the fluorescein ester, which can act as a substrate for nonspecific cellular esterases to liberate fluorescein that only diffuses slowly from intact, metabolically active cells. Loss of this fluorochromasia has been shown to correlate with other indicators of cell damage. Ethidium bromide is a red fluorescent compound that binds to nuclear material and is used to visualize damaged cells that have not

formed or retained fluorescein. Damaged cells that have lost fluorescein appear red, whereas in intact cells the green fluorescence of the fluorescein masks the red fluorescence of ethidium bromide.

1.5 Quality Criteria (to be defined)

1.6 Description of the Test Method
1.6.1 Preparations
A cell line (L-929 cell line) is used.

1.6.2 Test Conditions
Number of Cultures
Five replicates for each experimental point are used.

Use of Negative and Positive Controls
(to be defined)

Exposure Concentrations
(to be defined)

Culture Conditions
(to be defined)

Metabolic Activation
(most chemicals require metabolic activation)

1.6.3 Procedure
1.6.3.1 Preparation of Cultures
(to be defined)

1.6.3.2 Treatment of Cultures with the Test Substance
Cells are maintained in continuous suspension at an appropriate density and treated with test material. After mixing of cell suspension with medium containing fluorescein diacetate and ethidium bromide, an aliquot of the dye/cell suspension is placed under an inverted microscope and the cells examined under epifluorescent illumination. Scoring is made by an image analyzer that counts the number of green and red fluorescent cells.

1.6.3.3 Analysis
The toxic effect is expressed as a DDS_{50} value, i.e., the concentration of test chemical required to damage 50% of the cell population. DDS_{50} values are calculated by linear regression analysis of the data (method of least squares).

2. DATA

3. REPORTING
3.1 Test Report
The test report shall, if possible, include the following information:

* test conditions: detailed description of treatment and sampling schedule, dose levels, toxicity data, negative and positive controls;

- dose/effect relationship when possible;
- statistical evaluation;
- discussion of the results;
- interpretation of the results.

3.2 Evaluation and Interpretation
(to be defined)

4. ALTERNATIVE TO ANIMAL TEST
This method may be used in the screening for eye irritant chemicals.

BIBLIOGRAPHY

Gettings, S.D., J. J. Teal, D. M. Bagley, J. L. Demetrulias, L. C. Di Pasquale, K. L. Hintze, M. G. Rozen, S. L. Weise, M. Chudkowski, K. D. Marenus, W. J. W. Pape, M. Roddy, R. Schnetzinger, P. M. Silber, S. M. Glaza and P. J. Kurtz, The CTFA evaluation of alternatives program: An evaluation of *in vitro* alternatives to the Draize primary eye irritation test (Phase 1) Hydro-alcoholic formulations; (Part 2) Data analysis and biological significance, *In Vitro Toxicology*, Vol. 4, No. 4, p. 247, 1991.

Scaife, M. C., An *in vitro* cytotoxicity test to predict the ocular irritation potential of detergents and detergent products, *Food and Chemical Toxicology*, Vol. 23, No. 2, p. 253, 1985.

DYE TRANSFER ASSAY FOR ANALYSIS OF GJIC

1. METHOD

1.1 Introduction, 1.2 Definition, and 1.3 Reference Substances (to be defined)

1.4 Principle of the Test Method
The dye transfer assay for analysis of gap junctional intercellular communications (GJIC) is a cytotoxic test used to identify alteration of cell-cell communications (e.g., disturbance of intermediate filament networks) on primary cultures exposed to test chemicals. Since GJIC, an important mode of cell-cell exchange of molecules, may become aberrant in the carcinogenic process, screening tests for potential promoters based on GJIC inhibition may be employed. GJIC measurements are performed by microinjection of a fluorescent dye into single cells at the colony periphery and scoring dye transfer to surrounding cells.

1.5 Quality Criteria (to be defined)

1.6 Description of the Test Method
1.6.1 Preparations
Test chemical is dissolved in DMSO. Primary cultures (mouse skin epidermal keratinocytes; human hair follicle epidermal keratinocytes) are used.

1.6.2 Test Conditions
Number of Cultures
Triplicate cultures are used for each experimental point; each experiment is performed at least twice.

Use of Negative and Positive Controls
The solvent is used as a negative control.

Exposure Concentrations
   (to be defined)

Culture Conditions
   Appropriate culture medium, pretreatment time, dosing duration, and pretreated culture vessels are used.

Metabolic Activation
   (most chemicals require metabolic activation)

1.6.3 Procedure
1.6.3.1 Preparation of Cultures
Primary Cultures

   Mouse skin epidermal keratinocytes (MEKs) cultures are prepared from the dorsal skin mice. Typical cell yields are $15–30 \times 106$ cells/dorsal skin, with viabilities of 60 to 80% as determined by tripan blue exclusion. Cells are seeded onto FAV-coated dishes (Falcon) in 4 ml medium at a density of 20×106 viable cells/dish. After 24 h, cultures are re-fed with fresh medium and used for dye transfer assay 2 to 3 d later. FAV (fibronectin-albumin-collagen) solution contains 10 µl bovine fibronectin/ml (Sigma Chemical Co., St. Louis, MO, USA), 0.1 mg bovine serum albumin/ml (Sigma), 30 µl collagen/ml (Collagen Corp., Palo Alto, CA, USA) and 20 mM-HEPES buffer (Sigma) in $Ca^{2+}Mg^{2+}$ free phosphate buffered saline (Gibco, Grand Island, NY, USA).

   MEK cells are maintained in low calcium (LCM) basal essential medium prepared from individual ingredients (Sigma), without calcium and with hormone supplements. Calcium chloride is added to give a final calcium concentration of 0.05 mM.

   Single hairs are plucked gently from healthy volunteers using sterile forceps. The proximal end of each hair is cut into a length of 2 to 3 mm and, with the hair bulb still intact, is rinsed in medium and then placed in a drop of medium on the surface of a 60 mm plastic culture dish (Falcon), which has been coated with FAV solution containing 10 µl bovine fibronectin/ml (Sigma Chemical Co., St. Louis, MO, USA), 0.1 mg bovine serum albumin/ml (Sigma), 30 µl collagen/ml (Collagen Corp., Palo Alto, CA, USA) and 20 mM-HEPES buffer (Sigma) in $Ca^{2+}Mg^{2+}$free phosphate buffered saline (Gibco, Grand Island, NY, USA). After a 24-h attachment period, 4 ml medium is carefully added and the cultures are maintained for about 2 to 3 weeks with regular medium changes.

   Human hair follicle epidermal keratinocytes (HFC) cultures generally are maintained in high calcium medium (HCM) containing a standard free calcium concentration of about 1.2 mM-calcium. This is composed of 3 parts Dulbecco's modified Eagle's medium (low glucose; Gibco), 1 part Ham's F12 medium (Sigma), 10% fetal bovine serum (Orgenic Biologicals, Betha Emk, Israel), 5 µg insulin/ml (Sigma), 0.4 µg hydrocortisone/ml (Sigma), 0.135 mM-adenine (Sigma), 2 nM-triiodothyronine (Sigma), 0.1 nM-choleratoxin (Sigma), 10 ng epidermal growth factor/ml (Sigma), 10 µg transferrin/ml (Sigma), 100 U penicillin/ml, and 50 µg streptomycin/ml (Gibco).

1.6.3.2 Treatment of the Cultures with the Test Substance
Primary Cultures

   Chemical is tested for 1 to 24 h. GJIC measurements are performed in 2 to 3-day-old cultures (MEKs) or in 2-week-old cultures (colonies size is about 5 mm in diameter, HFC) by microinjection of the fluorescent dye Lucifer Yellow CH into single cells at the colony periphery and scoring dye transfer to surrounding cells. Injection needles are prepared from microfilament glass (A-M Systems, Everett, WA, USA) using a dual-step puller (Narishige Co., Tokyo, Japan);

needles are filled with a solution of 5% Lucifer Yellow CH (Sigma) in 0.33 M-lithium chloride and fixed in the condenser of an inverted microscope (Olympus Injectoscope IMT-2 SYF); individual cells are injected with the dye with the aid of an automatic pneumatic microinjector (Eppendorf Model 5242) and the extent of cell-cell spread of the dye is observed 10 to 15 min after injection (15 to 30 independent injections). For HFC, cells of older colonies (3 weeks) are more easily injected if the cultures are maintained in low calcium medium (LCM) for 48 h beforehand. This is prepared from individual ingredients (Sigma) without calcium and with hormone supplements: calcium chloride is added to give a final concentration of 0.05 mM.

1.6.3.3 Analysis
Values reported at each dose are means + SEM for 20 injection sites.

2. DATA

3. REPORTING
3.1 Test Report
The test report shall, if possible, include the following information:

- test conditions: detailed description of treatment and sampling schedule, dose levels, negative and positive controls;
- criteria for scoring dye transfer;
- dose/effect relationship when possible;
- statistical evaluation, if the case;
- discussion of the results;
- interpretation of the results.

3.2 Evaluation and Interpretation
(to be defined)

4. ALTERNATIVE TO ANIMAL TEST
This test method may be used in the screening for potential tumor promoter/carcinogenic chemicals.

BIBLIOGRAPHY
Swierenga, S. H. H., J. Fitzgerald, H. Yamasaki, C. Piccoli and M. Goldberg, Use of primary keratinocyte cultures from plucked human hairs for analysis of gap junctional intercellular communication, *Toxicology In Vitro*, Vol. 5, No. 5/6, p. 411, 1991.

ENUCLEATED EYE TEST (EET)

1. METHOD

1.1 Introduction, 1.2 Definition, and 1.3 Reference Substances (to be defined)

1.4 Principle of the Test Method
EET, an *ex vivo* test, uses tissues taken from humanely killed animals and most nearly mimics the *in vivo* situation, having the advantage that it accommodates aspects of absorption and penetration through the corneal surface. The endpoints used for the assessment of eye irritation are corneal swelling, corneal opacity, and the degree and persistence of fluorescein

staining. The technique does not necessarily reduce the number of animals used per test, but eliminates potential trauma.

1.5 Quality Criteria (to be defined)

1.6 Description of the Test Method
1.6.1 Preparations

Test chemicals (both solids and liquids) are tested undiluted with some exceptions. Rabbit eyes are used.

1.6.2 Test Conditions
Number of Cultures

The test substance is tested on five eyes while one serves as control.

Use of Negative and Positive Controls

A negative control is used.

Exposure Concentrations

(to be defined)

Culture Conditions

Appropriate instruments (hand slit-lamp or opthasonic pachometer for corneal swelling examination; clamps and superfusion apparatus) are used.

1.6.3 Procedure
1.6.3.1 Preparation of Cultures
Rabbit Eyes

Rabbits are used as eye donors. Before death, the animals corneal thickness is measured. They are killed by an overdose of anesthetic or with Euthesate (Apharmo), administered via the marginal ear vein. Immediately after death, the eye is dissected. This procedure takes about 2 min. Next, the nictitating membrane is firmly drawn away from the eyeball with surgical forceps and held in this position during the entire dissection. The conjunctivae between the nictitating membrane and the eyeball are then cut with fine, bent scissors. Next, the extraorbital muscles, optic nerve, and remainder of the conjunctivae are cut, and the eyeball is removed from the orbit. Dissections are done with extreme care to avoid any touching of the surface of the cornea. Cutting the optic nerve too close to the eyeball, which could result in rupture and loss of intraocular pressure, is also avoided. Immediately after dissection, if necessary, the enucleated eye is rinsed with isotonic saline at about 32°C to remove possible blood-remains, hairs, and dust particles. The isolated eye is placed in the clamp with the cornea positioned vertically. The clamp holding the eye is placed in the superfusion chamber; the eyes are examined immediately after they are placed in the superfusion apparatus (after an equilibration time of 30 to 45 min) to ensure that they are not damaged during dissection.

Fluorescein sodium 2% (w/v) is applied to the surface of the cornea for a few seconds and then rinsed off with 5 to 10 ml isotonic saline at about 32°C. Corneal thickness is measured using a depth-measuring device. An accurate measurement is taken at the corneal apex. Eyes with a corneal thickness plus or minus 10% of the average corneal thickness of the six eyes, or that are stained with fluorescein, indicating the cornea to be permeable, or that showed any other signs of damage, are rejected. Following an equilibration period of 45 to 60 min, the eyes are reexamined according to the same procedure as mentioned above and the corneal thickness of each eye is recorded (base-line). During reexamination, fluorescein application is not repeated.

1.6.3.2 Treatment of the Cultures with the Test Substance
Rabbit Eyes

At time t = 0, immediately after the reexamination, the test substance is applied to the eye. Liquid materials are applied to the eye at the center of the cornea in an amount of 0.1 ml from a 1 ml syringe. The eye is left in contact with the test substance for 10 sec. Solids, if necessary, are first ground to a fine powder and subsequently tested by applying 25 to 100 mg to the cornea in such a way that the entire cornea is covered. After application, the test substance is left in contact with the cornea for 10 sec. Directly thereafter, the corneal surface is rinsed thoroughly with approximately 20 ml of isotonic saline at about 32°C. Superfusion is restarted immediately after the eyes are rinsed. If necessary, an extra rinsing is performed at the 30-min reading.

The different endpoints are examined at various times:

- corneal opacity at 30, 75, 120, 180, and 240 min, after the treatment; or at 60, 120, 180, 240, and 300 min, after the treatment; or at 30 and 240 min after the treatment;
- corneal swelling at 30, 75, 120, 180, and 240 min after the treatment; or 60, 120, 180, 240, and 300 min after the treatment;
- fluorescein retention by the cornea epithelium is reassessed using fluorescein at 30 and 240 min after the treatment; or only at 240 min after the treatment.

Following the last examination at 240 min after treatment, the eyes are taken from the clamps and fixed in about 25 ml Bouin's fixative for possible future histopathological examinations.

1.6.3.3 Analysis

The following criteria and coring systems are applied for the assessment of possible effects:

Corneal Swelling

Corneal swelling, expressed as a percentage, is calculated according to the following formula:

$$\frac{(\text{Corneal thickness at time } t - \text{Corneal thickness at } t = 0)}{\text{Corneal thickness at } t = 0} \times 100\%$$

Fluorescein Retention (epithelial damage)

0 = no fluorescein retention
1 = small number of cells retaining fluorescein
2 = individual cells and areas of the cornea retaining fluorescein
3 = large areas of the cornea retaining fluorescein

Corneal Opacity

Opacity degree of density (area most dense taken from scoring).

0 = no opacity
1 = scattered or diffuse areas, details of iris clearly visible
2 = easily discernible translucent area, details of iris slightly obscured
3 = severe corneal opacity, no details of iris visible, size of pupil barely discernible
4 = complete corneal opacity, iris invisible

The swelling, fluorescein retention and opacity of the cornea are taken into account together for the estimation of the eye irritation potential. The chemicals arc divided into four categories:

I   = no effect
II   = slight effect
III   = moderate effect
IV   = severe effect

The three endpoints are evaluated in according with the following formulae:

Corneal Swelling

IV = >26% swelling before 75 min or 32% swelling after 75 min
III = >12% swelling before 75 min or >18% and <26% swelling at any time
II = >5% and <12% swelling at any time
I   = <5% swelling at any time

Fluorescein Retention Score at 240 Min

IV = 2.6 to 3.0
III = 1.6 to 2.5
II = 0.6 to 1.5
I   = 0.0 to 0.5

Corneal Opacity (Mean Maximum Score)

IV = 2.6 to 4.0
III = 1.6 to 2.5
II = 0.6 to 1.5
I   = 0.0 to 0.5

In the alternative, the percentage of corneal swelling is calculated and then the result is adjusted according to corneal fluorescein retention or opacity*:

IV = >20% swelling within 1 h or if corneal opacity is visible to the naked eye
III = >20% swelling within 2 h
II = >20% swelling by 5 h
I   = <20% swelling at any time

a) * = one or more eyes intensely stained by fluorescein (i.e., a bright green color completely staining the cornea) for >1 h, increase by one grade the irritation grading allocated on the basis of corneal swelling;

b) * = four or more eyes faintly stained (i.e., a pale green color either partially or completely staining the cornea) for 30 min, increase by one grade the irritation grading allocated on the basis of corneal swelling.

In the alternative, if corneal swelling at 4 h is the main factor:

IV = >90% swelling at 4 h or if corneal opacity score >3
III = 45 to 90% swelling at 4 h or if corneal opacity score >2
II = 30 to 45% swelling at 4 h
I   = <30% swelling at 4 h

2. DATA

3. REPORTING
3.1 Test Report
Animal strain and size are mentioned.

3.2 Evaluation and Interpretation
(to be defined)

4. ALTERNATIVE TO ANIMAL TEST
This method may be used in the screening for potential eye irritant chemicals.

BIBLIOGRAPHY

Commission of the European Communities, Collaborative study on the evaluation of alternative methods to the eye irritation test — Part I, Doc. XI/632/91 — V/E/1/131/91, Brussels, p. 22, 1991.

Commission of the European Communities, Collaborative study on the evaluation of alternative methods to the eye irritation test — *Part II*, Doc. XI/632/91 — V/E/1/131/91, Brussels, p. 242, 1991.

EPIDERMAL SLICE TECHNIQUE FOR SKIN CORROSIVE POTENTIAL

1. METHOD

1.1 Introduction, 1.2 Definition, and 1.3 Reference Substances (to be defined)

1.4 Principle of the Test Method
The Epidermal Slice Technique is an *in vitro* assay used to identify chemical agents with a marked toxic potential to the skin. It represents an *in vitro* model for predicting chemicals that are corrosive to the skin. *In vivo* data indicated that corrosive chemicals exert a physico-chemical as well as a biological effect on skin tissue. This physicochemical effect would result in a direct lysis or degradation of normal stratum corneum, which in turn could be monitored as a reduction in the electrical resistance of skin slices.

1.5 Quality Criteria (to be defined)

1.6 Description of the Test Method
1.6.1 Preparations
Chemicals are applied as such except for solids and waxes when a 50% (w/v) formulation is prepared in either ethanol, acetone, or dimethylformamide.
Epidermal slices (rat epidermal slices) are used.

1.6.2 Test Conditions
Number of Cultures
A minimun of three skin slices are used for the assessment of each chemical.

Use of Negative and Positive Controls
Untreated rat epidermal skin slices are used as negative controls.

Exposure Concentrations
(to be defined)

Culture Conditions
Appropriate instruments are used for the test procedure.

1.6.3 Procedure
1.6.3.1 Preparation of Cultures
Tissue Explant

Animals are anesthetized (3% Fluothane) and the dorsal and flank hairs carefully removed using fine clippers. At least 48 h after hair clipping, animals are killed and the dorsal skin is removed as a single pelt; excess fat is cut away and the remaining skin placed over a cork saddle. An appropriate apparatus for the *in vitro* epidermal slice model is used. Two epidermal slices (18 mm × 80 mm) are placed, stratum corneum uppermost, over a rubber "O" ring. A purpose-designed PTFE tube is press-fitted onto the slices and excess tissue is trimmed away. The epidermal slices attached to the PTFE tubes are suspended in physiological saline and maintained at ambient temperature (20°C).

1.6.3.2 Treatment of the Cultures with the Test Substance

Each test chemical (0.3 ml) is placed onto the stratum corneum of the skin slice. Following a contact of 4 h, chemical is removed with a jet of warm water (40 to 50°C); electrical resistance is measured 20 h later, 24 h after the initial application. The epidermal slice is kept in isotonic saline at ambient temperature. Electrical resistance of skin slices is measured by an a.c. half-bridge apparatus. Immediately before measurement of electrical resistance, isotonic saline (3 ml) is added to the stratum corneum surface of the skin.

1.6.3.3 Analysis

The electrical resistance of untreated rat epidermal skin slices or skin discs ranges from 6 to 20 skin kΩ disc; an electrical resistance value of 4 kW/skin disc (3.2 kW/cm²) has been selected as a threshold value for a positive effect in this *in vitro* model: chemicals reducing electrical resistance below 4 kW/skin disc *in vitro* would be predicted to induce a corrosive lesion *in vivo* using conventional animal protocols.

2. DATA

3. REPORTING
3.1 Test Report
Animal species and strains must be mentioned.

3.2 Evaluation and Interpretation
(to be defined)

4. ALTERNATIVE TO ANIMAL TEST
This method may be used for the screening of potential skin irritant chemicals.

BIBLIOGRAPHY

Botham, P. A., T. J. Hall, R. Dennett, J. C. McCall, D. A. Basketter, E. Whittle, M. Cheeseman, D. J. Esdaile and J. Gardner, The skin corrosivity test *in vitro*. Results of an inter-laboratory trial, *Toxicology In Vitro*, Vol. 6, No. 3, p. 191, 1992.

Commission of the European Communities, Collaborative study on the relationship between "*in vivo*" primary irritation and "*in vitro*" experimental models, Doc. CEC/V/E/3/Lux/157/188 Rev. 1, Brussels, 1989.

Oliver, G. J. A., M. A. Pemberton and C. Rhodes, An *in vitro* model for identifying skin-corrosive chemicals. I. Initial validation, *Toxicology In Vitro*, Vol. 2, No. 1, p. 7, 1988.

ESCHERICHIA COLI — REVERSE MUTATION ASSAY
(92/69/EEC DIR.)

1. METHOD

1.1 Introduction and 1.2 Definition
None.

1.3 Reference Substances
None.

1.4 Principles of the Test Method

The *Escherichia coli* tryptophan (trp) reversion system is a microbial assay that measures trp⁻ → trp⁺ reversion by chemicals that cause base changes in the genome of the organism.

Bacteria are exposed to test chemicals with and without metabolic activation. After a suitable period of incubation on minimal medium, revertant colonies are counted and compared to the number of spontaneous revertants in an untreated and/or solvent control culture.

1.5 Quality Criteria
None.

1.6 Description of the Test Method

The following methods may be used to perform the assay: (1) the preincubation method; and (2) the direct incorporation method in which bacteria and test agent are mixed in overlay agar and poured over the surface of a selective agar plate.

1.6.1 Preparation
1.6.1.1 Bacteria

Bacteria are grown at 37°C up to late exponential or early stationary phase of growth. Approximate cell density should be 10^8 to 10^9 cells per milliliter.

1.6.1.2 Metabolic Activation

Bacteria should be exposed to the test substance both in the presence and absence of an appropriate metabolic activation system. The most commonly used system is a cofactor-supplemented postmitochondrial fraction prepared from the liver of rodents treated with enzyme-inducing agents.

1.6.2. Test Conditions
Tester Strains

Three strains, WP2, WP2 uvr A, and WP2 uvr A pKM 101, should be used. Recognized methods of stock culture preparations and storage are to be used. The growth requirements and the genetic identity of the strains, their sensitivity to UV radiation or mitomycin C, and the resistance to ampicillin in strain WP2 uvr A pKM 101 have to be checked. The strains should also yield spontaneous revertants within the frequency ranges expected.

Media

An appropriate medium for the expression and selection of mutants is used with an adequate overlay agar.

Use of Negative and Positive Controls

Concurrent untreated and solvent controls have to be performed. Positive controls have to be conducted also for two purposes:

1. To confirm the sensitivity of bacterial strains.
   Methyl methane sulfonate, 4-nitroquinoline oxide, or ethylnitrosourea may be used as positive controls for tests without metabolic activation.
2. To ensure the activity of the appropriate metabolizing systems.
   A positive control for the activity of one (the) metabolizing system for all strains is 2-aminoanthracene. When available, a positive control of the same chemical class as the chemical under test should be used.

Amount of Test Substance per Plate

At least five different amounts of test chemical are tested, with half-log intervals between plates. Substances are tested up to the limit of solubility or toxicity. Toxicity is evidenced by a reduction in the number of spontaneous revertants, a clearing of the background lawn, or by degree of survival of treated cultures. Nontoxic chemicals should be tested to 5 mg per plate before considering the test substance negative.

Incubation Conditions

Plates are incubated for 48 to 72 h at 37°C.

1.6.3 Procedure

For the direct plate incorporation method without enzyme activation, the chemical and 0.1 ml of a fresh bacterial culture are added to 2.0 ml of overlay agar. For tests with metabolic activation, 0.5 ml of liver enzyme activation mixture containing an adequate amount of postmitochondrial fraction is added to the agar overlay after the addition of test chemical and bacteria. The contents of each tube are mixed and poured over the surface of a selective agar plate. Overlay agar is allowed to solidify and plates are incubated at 37°C for 48 to 72 h. At the end of the incubation period, revertant colonies per plate are counted.

For the preincubation method, a mixture of test chemical, 0.1 ml of a fresh bacterial culture and an adequate amount of liver enzyme activation mixture or the same amount of buffer is preincubated before adding 2.0 ml of overlay agar. All other procedures are the same as for the incorporation method.

All plating for both methods is done at least in triplicate.

2. DATA

The numbers of revertant colonies per plate are reported for both control and treated series. Individual plate counts, the mean number of revertant colonies per plate and standard deviations should be presented for the tested chemical and the controls. All results are confirmed in an independent experiment. Data should be evaluated using appropriate statistical methods.

Data should be evaluated using appropriate statistical methods.

At least two independent experiments are conducted. It is not necessary to perform the second one in an identical way to the initial experiment. Indeed, it may be preferable to alter certain test conditions in order to obtain more useful data.

3. REPORTING
3.1 Test Report

The test report shall, if possible, include the following information:

- bacteria, strain used;
- test conditions: dose levels, toxicity, composition of media; treatment procedures (preincubation incubation); liver enzyme activation mixture; reference substances, negative controls;
- individual plate count, the mean number of revertant colonies per plate, standard deviation, dose/effect relationship when possible;
- discussion of the results;
- interpretation of the results.

3.2 Evaluation and Interpretation

There are several criteria for determining a positive result, one of which is a statistically significant dose-related increase in the number of revertants. Another criterion may be the detection of a reproducible and statistically significant positive response for at least one of the test points.

A test substance producing neither a statistically significant dose-related increase in the number of revertants nor a statistically significant and reproducible positive response at any one of the test points is considered nonmutagenic in this system.

Positive results from the *E. coli* reverse mutation assay indicate that a substance induces mutations in the genome of this organism. Negative results indicate that under the test conditions, the test substance is not mutagenic in *E. coli*.

The *E. coli* reverse mutation assay may be especially suited to testing some classes of chemicals such as hydrazines, nitrofurans, and nitrosamines.

4. ALTERNATIVE TO ANIMAL TEST

This method is used for the identification of mutagenic chemicals.

BIBLIOGRAPHY

Annex to Commission Directive 92/69/EEC, 31 July 1992, Adapting to technical progress for the seventeenth time Council Directive 67/548/EEC on the approximation of laws, regulations and administrative provisions relating to the classification, packaging and labelling of dangerous substances, *Official Journal of the European Communities,* No. L383A, Vol. 35, p. 1, 1992.

Brusick, X. X., V. F. Simmon, H. D. Rosenkranz, V. A. Ray and R. S. Stafford, An evaluation of the *Escherichia coli* WP2 and WP2 uvrA Reverse Mutation Assay, *Mutation Research,* Vol. 76, p. 169, 1980.

Note: The *Salmonella typhimurium* and *Escherichia coli* reverse mutation assays are being combined at present by OECD experts in one single guideline.

EYTEX® ASSAY

1. METHOD

1.1 Introduction, 1.2 Definition, and 1.3 Reference Substances (to be defined)

1.4 Principle of the Test Method

The EYTEX® method was developed by *In Vitro* International (IVI), Irvine, CA, USA. It is an *in vitro* test that can be used to reduce the need for the *in vivo* Draize rabbit eye test. The EYTEX® System is based on alterations in the conformation and hydration of an ordered macromolecular matrix, including several molecules that contribute to the overall response of the protein matrix to a diverse array of test compounds, such as bases, salts, solvents, surfactants, lubricants, preservatives, emulsions, chemicals, and formulations from diverse classes and with different ranges of toxicity, representing various mechanisms of ocular toxicity. The reagent has been developed and optimized over the years, and the complex mixture seems to react to irritants in the same manner as does the cornea of the eye. Quantification of the EYTEX® method is based on measurement of changes in the optical density (OD) of the matrix that occur when the matrix is exposed to samples. The resultant turbidity, which is directly proportional to the irritation of the sample, is compared with that produced by eye irritant standards of known Draize score. That is, the EYTEX®/Draize equivalent (EDE) score is determined from a calibration curve. The result can be used to predict *in vivo* ocular irritation. Samples having different characteristics require the use of different protocols: EYTEX® standard assay (STD), membrane partition assay (MPA), rapid membrane assay (RMA), upright membrane assay (UMA), alkaline membrane assay (AMA), and high sensitivity assay (HSA).

STD assay is designed for nonopaque, water-soluble or miscible materials; MPA assay is designed for opaque, intensely colored/pigmented, water insoluble, immiscible materials; RMA assay is designed for ethoxylated and amphoteric surfactants, formulations containing these surfactant types or high surfactant concentrations, and products not qualified with the STD or MPA assay; UMA assay is designed as an improved MPA assay; AMA assay is designed for chemicals with pH > 8; HSA assay is designed for low irritation samples.

1.5 Quality Criteria (to be defined)

1.6 Description of the Test Method
1.6.1 Preparations
All protocols use the same matrix mixture of extracted and purified protein from Jack beans (*Canavalia ensisormis*), which is a lyophilized powder containing plant globulins, plant albumin, plant ovalbumin, plant mucopolysaccharides, plant carbohydrate, plant triglyceride, plant cholesterol, and plant saponins, along with buffer salts, amino acids, and preservatives. The EYTEX® reagent is reconstituted by the addition of distilled water. An oligomeric protein with a molar mass of approximately 300,000 g/mol is the major active component of the reagent. This oligomer, characterized by 12 subunits, associates itself into strands that are then incorporated into a gel network.

1.6.2 Test Conditions
Use of Negative and Positive Control
   (to be defined)

1.6.3 Procedure
1.6.3.1 Preparation of the EYTEX® Reagent
   The powder is reconstituted by addition of distilled water containing 0.1% (w/v) sodium azide as a preservative to produce a concentrated solution buffered at pH 9.

1.6.3.2 Test Procedure
The EYTEX® Protocols
   STD assay — samples are directly in contact with the EYTEX® reagent; the incubation time is 1 h at 25°C.
   MPA assay — samples are placed in cups formed by the membrane, which is permeable to molecules of molecular weight 16,000 or below, which separates samples from the cuvette chamber. The EYTEX® reagent or diluent is added to the cuvette. The membrane cup and

sample are placed in the cuvette, and are sealed with a cap. The capped system is mixed by rotation for 24 h at 25°C. The assay incubation is performed with the cuvette in an inverted position. This positioning allows maximal contact of reagent with the membrane cup surface. Low molecular weight materials can diffuse between the sample and reagent compartments, and chemical irritants can interact with the EYTEX® reagent.

RMA assay — is used when products cannot be qualified by the STD, MPA, or UMA protocols. This protocol corrects for the interference of test sample with the reagent system. Specific features are the use of the increased threefold concentration of activator reagent and a shortened incubation time of 5 h at 25°C. Also, to hold the sample, it incorporates a modified semipermeable membrane cup attached to a plastic ring, termed a "bullet." Its use permits the sample cuvette to be put in an upright position during assay incubation, which optimizes assay development.

UMA assay — is an improvement on the MPA, overcoming handling and leakage problems by replacing the membrane cup with a smaller membrane fixed in a plastic ring, termed a bullet. The incubation time is 24 h at 25°C.

AMA assay — is used, when necessary, for very alkaline substances (pH > 8). It is an MPA protocol in which the use of the activator reagent is omitted. The activator is an acidic buffered solution (pH 3), which will decrease the alkalinity associated with an alkaline test sample. However, the alkalinity of a substance is considered to be a component of its eye irritation potential. Omitting the activator therefore provides for maximum assay sensitivity to samples with high pH. The incubation time is 24 h at 25°C.

HSA assay — the ratio of the test sample to the active component of the EYTEX® reagent is changed to amplify the response of test materials with low irritation. This increased response reduces the percent variability contributed by the system components in the final result. Better and more accurate calibration from *in vivo* Draize scores 0 to 2, to 8 to 16, is included to improve accuracy. There are four calibrators, instead of two, to define the relationship of optical density to Draize equivalent. This permits a better definition of nonirritant materials with Draize equivalents from 0 to 3. The HSA is a specialized protocol for low irritation samples. It will not qualify test samples with high surfactant concentrations, low and high pH, or reactive solvents.

A set of calibrators defines the relationship of turbidity produced in the reagent to the Draize score. All the OD readings are used to determine an *in vitro* irritation classification, based on a calibrator curve. The EDE is obtained by reading across from the OD for the sample to the calibration curve and then extending a line down to the Draize equivalent scale.

Qualification

The EYTEX® system requires qualification of both the assay and the sample data. Assay qualification is necessary to show that the assay has been performed correctly according to the standard procedures of the EYTEX® — directions for use (DFU) with calibrators and quality control (QC) samples. For sample qualification, data must satisfy all of the following criteria:

1. the sample blank must be less than 0.5 OD units. For ease of use, the EYTEX® DFU suggests using OD × 1000, i.e., 500;
2. the net EYTEX® response must be greater than zero;
3. there must be no significant inhibition;
4. the curve shape of the dose-response assay is very important, and must be flat or increasing for three consecutive increases in sample volume. Allowable ranges of changes of OD for flat or increasing curve shape are given in the EYTEX® DFU.

A similar set of criteria are obtained in the DFU for sample blanks.

Calibrators

These are pure chemicals with known *in vivo* results which have been selected to cover the full range of Draize scores. They are measured in each assay and used to prepare the calibration curve of net EYTEX® response vs. Draize equivalent. The calibrators must fall within prespecified limits for the assay to be qualified.

Control Samples

Samples of known EDE are run with each assay. Results for these samples must fall within prespecified limits for the assay to be qualified.

Net EYTEX® Response

The net OD for the test sample is obtained after subtracting the OD of the sample blank from the sample reading.

Diluent

A buffer solution is used with the sample in place of EYTEX® reagent to provide a sample blank reading.

Activator

A buffer solution is added to the reconstituted EYTEX® reagent just before use, to enhance the sensitivity of the reagent. The STD, MPA, and UMA protocols require 1× activator level (0.5 ml in 25 ml of reagent), while the RMA protocol requires 3× activator level (1.5 ml in 25 ml of reagent).

Incubation Time

After adding a sample to the activated EYTEX® reagent, the turbidity due to any irritation takes time to develop. Incubation times at 25°C have been optimized to ensure maximum response for each protocol.

Dose-Response Curve

The net EYTEX® response vs. the volume of sample is plotted, for two qualified results on different samples.

Inhibition

The apparent reduction in OD with increasing dose of sample may be due to the solubilization of the coagulating EYTEX® reagent by the sample itself.

Inhibition Check (IC)

Inhibition is suspected, if the net EYTEX® response for a sample is less than that for the middle of the three calibrators run during the assay. If this is the case, an IC reagent, which is a known irritant, is added to the samples with low responses. Inhibition is indicated, if, after incubation for 10 min, there is an insufficient increase in OD. If the OD has increased to a value higher than that of the middle calibrator, CR2, then the IC has resulted in a pass. All other results must be considered as failures.

Interference

Interference is the term used by IVI for a nonqualified dose-response curve, but where the IC still shows a large increase in OD, i.e., a pass. Unlike inhibition, interference does not always exhibit a net EYTEX® response of less than the middle calibrator, CR2. It is recognized more by the shape of the dose-response curve.

1.6.3.3 Analysis

All optical density readings are used to determine an EDE based on a calibration curve of calibrators with known *in vivo* results.

Example: the cationic detergent benzalkonium chloride (BAC) is chosen as a reference standard: this compound exhibits a linear dose-response relationship in the EYTEX® test system, whether measured as optical density or as turbidity. Furthermore, *in vivo* measurements of ocular irritation are available for a range of concentrations of BAC: these data are used to assign irritation classifications to ranges of BAC concentrations. The ocular irritation of an unknown sample is then estimated by comparison of the optical density or turbidity observed at a given concentration (less correction for blank readings) to the BAC calibration curve. The concentration of BAC required to achieve an optical density or turbidity equivalent to that of the unknown is converted to an irritation classification.

EDE Scoring Scale (according to Gordon & Bergman Scale)

Scoring Range	Irritation Classification
0–1	Nonirritant
1–5	Very slight
5–20	Very mild
20–30	Mild
30–50	Low moderate
50–70	High moderate
>70	Severe

EDE Scoring Scale

Scoring Range	Predicted *In Vivo* Classification
0–15	Minimal
15–19	Minimal/Mild
19–22	Mild
22–25	Mild/Moderate
25–33	Moderate
33–35	Moderate/severe
35–45	Severe
>45	Severe/Extreme

EYTEX® Irritation Equivalent (EIE) Scoring Scale (compared to modified Kay & Calandra Scale)

Scoring Range	Irritation Judgment
0–3	Non/minimal
3.1–16	Minimal
16.1–26	Mild
26.1–50	Moderate
>50	Severe

EES Scoring Scale (compared to modified Kay & Calandra Scale)

EES Scoring Range	Irritation Classification
≤22	Nonirritating
>22–≤33	Irritating
>33	Severely irritating

Statistical Analysis

The results of EYTEX® and *in vivo* testing are compared whenever there is at least one result with the Draize method at the same concentration for which there is an *in vitro* EYTEX®

result. A full correlation value of 1.0 is assigned when a test substance receives an identical irritation classification by the two methods. A partial correlation value of 0.5 is assigned when the EYTEX® result is within one classification of the *in vivo* result. In some cases, there is disagreement within the literature as to the Draize classification of a test substance: correlation values of 0.75 are assigned when examples of both fully and partially correlated data are available. Results differing by more than one classification are assigned a correlation value of 0. Thus, if the results are expressed as follows:

A = number of samples with full correlation;
B = number of samples with partial correlation;
C = number of samples with both full and partial correlation results;
D = number of samples with zero correlation,

then the percent correlation is calculated as:

$$\% \text{ Correlation} = 100 \times (A + 0.5 \times B + 0.75 \times C)/(A + B + C + D).$$

2. DATA

3. REPORTING
3.1 Test Report
The test report shall, if possible, include the following information:

- test conditions: detailed description of treatment and sampling schedule, dose levels, toxicity data, negative and positive controls,
- dose/effect relationship when possible,
- statistical evaluation,
- discussion of the results,
- interpretation of the results.

3.2 Evaluation and Interpretation
(to be defined)

4. ALTERNATIVE TO ANIMAL TEST
This method may be used in the screening for potential eye irritant chemicals.

BIBLIOGRAPHY

Courtellemont, P., P. Hebert and G. Redziniak, Evaluation of the EYTEX® System as a screening method for ocular tolerance: Application to raw materials and finished products, *ATLA*, Vol. 20, p. 466, 1992.

Gettings, S.D., J. J. Teal, D. M. Bagley, J. L. Demetrulias, L. C. Di Pasquale, K. L. Hintze, M. G. Rozen, S. L. Weise, M. Chudkowski, K. D. Marenus, W. J. W. Pape, M. Roddy, R. Schnetzinger, P. M. Silber, S. M. Glaza and P. J. Kurtz, The CTFA evaluation of alternatives program: An evaluation of *in vitro* alternatives to the Draize primary eye irritation test (Phase 1) Hydro-alcoholic formulations; (Part 2) Data analysis and biological significance, *In Vitro Toxicology*, Vol. 4, No. 4, p. 247, 1991.

Gordon, V. C., EYTEX® third generation, in *In Vitro Toxicology: Mechanisms and New Technology*, Vol. 8, Goldberg, A. M., Ed., Mary Ann Liebert, New York, 1991, p. 241.

Gordon, V. C., The scientific basis of the EYTEX® System, *ATLA*, Vol. 20, p. 537, 1992.

Gordon, V. C. and H. C. Bergman, The EYTEX®-MPA System: An *in vitro* method for evaluation of ocular safety, in *Progress in In Vitro Toxicology*, Vol. 6, Goldberg, A. M., Ed., Mary Ann Liebert, New York, 1988, p. 309.

Gordon, V. C. and H. C. Bergman, EYTEX®: An *in vitro* method for evaluation of ocular irritation, *In Vitro Toxicology: Approaches to Validation,* Vol. 5, Goldberg, A. M., Ed., Mary Ann Liebert, New York, 1987, p. 293.

Gordon V. C., C. P. Kelly and H. C. Bergman, Applications of the EYTEX® method, *Toxicology In Vitro,* Vol. 4, No. 4/5, p. 314, 1990.

Kruszewski, F. H., L. H. Hearn, K. T. Smith, J. J. Teal, V. Gordon and M. S. Dickens, Application of the EYTEX® System to the evaluation of cosmetic products and their ingredients, *ATLA,* Vol. 20, p. 146, 1992.

Martin, C. G., Qualification of the EYTEX® data: A user's guide, *ATLA,* Vol. 21, p. 239, 1993.

O'Brien, K. A. F., M. B. Dixit, J. C. McCall, P. A. Botham and R. W. Lewis, An interlaboratory assessment of the EYTEX® System, *Toxicology In Vitro,* Vol. 6, No. 6, p. 549, 1992.

Regnier, J. F., C. Imbert and J. C. Boutonnet, Evaluation of the EYTEX® System as a screening method for the ocular irritation of chemical products, *ATLA,* Vol. 22, p. 32, 1994.

GENE MUTATION TEST
(*SACCHAROMYCES CEREVISIAE*) (87/302/EEC DIR.)

1. METHOD

1.1 Introduction and 1.2 Definition
None.

1.3 Reference Substances
None.

1.4 Principle of the Test Method

A variety of haploid and diploid strains of the yeast *Saccharomyces cerevisiae* can be used to measure the production of gene mutations induced by chemical agents with and without metabolic activation.

Forward mutation systems in haploid strains, such as the measurement of mutation from red, adenine-requiring mutants (ade-1, ade-2) to double adenine-requiring white mutants and selective systems such as the induction of resistance to canavnaine and cycloheximide, have been utilized.

The most extensively validated reverse mutation system involves the use of the haploid strain XV 185–14C which carries the ochre nonsense mutations ade 2–1, arg 4–17, lys 1–1, and trp 5–48, which are reversible by base substitution mutagens that induce site specific mutations or ochre suppressor mutations. XV 185–14C also carries the his 1–7 marker, a missense mutation reverted mainly by second site mutations, and the marker hom 3–10, which is reverted by frameshift mutagens. In diploid strains of *S. cerevisiae,* the only extensively used strain is D_7, which is homozygous for ilv 1–92.

1.5 Quality Criteria
None.

1.6 Description of the Test Method
1.6.1 Preparations

Solutions of test chemicals and control should be prepared just prior to testing, using an appropriate vehicle. In the case of organic compounds that are not water soluble, not more than a 2% solution v/v of organic solvents such as ethanol, acetone, or dimethylsulfoxide (DMSO) should be used. The final concentration of the vehicle should not significantly affect cell viability and growth characteristics.

Metabolic Activation

Cells should be exposed to test chemicals both in the presence and absence of an appropriate exogenous metabolic activation system.

The most commonly used system is a cofactor supplemented postmitochondrial fraction from the livers of rodents pretreated with enzyme inducing agents. The use of other species, tissues, postmitochondrial fractions, or procedures also may be appropriate for metabolic activation.

1.6.2 Test Conditions

Tester Strains

The haploid strain XV 185–14C and the diploid strain D_7 are the most used in gene mutation studies. Other strains also may be appropriate.

Media

Appropriate culture media are used for the determination of survival and mutant numbers.

Use of Negative and Positive Controls

Positive, untreated, and solvent controls should be performed concurrently. Appropriate positive control chemicals should be used for each specific mutational endpoint.

Exposure Concentration

At least five adequately spaced concentrations of the test substance should be used. For toxic substances, the highest concentration tested should not reduce survival below 5 to 10%. Relatively water-insoluble substances should be tested up to their limit of solubility, using appropriate procedures. For freely water-soluble nontoxic substances, the upper concentration should be determined on a case-by-case basis.

Incubation Conditions

The plates are incubated 4 to 7 d at 28 to 30°C in the dark.

Spontaneous Mutation Frequencies

Subcultures should be used with spontaneous mutation frequencies within the accepted normal range.

Number of Replicates

At least three replicate plates should be used per concentration for the assay of prototrophs produced by gene mutation and for cell viability. In the case of experiments using markers such as hom 3–10 with a low mutation rate, the number of plates used must be increased to provide statistically relevant data.

1.6.2 Procedure

Treatment of *S. cerevisiae* strains usually is performed in a liquid test procedure involving either stationary or growing cells. Initial experiments should be carried out on growing cells: 1 to 5×10^5 cells/ml are exposed to the test chemical for up to 18 h at 28 to 37°C with shaking; an adequate amount of metabolic activation system is added during treatment when appropriate. At the end of the treatment, cells are centrifuged, washed and seeded upon an appropriate culture medium. After incubation, plates are scored for survival and the indication of gene mutation.

If the first experiment is negative, then a second experiment should be performed using stationary phase cells. If the first experiment is positive it is confirmed in an appropriate independent experiment.

2. DATA

Data should be presented in tabular form indicating the number of colonies counted, number of mutants, survival and mutant frequency. All results should be confirmed in an independent experiment. The data should be evaluated using appropriate statistical methods.

3. REPORTING

3.1 Test Report

The test report shall, if possible, contain the following information:

- strain used;
- test conditions: stationary phase or growing cells. composition of media, incubation temperature and duration, metabolic activation system;
- treatment conditions: exposure levels, procedure and duration of treatment, treatment temperature, positive and negative controls;
- number of colonies counted, number of mutants, survival and mutant frequency, dose/response relationship if applicable, statistical evaluation of data;
- discussion of results;
- interpretation of results.

3.2 Evaluation and Interpretation

There are several criteria for determining a positive result, one of which is a statistically significant dose-related increase in the number of mutants as well as in the mutant frequency.

Another criterion may be based upon the detection of a reproducible and statistically significant positive response for at least one of the test substance concentrations. A test substance producing neither a statistically significant dose-related increase in the mutant frequency, nor a statistically significant and reproducible positive response at any one of the test substance concentrates is considered nonmutagenic in this system. Both biological and statistical significance should be considered together in this evaluation.

4. ALTERNATIVE TO ANIMAL TEST

This test is used for the identification of mutagenic chemicals.

BIBLIOGRAPHY

Commission Directive 87/302/EEC, 18 November 1987, Adapting to technical progress for the ninth time Council Directive 67/548/EEC on the approximation of laws, regulations and administrative provisions relating to the classification, packaging and labelling of dangerous substances, *Official Journal of the European Communities,* No. L133, Vol. 31, p.1, 1988.

Zimmermann, F. K., R. C. Von Borstel, E. S. Von Halle, J. M. Parry, D. Siebert, G. Zetterberg, R. Barale and N. Loprieno, Testing of chemicals for genetic activity with *Saccaromyces cerevisiae, Mutation Research,* Vol. 133, p. 199, 1984.

HET-CAM TEST

1. METHOD

1.1 Introduction, 1.2 Definition, and 1.3 Reference Substances (to be defined)

1.4 Principle of the Test Method

The hen's egg test (HET), extended to include chorioallantoic membrane (CAM) of fertilized egg, may be used as a mucous-membrane irritation test. This vascular membrane is provided with a circulatory system without any nervous connection to the living embryo and so allows examination of the immediate vascular change or reactions induced by chemicals (hyperemia, hemorrhage, and coagulation); these phenomena are similar to those assessed in *in vivo* eye irritation test. This assay has been suggested to have a limited use for screening compounds for their irritative potential to eye.

1.5 Quality Criteria (to be defined)

1.6 Description of the Test Method

1.6.1 Preparations

Hen's egg chorioallantoic membrane is used.

1.6.2 Test Conditions

Number of Cultures

Four to six eggs for each experimental point are used.

Use of Negative and Positive Controls

As negative control, two eggs, treated with vehicle only, are used.

Exposure Concentrations

(to be defined)

Culture Conditions

Some limitations about eggs: Defective eggs are discarded; only eggs weighing 50 to 60 g are used.

1.6.3 Procedure

1.6.3.1 Preparation of Cultures

Hen's Egg: The hen's eggs are put in incubator trays (Marsh Roll-X, Robin Haigh Incubators) with the large ends up; the trays are placed in the incubator, which automatically rotates and is maintained at an optimum temperature of $37.5 \pm 0.5°C$ and a relative humidity of $62.5 \pm 7.5\%$. The eggs are scored on day 5 of incubation and every day thereafter; nonviable embryos are removed. On day 10 of incubation, the egg shell is scratched around the air cell by a dentist's rotary saw (Drillmaster Junior A400, Microflame Ltd.) and then pared off. After careful removal of the inner egg membranes, the vascular CAM is exposed.

1.6.3.2 Treatment of the Cultures with the Test Substance

Hen's Egg: Test chemicals are dropped onto the membrane: 0.2 ml in the case of liquid test chemicals; 0.1 g in the case of solid test chemicals (the CAM is irrigated after 20 sec with 5 ml of warm water). The reactions are observed, scored, and classified at 0.5, 2, and 5 min (300 sec) after treatment.

1.6.3.3 Analysis

The test system measures inflammation (hyperemia), hemorrhages, and corrosiveness (coagulation) by examining CAM, the blood vessels, including the capillary system, and the albumen. The exact starting time of each reaction is observed and recorded, and the grade of effect scored. The time of each observation is the duration since dosing for liquids, or the duration since rinsing for solids.

Scoring Scheme for Irritation Testing

Effect	Score 0.5 min	2 min	5 min
Hyperemia	5	3	1
Hemorrhage	7	5	3
Coagulation	9	7	5

The numerical time-dependent scores are summed to give a single numerical value indicating the irritation potential of the test substances on a scale with a maximum value of 21.

Classification of Cumulative Scores

Cumulative Score	Irritation Assessment
0–0.9	Practically none
1–4.9	Slight
5–8.9	Moderate
9–21	Strong

The mean value obtained is transformed to standard format by use of the calculation below:

$$\text{Irritation index} = (301 - \text{starting time of hemorrhage}) \times 5/300$$
$$+ (301 - \text{starting time of lysis}) \times 7/300$$
$$+ (301 - \text{starting time of coagulation}) \times 9/300$$

2. DATA

3. REPORTING
3.1 Test Report
Animal strains must be mentioned.

3.2 Evaluation and Interpretation
(to be defined)

4. ALTERNATIVE TO ANIMAL TEST
It may be used in the screening for potential eye irritant chemicals.

BIBLIOGRAPHY

Bagley, D. M., L. H. Bruner, O. De Silva, M. Cottin, K. A. F. O'Brien, M. Uttley and A. P. Walker, An evaluation of five potential alternatives *in vitro* to the rabbit eye irritation test *in vivo*, *Toxicology In Vitro*, Vol. 6, No. 4, p. 275, 1992.

Commission of the European Communities, Collaborative study on the evaluation of alternative methods to the eye irritation test — Part 1, Doc. XI/632/91 V/E/1/131/91, Brussels, 1991.

Commission of the European Communities, Collaborative study on the evaluation of alternative methods to the eye irritation test — Part II, Doc. XI/632/91 V/E/1/131/91, Brussels 1991.

De Silva, O., A. Rougier and K. G. Dossou, The HET-CAM test: A study of the irritation potential of chemicals and formulations, *ATLA*, Vol. 20, p. 432, 1992.

Gettings, S. D., J. J. Teal, D. M. Bagley, J. L. Demetrulias, L. C. Di Pasquale, K. L. Hintze, M. G. Rozen, S. L. Weise, M. Chudkowski, K. D. Marenus, W. J. W. Pape, M. Roddy, R. Schnetzinger, P. M. Silber, S. M. Glaza and P. J. Kurtz, The CTFA evaluation of alternatives program: An evaluation of *in vitro* alternatives to the Draize primary eye irritation test (Phase 1) Hydro-alcoholic formulations; (Part 2) Data analysis and biological significance, *In Vitro Toxicology*, Vol. 4, No. 4, p. 247, 1991.

INVITTOX **Protocol,** No. 15, February 1990.

INVITTOX **Protocol,** No. 47, January 1992.

Kalweit, S., R. Besoke, I. Gerner and H. Spielmann, A national validation project of alternative methods to the Draize rabbit eye test, *Toxicology In Vitro*, Vol. 4, p. 702, 1990.

Lawrence, R. S., D. M. Ackroyd and D. L. Williams, The chorioallantoic membrane in the prediction of eye irritation potential, *Toxicology In Vitro*, Vol. 4, No. 4–5, p. 321, 1990.

Luepke, N. P., HET-Chorionallantois-Test: An alternative to the Draize rabbit eye test, in *In Vitro Toxicology*, Vol. 3, Goldberg, A. M., Ed., Mary Ann Liebert, New York, 1985, p. 592.

Lüpke, N. P., Hen's Egg Chorioallantoic Membrane Test for irritation potential, *Food & Chemical Toxicology*, Vol. 23, No. 2, p. 287, 1985.

Rougier, A., M. Cottin, O. De Silva, R. Roguet, P. Catroux, A. Toufic and K. G. Dossou, *In vitro* methods: Their relevance and complementarity in ocular safety assessment, *Lens and Eye Toxicity Research*, Vol. 9, No. 3/4, p. 229, 1992.

Spielmann, H., I. Gerner, S. Kalweit, R. Moog, T. Wirnsberger, K. Krauser, R. Kreiling, H. Kreuzer, N. P. Lüpke, H. G. Miltenburger, N. Muller, P. Murmann, W. Pape, B. Siegemund, J. Spengler, W. Steiling and F.J. Wiebel, Interlaboratory assessment of alternatives to the Draize eye irritation test in Germany, *Toxicology In Vitro*, 5, No. 5/6, p. 539, 1991.

Sterzel, W., N. P. Lüpke, S. Wallat and W. Holtmann, Validierung von Ersatzmethoden für Tierversuche zur Prüfung auf lokale Verträglichkeit. Teil 3: *In vitro* — Untersuchungen mit bebrüteten Hühnereiern — Abschlußbericht. BMFT-Projekt: 03 8640 9, Bundesministerium für Forschung und Technologie, Düsseldorf, 1987.

IN VITRO ACUTE HEPATOTOXICITY TEST

1. METHOD

1.1 Introduction, 1.2 Definition, and 1.3 Reference Substances (to be defined)

1.4 Principle of the Test Method

The liver slice system is a convenient *in vitro* acute toxicity test in which the environmental conditions of the hepatocytes are conserved and resemble those of the intact animal. It can be used for primary screening of hepatotoxic agents, for testing potential antidotes against hepatotoxins and for demonstration of species and age differences in the toxicity of various substances. Several biochemical parameters (LDH leakage, ATP content, protein synthesis, and secretion) are measured.

1.5 Quality Criteria (to be defined)

1.6 Description of the Test Method
1.6.1 Preparations

Chemicals are dissolved in warmed propylene glycol. Liver slices from male rats and mice of various age groups are used.

1.6.2 Test Conditions
Number of Cultures

At least two experiments are performed.

Use of Negative and Positive Controls

The zero time values, determined in slices at the beginning of incubation (max. 5 sec), are used as negative controls.

Exposure Concentrations

(to be defined)

Culture Conditions

Appropriate instruments are used to prepare and incubate tissue samples; up to 120 slices are obtained from one rat liver.

1.6.3 Procedure
1.6.3.1 Preparation of Cultures
Tissue Slices

Male rats or mice of different age groups are killed by a blow on the head after ether anesthesia. Liver lobes are removed and sliced into small pieces of about 0.5 × 0.5 mm. The slices are incubated for 1 h in an Erlenmeyer flask containing Krebs Ringer Heps (KRH) medium (2.5 mM-Hepes pH 7.4, 118 mM-NaCl, 2.85 mM-KCl, 2.5 mM-CaCl$_2$, 1.15 mM-KH$_2$PO$_4$, 1.18 mM-MgSO$_4$, 5.0 mM β-hydroxybutyrate and 4.0 mM glucose) and washed every 10 min with this medium. The slices are then divided into small portions and are incubated in a 20-ml capped glass beaker containing 2 ml of KRH medium. The beakers are maintained at 37°C in a rotary water-bath shaker (G-76) with oxygen aeration every 10 min. The slices are incubated for a further hour prior to exposure to the test agent.

Male rats are provided with a standard diet and water ad libitum. The rats are anesthetized with sodium pentobarbital (ip, 60 mg/kg body weight). The livers are excised through a midventral incision, rinsed, and immediately immersed in ice-cold Krebs-Henseleit buffer, pH 7.4. Tissue cylinders are prepared with a sharpened metal tube of 1 cm outer diameter mounted on a motor that turned and advanced the metal tube into the liver lobes, which are spread out on a rubber support. Following the preparation of 10 to 15 tissue cylinders, liver slices (250 μm thickness) are prepared using a mechanical tissue slicer containing ice-cold, oxygenated (95/5 O$_2$/CO$_2$) Krebs-Henseleit buffer pH 7.4, supplemented with 25 mM-glucose. The first and last slices that contain the Glisson capsule are discarded. The slices are pooled in oxygenated Optimem medium (Gibco) supplemented with 2% Ultroser G (Gibco) at room temperature before their incubation.

Liver slices are then deposited two by two on methylcellulose membranes (2.5 × 3 cm; 5 μm pore size, Millipore). An incubation system is designed to allow adequate exposure of both surfaces of the slices to dissolved oxygen and to nutrients in the culture medium: it consists of two lanes of incubation running in parallel. Culture medium is pumped at a constant flow rate through a multichannel peristaltic pump into a preconditioning reservoir where it is oxygenated by bubbling 95% O$_2$/5% CO$_2$. The mediun emerges into the lane of incubation that contains the liver slices resting on methylcellulose membranes. Up to four incubation systems can be used in parallel, thus allowing eight different conditions to be studied at the same time. The medium and the slices from each lane can be collected and assayed for metabolites, enzymes and other biochemical components. The Optimem culture medium is supplemented with 2% Ultroser G, 100 IU penicillin/ml (Gibco), 0.1 mg streptomycin/ml (Gibco), and glucose to obtain a final concentration of 28 mM. The temperature in the incubation chamber is maintained at 37°C by a thermoregulator.

1.6.3.2 Treatment of the Cultures with the Test Substance
Tissue Slices

Treatment time is 120 min: then LDH is determined in the slice medium. The total enzyme level is measured following slice homogenization (Kinematica homogenizer) and centrifugation (10,000 g for 3 min). For testing a potential antidote, it is added 20 min after hepatotoxin application.

Several analytical procedures are monitored during a 20-h incubation period with test chemicals:

- Lactate dehydrogenase leakage: Aliquots of the culture medium are analyzed.
- Protein synthesis: The slices are incubated in the presence of [^{14}C]leucine (393 µCi/mmol, Radiochemical Center Amersham). They are removed from the incubation system at the appropriate times, immediately washed three times in ice-cold 0.9% NaCl and homogenized in 1 ml 2% perchloric acid by sonication (Braunsonic 300S; 60W, 20s). The omogenate is centrifuged at 11,000 g for 5 min (Beckman microfuge). The pellets are washed by suspension and recentrifugation in 2% perchloric acid and then in H$_2$O, and finally dissolved by sonication in 1 ml 0.3 N-NaOH. The incorporation of [^{14}C]leucine into acid-precipitable protein is determined in a 0.75-ml aliquot of the dissolved pellet after neutralization with 0.25 ml of 1 N-HCl. Results are expressed as cpm/mg slice protein.
- Protein secretion: Protein secretion is evaluated by measuring the incorporation of [^{14}C]leucine into acid-precipitable medium proteins. Results are expressed as cpm/ml medium.
- ATP content: ATP levels are evaluated in the supernatant from the centrifugation in the Beckman microfuge and measured spectrophotometrically. Preincubation values for ATP content are determined on freshly isolated slice (S value). Results are expressed as nmol/mg slice protein.

1.6.3.3 Analysis
Data are expressed:

- as percentages of the control value at the same incubation time;
- by subtracting zero time value (5 sec of exposure) from the determined value and calculating the ratio between the value obtained and that of the total enzyme activity.

2. DATA

3. REPORTING
3.1 Test Report
Animal species, strains, culture, and treatment time conditions must be reported.

3.2 Evaluation and Interpretation
(to be defined)

4. ALTERNATIVE TO ANIMAL TEST
This method may be used in the screening for potential toxic chemicals.

BIBLIOGRAPHY
Goethals, F., D. Deboyser, V. Lefebvre, I. De Coster and M. Roberfroid, Adult rat liver slices as a model for studying the hepatotoxicity of vincaalkaloids, *Toxicology In Vitro,* Vol. 4, No. 4/5, p. 435, 1990.

INVITTOX Protocol No. 42, January 1992;

Wormser, U. and S. Ben-Zakine, The liver slice system: An *in vitro* acute toxicity test for assessment of hepatotoxins and their antidote, *Toxicology In Vitro,* Vol. 4, No. 4/5, p. 449, 1990.

IN VITRO MAMMALIAN CELL GENE MUTATION TEST
(87/302/EEC DIR.)

1. METHOD

1.1 Introduction, 1.2 Definition, and 1.3 Reference Substances
None.

1.4 Principle of the Test Method

Mammalian cell culture systems may be used to detect mutations induced by chemical substances. Widely used cell lines include L5178Y mouse lymphoma cells and the CHO and V-79 lines of Chinese hamster cells. In these cell lines the most commonly used systems measure mutations at the thymidine kinase (TK), hypoxanthine guanine phosphoribosyl transferase (HPRT) and Na^+/K^+ ATPase loci. The TK and HPRT mutational systems detect base-pair mutations, frameshift mutations and small deletions; the Na^+/K^+ system detects base-pair mutations only.

Cells deficient in TK, due to the forward mutation $TK^+ \rightarrow TK^-$, are resistant to bromodeoxyuridine (BrdU), fluorodeoxyuridine (FdU) or trifluorothymidine (TFT) since these antimetabolites are not incorporated into cellular nucleotides by the "salvage" enzyme system TK; the nucleotides needed for cellular metabolism are obtained solely from *de novo* synthesis. However, in the presence of TK, BrdU, FdU, and TFT are incorporated into the nucleotides, resulting in inhibition of cellular metabolism and cytotoxicity. Thus, the mutant cells are able to proliferate in the presence of BrdU, FdU, or TFT, whereas the normal cells, which contain TK, are not. Similarly, cells deficient in HPRT are selected by resistance to 8-azaguanine (AG) or 6-thioguanine (TG). Cells with altered Na^+/K^+ ATPase are selected by resistance to ouabain.

Cytotoxicity is determined by measuring the effect of the test material on colony-forming abilities (cloning efficiency) or growth rates of the cultures. Mutant frequency is determined by seeding known numbers of cells in medium containing the selective agent to detect mutant cells, and in medium without selective agent to determine the surviving cells. After a suitable incubation period, colonies are counted. Mutant frequencies are calculated from the number of mutant colonies corrected for cell survival.

1.5 Quality Criteria
None.

1.6 Description of the Test Method
1.6.1 Preparations
Cells

A variety of cell lines are available for use in this assay. These include subclones of L5178Y, CHO cells, or V-79 cells with a demonstrated sensitivity to chemical mutagens, a high cloning efficiency and a low spontaneous mutation frequency. Cells may be periodically checked for karyotype stability and should be checked for mycoplasma contamination. Other cell types may be used providing their validity as an assay for chemically induced gene mutations can be fully documented.

Medium

Appropriate culture media and incubation conditions (e.g., temperature, culture vessels used, CO_2 concentrations and humidity) should be used. Media and sera should be chosen according to the selective systems and cell type used in the assay.

Test Substance

Test substances may be prepared in culture media or dissolved or suspended in appropriate vehicles prior to treatment of the cells. The final concentration of the vehicle in the culture system should not affect cell viability or growth rate.

Metabolic Activation

Cells should be exposed to the test substance both in the presence and absence of an appropriate exogenous mammalian metabolic activation system. Alternatively, where cell types with intrinsic metabolic activity are used, the rate and nature of the activity should be known to be appropriate to the chemical class being tested.

1.6.2 Test Conditions
Use of Negative and Positive Controls

Positive controls, using both a direct acting compound and a compound requiring metabolic activation, should be included in each experiment; a negative (vehicle) control also should be used.

The following are examples of substances that might be used as positive controls:

- Direct acting compounds
  - ethylmethanesulfonate
  - hycanthone
- Indirect acting compounds
  - acetylaminofluorene
  - 7,12-dimethylbenzanthracene
  - N-nitrosodimethylamine

When appropriate, an additional positive control of the same chemical class as the chemical under test could be included.

Exposure Concentrations

Several concentrations of the test substance should be used. These concentrations should yield a concentration-related toxic effect, the highest concentration producing a low level of survival and the survival in the lowest concentration being approximately the same as that in the negative control.

Relatively water-insoluble substances should be tested up to the limit of solubility using appropriate procedures. For freely water-soluble nontoxic substances, the upper test substance concentration should be determined on a case-by-case basis.

1.6.3 Procedure

The number of cells used per culture should be related to the spontaneous mutation frequency; a general guide is to use a number of viable cells that is ten times the inverse of the spontaneous mutation frequency.

Cells should be exposed for a suitable period of time; in most cases 2 to 5 h is effective. Cells without sufficient intrinsic metabolic activity should be exposed to the test substance in the presence and absence of an appropriate metabolic activation system. At the end of the exposure period, cells are washed free of test substance and cultured to determine viability and to allow for expression of the mutant phenotype.

At the end of the expression period, which should be sufficient to allow near optimal phenotypic expression of induced mutants, the cells are grown in medium with and without selective agents for the determination of numbers of mutants and viability. All results are confirmed in an independent experiment.

2. DATA

Data should be presented in tabular form. Inhibition of tumor cell attachment individual plate counts for the test substance and controls should be presented for both mutation induction and survival. The mean number of colonies per plate and the standard deviation should also be given. Mutation frequency should be expressed as number of mutants per number of surviving cells. Survival and cloning efficiencies are expressed as a percentage of the control level.

Data should be evaluated using appropriate statistical methods.

3. REPORTING
3.1 Test Report

The test report shall, if possible, contain the following information:

- cell line used, number of cell cultures, methods for maintenance of cell cultures;
- test conditions: composition of media, CO_2 concentration, concentration of test substance, vehicle used, incubation temperature, incubation time, length of expression period (including number of cells seeded and subcultures and feeding schedules, if appropriate), duration of treatment, cell density during treatment, type of mammalian metabolic activation system used, positive and negative controls, selective agent used;
- rationale for dose selection;
- method used to enumerate numbers of viable and mutant cells;
- statistical evaluation;
- discussion of results;
- interpretation of results.

3.2 Evaluation and Interpretation

There are several criteria for determining a positive result, one of which is a statistically significant concentration-related increase in the mutant frequency. Another may be based upon detection of a reproducible and statistically significant positive response for at least one of the test substance concentrations.

Positive results for an *in vitro* mammalian cell gene mutation test indicate that a substance induces gene mutations in the cultured mammalian cells used. Negative results indicate that, under the test conditions, the test substance does not induce gene mutations in the cultured mammalian cells used.

4. ALTERNATIVE TO ANIMAL TEST

This method is used for the identification of mutagenic chemicals.

BIBLIOGRAPHY

Commission Directive 87/302/EEC, 18 November 1987, Adapting to technical progress for the ninth time Council Directive 67/548/EEC on the approximation of laws, regulations and administrative provisions relating to the classification, packaging and labelling of dangerous substances, *Official Journal of the European Communities,* No. L133, Vol. 31, p. 61, 1988.

Clive, D. R, R. McCuen, J. F. S. Spector, C. Piper and K. H. Mavournin, Specific gene mutations in L5178Y cells in culture, *Mutation Research,* Vol. 15, p. 225, 1983.

Hsie, A. W., D. A. Casciano, D. B. Coug, D. F. Krahn, J. P. O'Neal and B.L. Whitfield, The use of Chinese hamster ovary cells to quantify specific locus mutation and to determine mutagenicity of chemicals, *Mutation Research,* Vol. 6, p. 193, 1981.

Note: The updating of this methodology is in progress at the OECD.

IN VITRO MAMMALIAN CELL TRANSFORMATION TEST
(87/302/EEC DIR.)

1. METHOD

1.1 Introduction and 1.2 Definition

1.3 Reference Substances
None.

1.4 Principle of the Test Method

Mammalian cell culture systems may be used to detect phenotypic changes *in vitro* induced by chemical substances associated with malignant transformation *in vivo*. Widely used cells include C3H/10T$^1/_2$, BALB 3T3 clone A31, BALB 3T3 clone A31-1-1, SHE, and Fischer rat; the tests rely on changes in cell morphology, focus formation, or changes in anchorage dependence in semisolid agar. Less widely used systems exist that detect other physiological or morphological changes in cells following exposure to carcinogenic chemicals. None of the *in vitro* test endpoints has an established mechanistic link with cancer. Some of the test systems are capable of detecting tumor promotors. Cytotoxicity may be determined by measuring the effect of the test material on colony-forming abilities (cloning efficiency) or growth rates of the cultures. The measurement of cytotoxicity is to establish that exposure to the test chemical has been toxicologically relevant but cannot be used to calculate transformation frequency in all assays since some may involve prolonged incubation and/or replating.

1.5 Quality Criteria
None.

1.6 Description of the Test Method
1.6.1 Preparations
Cells

A variety of cell lines or primary cells are available depending on the transformation test being used. The investigator must ensure that the cells in the test being performed exhibit the appropriate phenotypic change after exposure to known carcinogens and that the test, in the investigator's laboratory, is of proven and documented validity and reliability.

Medium

Media and experimental conditions should be used that are appropriate to the transformation assay in use.

Test Substance

Test substances may be prepared in culture media or dissolved or suspended in appropriate vehicles prior to treatment of the cells. The final concentration of the vehicle in the culture system should not affect cell viability, growth rate or transformation incidence.

Metabolic Activation

Cells should be exposed to the test substance both in the presence and absence of an appropriate metabolic activation system. Alternatively, when cell types are used that possess intrinsic metabolic activity, the nature of the activity should be known to be appropriate to the chemical class being tested.

1.6.2 Test Conditions
Use of Negative and Positive Controls
Positive controls, using both a direct-acting compound and a compound requiring metabolic activation should be included in each experiment; a negative (vehicle) control also should be used.

The following are examples of substances that might be used as positive controls:

- direct-acting chemicals
  - ethylmethanesulfonate
  - b-propiolactone
- compounds requiring metabolic activation
  - 2-acetylaminofluorene
  - 4-dimethylaminoazobenzene
  - 7,12-dimethylbenzanthracene

When appropriate, an additional positive control of the same chemical class as the compound under test should be included.

Exposure Concentrations
Several concentrations of the test substance should be used. They should yield a concentration-related toxic effect, the highest one producing a low level of survival and the survival in the lowest one being approximately the same as that in the negative control. Relatively water-insoluble substances should be tested up to the limit of solubility using appropriate procedures. For freely water-soluble nontoxic substances the upper test substance concentration should be determined on a case-by-case basis.

1.6.3 Procedure
Cells should be exposed for a suitable period of time depending on the test system in use, and this may involve redosing accompanied by a change of medium (and if necessary, fresh metabolic activation mixture) if exposure is prolonged. Cells without sufficient intrinsic metabolic activity should be exposed to the test substance in the presence and absence of an appropriate metabolic activation system. At the end of the exposure period, cells are washed free of test substance and cultured under conditions appropriate for the appearance of the transformed phenotype being monitored and the incidence of transformation determined. All results are confirmed in an independent experiment.

2. DATA
Data should be presented in tabular form and may take a variety of forms according to the assay being used, e.g., plate counts, positive plates, or numbers of transformed cells. Where appropriate, survival should be expressed as a percentage of control levels and transformation frequency expressed as the number of transformants per number of survivors. Data should be evaluated using appropriate statistical methods.

3. REPORTING
3.1 Test Report
The test report shall, if possible, contain the following information:

- cell type used, number of cell cultures, methods for maintenance of cell cultures;
- test conditions: concentration of test substance, vehicle used, incubation time, duration and frequency of treatment, cell density during treatment, type of exogenous metabolic

activation system used, positive and negative controls, specification of phenotype being monitored, selective system used (if appropriate), rationale for dose selection;
- method used to enumerate viable and transformed cells;
- statistical evaluation;
- discussion of results;
- interpretation of results.

3.2 Evaluation and Interpretation

4. ALTERNATIVE TO ANIMAL TEST
This method may be used for the identification of potential carcinogenic chemicals.

BIBLIOGRAPHY

Dunkel, V. C., L. M. Schechtman, A. S. Tu, A. Sivak, R. A. Lubet and T. P. Cameron, Interlaboratory evaluation of the C3H/lOTl/2 cell transformation assay, *Environmental and Molecular Mutagenesis*, Vol. 12, p. 21, 1988.

Kakunaga, T. and J. D. Crow, Cell variants showing differential susceptibility to ultraviolet light-induced transformation, *Science*, Vol. 209, p. 505, 1980.

Matthews, E. J., J. W. Spalding and R. W. Tennant, Transformation of BALB/c-3T3 cells: V. Transformation responses of 168 chemicals compared with mutagenicity in Salmonella and carcinogenicity in rodent bioassays, *Environmental Health Perspectives Supplements*, Vol. 101 (Suppl. 2), p. 347, 1993.

Commission Directive 87/302/EEC, 18 November 1987, Adapting to technical progress for the ninth time Council Directive 67/548/EEC on the approximation of laws, regulations and administrative provisions relating to the classification, packaging and labelling of dangerous substances, *Official Journal of the European Communities*, No. L133, Vol. 31, p. 73, 1988.

Pienta, R. J., A hamster embryo cell model system for identifying carcinogens, in *Carcinogens, Identification and Mechanisms of Action*, Griffin, A. C. and C. R. Shaw, Eds., Raven Press. New York. 1979, p. 121.

Sheu, C. W., S. N. Dobras, I. Rodriguez, J. K. Lee and P. P. Fu, Transforming activity of selected polycyclic aromatic hydrocarbons and their nitro-derivatives in BALB/3T3 A31-1-1 cells, *Food and Chemical Toxicology*, Vol. 32, p. 611, 1994.

IN VITRO MAMMALIAN CYTOGENETIC TEST
(92/69/EEC DIR.)

1. METHOD

1.1 Introduction, 1.2 Definition, and 1.3 Reference Substances
None.

1.4 Principle of the Test Method
The *in vitro* cytogenetic test is a short-term mutagenicity test for the detection of structural chromosomal aberrations in cultured mammalian cells. Cultures of established cell lines as well as primary cell cultures may be used. After exposure to test chemicals with and without a liver enzyme activation mixture (a cofactor supplemented postmitochondrial fraction), cell cultures are treated with spindle inhibitors, such as colchicine, to accumulate cells in a metaphase-like stage of mitosis (c-metaphase). Cells are harvested at appropriate times and chromosome preparations are made. Preparations are stained and metaphase cells are analyzed for chromosomal abnormalities.

1.5 Quality Criteria
None.

1.6 Description of the Test Method
1.6.1 Preparations

Test chemicals are prepared in culture medium or dissolved in appropriate vehicles prior to treatment of the cells. Established cell lines or cultures of primary cells are used, e.g., Chinese hamster cells and human lymphocytes.

1.6.2 Test Conditions
Number of Cultures

At least duplicate cultures are used for each experimental point.

Use of Negative and Positive Controls

Solvent (when the solvent is not the culture medium or water), liver enzyme activation mixture, liver enzyme activation mixture and solvent, and untreated controls are used as negative controls.

In each experiment a positive control is included; when liver enzyme activation mixture is used to activate the test chemical, a compound known to require metabolic activation must be used as a positive control.

Dose Level

At least three doses of the test compound over at least a one-log dose range are employed, the highest dose suppressing the mitotic activity by approximately 50%.

Culture Conditions

Appropriate culture medium, incubation conditions (e.g., temperature, culture vessels used, CO_2 concentrations, and humidity) are used.

1.6.3 Procedure
1.6.3.1 Preparation of Cultures

Established Cell Lines: Cells are generated from stock cultures (e.g., by trypsinization or by shaking off), seeded in culture vessels at appropriate density, and incubated at 37°C.

Human Lymphocytes: Heparinized whole blood is added to culture medium containing phytohemagglutinin, fetal calf serum and antibiotics and incubated at 37°C.

1.6.3.2 Treatment of the Cultures with the Test Substance

Treatment without Liver Enzyme Activation Mixture: All treatments shall cover the period of one whole cell cycle and fixation schemes shall ensure the analysis of first posttreatment mitoses of cells treated at different stages in the cycle. When the treatment does not cover the length of one whole cell cycle, multiple fixation times are chosen to sample cells that are in different stages of the cell cycle during the treatment, i.e., G_1, S, and G_2. The test chemical is added to cultures of established cell lines when they are in the exponential stage of growth. Human lymphocyte cultures are treated while they are in a semisynchronous condition. If the test chemical changes the cell cycle length, the fixation interval has to be changed accordingly.

Treatment with Liver Enzyme Activation Mixture: For the treatment, the test compound in combination with the activation system should be present for as long as possible without exerting a toxic effect on the cells. If, for toxicity reasons, this treatment does not cover the length of a whole cell cycle, multiple fixation times are chosen to sample cells that are in different stages of the cell cycle during the treatment, i.e., G_1, S, and G_2.

Harvesting Cells: Cell cultures are treated with the spindle inhibitor 1 to 2 h prior to harvesting. Each culture is harvested and processed separately for the preparation of chromosomes.

1.6.3.3 Chromosome Preparation

Chromosome preparations involve hypotonic treatment of the cells, fixation, spreading on slides, and staining.

Analysis

At least 100 well-spread metaphases per culture are analyzed for chromosomal aberrations. Slides are coded before analysis. In human lymphocytes, only metaphases containing 46 centromeres are analyzed. In established cell lines, only metaphases containing ±2 centromeres of the modal number are analyzed.

2. DATA

Data are presented in a tabular form. Chromatid-type aberrations (gaps, breaks, interchanges), chromosome-type aberrations (gaps, breaks, minutes, rings, dicentrics, polycentrics) and the number of aberrant metaphases (including and excluding gaps) are listed separately for all treated and control cultures. The data are evaluated by appropriate statistical methods.

3. REPORTING

3.1 Test Report

The test report shall, if possible, include the following information:

- cells used;
- test conditions: composition of medium, CO_2 concentration, incubation temperature, incubation time, dose levels, treatment time, duration of treatment with and concentration of the spindle inhibitor used, type of liver enzyme activation mixture used, positive and negative controls;
- number of cell cultures;
- number of metaphases analyzed (data given separately for each culture);
- mitotic index;
- type and number of aberrations given separately for each treated and control culture, modal number of chromosomes in established cell lines used;
- statistical evaluation;
- discussion of the results;
- interpretation of the results.

3.2 Evaluation and Interpretation

There are several criteria for determining a positive result, one of which is a statistically significant dose-related increase in the number of structural chromosomal aberrations. Another criterion may be the detection of a reproducible and statistically significant positive response for at least one of the test points.

A test substance producing neither a statistically significant dose-related increase in the number of structural chromosomal aberrations nor a statistically significant and reproducible positive response at any one of the test points is considered nonmutagenic in this system.

Positive results from the *in vitro* cytogenetic test indicate that a substance induces chromosomal aberrations in cultured mammalian somatic cells. Negative results indicate that under the test conditions, the test substance does not induce chromosomal aberrations in cultured mammalian somatic cells.

4. ALTERNATIVE TO ANIMAL TEST

This method is used for the identification of clastogenic chemicals.

BIBLIOGRAPHY

Annex to Commission Directive 92/69/EEC, 31 July 1992, Adapting to technical progress for the seventeenth time Council Directive 67/548/EEC on the approximation of laws, regulations and administrative provisions relating to the classification, packaging and labelling of dangerous substances, *Official Journal of the European Communities,* No. 383A, Vol. 35, p. 148, 1992.

Ishidate, M. Jr. and S. Odashima, Chromosome tests with 134 compounds on Chinese hamster cells *in vitro* — A screening for chemical carcinogens, *Mutation Research,* Vol. 48, p. 337, 1977.

Matsuoka, A., M. Hayaishi and M. Ishidate, Chromosomal aberration tests on 29 chemicals combined with S9 mix *in vitro, Mutation Research,* Vol. 66, p. 277, 1979.

Note: The updating of this methodology is in progress at the OECD.

IN VITRO MEASUREMENT OF INFLAMMATORY MEDIATORS

1. METHOD

1.1 Introduction, 1.2 Definition, and 1.3 Reference Substances (to be defined)

1.4 Principle of the Test Method

This *in vitro* methodology has been performed in order to evaluate the cutaneous irritative potential of chemicals. The test is based on the measurement of production and secretion of two inflammatory mediators (IL1α and PGE$_2$) revealed by radioimmunoassay.

1.5 Quality Criteria (to be defined)

1.6 Description of the Test Method
1.6.1 Preparations
Test chemicals are dissolved in medium.
Primary cultures (human keratinocytes) are used.

1.6.2 Test Conditions
Number of Cultures
Three independent cultures are used for each experimental point.

Use of Negative and Positive Controls
Negative control is used.

Exposure Concentrations
A range between nonlethal and lethal concentrations is used.

Culture Conditions
As various factors (mechanical disruption of the confluent monolayer, plating keratinocytes under serum-free conditions and low cell differentiation) act to stimulate IL1 production, strict experimental conditions are required; in the same way PGE$_2$ production decreases in confluent keratinocyte cultures.

Metabolic Activation
(most chemicals require metabolic activation)

1.6.3 Procedure
1.6.3.1 Preparation of Cultures
Primary Cultures

Human skin specimens, obtained from plastic surgery procedures, are used. Human keratinocytes preparations are made from electrokeratomed strips of skin 0.5 mm thick. The strips are cut into small pieces, incubated in antibiotic solution (gentamicin 0.16 mg/ml, penicillin 100 U/ml, streptomycin 100 μg/ml), then placed in 0.2% trypsin-EDTA in calcium- and magnesium-free PBS overnight at 4°C. The epidermis is peeled from the dermis and epidermal sheets are triturated. Cell suspensions then are passed through a nylon gauze to remove debris and large cell clumps. Cells are centrifuged and resuspended in culture medium (modified Eagle's medium) supplemented with 10% FCS, 50 U/ml penicillin, 50 μg/ml streptomycin, 2.5 μg/ml amphotericin, 1 mM Na-pyruvate, and 2 mM glutamine. Primary cultures are initiated by inoculating 2×10^5 viable cells per cm^2 into 35 mm diameter Nunc plastic culture dishes containing 2 ml culture medium. The cultures are grown in a humidified incubator at 37°C in an atmosphere containing 5% CO_2. The media are changed every 2 to 3 d.

1.6.3.2 Treatment of the Cultures with the Test Substance
Primary Cultures

Physical agent: Before irradiation, subconfluent culture media are eliminated and cells are washed twice with 1 ml PBS. After irradiation, fresh medium is added and cells are cultured over 24 h.

Chemical agent: Subconfluent cultures receive 1 ml fresh medium with various concentrations of test chemical for a 24-h incubation period.

Sample preparation: Culture media are collected, centrifuged to eliminate detached cells, and the supernatants are stored at –80°C until the determination of the two mediators in the extracellular compartment. In order to measure intracellular mediators, 2 ml fresh medium are added on the cellular sheet and immediately frozen in liquid nitrogen. Frozen cells are harvested mechanically and sonicated with a cell disruptor Sonifier B-20 (Bioblock Scientific Co.). Cell lysates are centrifuged at 5000 g for 30 min and the supernatants are stored at –80°C. IL1a and PGE_2 are evaluated in the extracellular (culture medium) and intracellular (cell lysate) compartments using radioimmunoassay (RIA, Radiochemical Centre, Amersham).

1.6.3.3 Analysis
(to be defined)

2. DATA

3. REPORTING
3.1 Test Report
Cell culture and treatment time conditions must be reported.

3.2 Evaluation and Interpretation
(to be defined)

4. ALTERNATIVE TO ANIMAL TEST
This method may be used in the screening for potential skin irritant chemicals.

BIBLIOGRAPHY

Cohen, C., G. Dossou, A. Rougier and R. Roguet, Measurement of inflammatory mediators produced by human keratinocytes *in vitro*, a predictive assessment of cutaneous irritation, *Toxicology In Vitro*, Vol. 5, No. 5/6, p. 407, 1991.

IN VITRO PERCUTANEOUS ABSORPTION ASSAY

1. INTRODUCTION

A variety of methods are used to examine *in vitro* skin penetration; an overview of these is given here.

2. DIFFUSION CELLS

There are many types and designs of diffusion cells suitable for use in *in vitro* experiments. Cells must be fabricated from nonreactive materials like glass, stainless steel, or transparent plastics (Plexiglas® or Teflon®). The stratum corneum of the skin faces the donor chamber and the dermal surface faces the receptor chamber fluid. By analysis of this receptor fluid, penetration of the test molecule through the skin is detected.

The existing horizontally or vertically orientated diffusion cells can be classified roughly into two different types, namely static or flow-through cells. They are usually based on the original static Franz cell system which now are most often used for applying a "finite dose." The skin is normally sandwiched between two halves of a glass chamber with the aid of O-rings or by overlapping the edge of the receptor compartment.

Variations of the static diffusion cells can be classified as either having air/fluid phase or fluid/fluid phase chambers. In the air/fluid system the epidermal surface of the skin is uncovered and normally exposed to ambient conditions. Such exposure allows volatile solvents to evaporate and chemicals may be precipitated on the surface. With volatile substances, the air flow in the donor chamber should be controlled carefully because the evaporation rate influences the penetration values. These diffusion cells more closely resemble the normal situation because the skin is exposed to ambient conditions and is not hydrated excessively.

In fluid/fluid systems of the chemical passing from one stirred fluid phase (the donor side) through the skin into a second fluid phase (the receptor side) is determined. Side-by-side two chamber diffusion cells are employed widely; in these the skin usually is oriented vertically to the two diffusion chambers. Typically, the amount of chemical which penetrates is small compared to the dose in the donor compartment; therefore this type of *in vitro* measurement has been referred to as the "infinite dose" technique. The fluid/fluid phase diffusion system represents occlusive exposure conditions.

In such an "infinite dose" experimental design nonphysiological alterations of the skin may be caused by excessive hydration or by solvent induced deterioration of the stratum corneum. The results of these investigations have, therefore, to be evaluated carefully when used for hazard assessment. This type of diffusion cell is probably not suited to the measurement of absorption rates after a period of 24 h since structural deterioration of the skin permeation barrier would lead to erroneous conclusions. In addition, skin surface temperature higher than 30°C must be avoided. Despite these limitations, this diffusion cell arrangement is useful for the measurement of fluxes and partition and diffusion coefficients is not recommended for measuring absorption from various formulations.

In static diffusion cells the small volumes of receptor solution drawn for analysis are replaced manually. In flow-through cells these volumes are replenished automatically. If low solubility of the penetrant in the receptor phase is a problem, the large volume and the continuous flow of the effluent may increase the amount of lipophilic chemical dissolved and thus improve the reliability of the data.

The donor compartment should allow easy access for delivery of the penetrant to the skin, should be stirred where possible and necessary, should be temperature controlled and allow the control of evaporation of volatile vehicles and penetrants. The receptor compartment should also be temperature controlled, have sufficient volume to maintain perfect skin conditions and stirred without obvious formation of boundary layers.

3. SKIN MEMBRANES

In *in vitro* skin penetration experiments, freshly excised skin (from laboratory animals or human surgery) or cadaver skin is used. Subcutaneous fat and any attached muscles should be carefully removed from the prepared skin areas. Human cadaver skin stored in airtight bags in the deep freezer up to 12 months can be used provided the integrity of the barrier is checked using ^{3}H-water as a probe.

Full or as split-thickness skin can be used. Split-thickness skin is especially recommended in animals like the rat, guinea pig, monkey, and pig, and in man where the thickness of whole skin is about 1 mm or more. Mouse skin, which is less than 500 µm thick, can be used as a whole. The dermatome is a widely used technique for preparation of split thickness skin of about 400 µm. It can be used with hairless and hairy skin and it does not adversely affect the viability of the membrane. Dermatomed skin must be used with highly hydrophobic compounds, where the aqueous dermis may represent a high diffusion barrier not apparent *in vivo*.

For separation of epidermis and dermis, several mechanical, thermal, and chemical techniques have been described. The epidermis can be removed readily with forceps after placing the skin samples on a hot plate for 2 min at 50°C or in a beaker of water at 60°C for 30 to 60 sec. This technique is particularly useful with human and hairless animal skin. Chemical separation by soaking skin samples in 2 *M* solutions of various anions like bromide, thiocyanate, and iodide, seems also to be effective with haired skin. Enzymatic separation using incubation with proteases like dispase, trypsin, pancreatin, or a bacterial collagenase is also effective. Protease incubations also have been used for preparation of isolated sheets of the stratum corneum of human cadaver skin.

4. RECEPTOR FLUID

The receptor fluid under the dermal side of the skin membrane has to fulfill two functions. It should maintain the integrity of the skin membrane during the experiment and it should act as an effective acceptor for the penetrating compound. For water soluble compounds, physiological saline buffered to pH 7.4 is recommended as the receptor phase. In case of lipophilic compounds (octanol/water partition coefficient $\geq 10^3$) the receptor phase needs to be altered to increase its ability to solubilize lipophilic molecules: the addition of four nonionic surfactants like polyethylene glycol oleyl-ether (6% in saline), methanol, ethanol, polyethyleneglycol, serum, or albumin to the buffer solution is described in the literature. It is necessary to ascertain that the receptor fluids used do not alter the permeability properties of the skin.

5. SKIN METABOLISM

Skin is capable of metabolizing endogenous and exogenous substances. The biotransformation reactions in the skin comprise metabolism, e.g., by oxidation, reduction, and hydrolysis (phase I) and conjugation, e.g., with glucuronic and sulfuric acid, glutathione, and methylation (phase II). Although the spectrum of reactions in the skin is similar to that in liver, the activity is much lower in the skin. To suppress bacterial growth and metabolism, an antibiotic is added to the receptor fluid.

In vitro percutaneous absorption studies with viable skin can indicate if a test substance may be toxified or detoxified during skin permeation. The various factors — such as area dose, vehicle, concentration, skin condition, mode of application (open vs. occlusion), etc. — influencing percutaneous absorption, and probably the extent of skin metabolism, make the finite dose technique best suited to mimic *in vivo* metabolic conditions. Quantitation of skin metabolism findings has to be interpreted with caution. Further investigations are necessary to assess how well *in vitro* absorption experiments with viable skin predict *in vivo* absorption in man.

6. TEMPERATURE

Because the absorption process relies on diffusion of molecules, the rate can be altered by changes in temperature. Skin should be maintained at a constant temperature; 30°C ± 1°C is recommended in Franz-type designs because this approximates normal skin temperature.

7. APPLICATION OF TEST SUBSTANCE

The "finite dose" technique allows varying amounts of material to be applied to the skin surface. In this way the experiment can provide data from a range of preparations such as powders, undiluted formulation, aqueous dilutions, and large and small volumes. The precise dose will inevitably depend on the data required. Solids or samples with a high viscosity can be applied to the skin on a weight basis using a rod; liquids usually are applied by volume using a syringe.

8. SAMPLING AND ANALYSIS

Samples of the receptor fluids, of a size determined by the assay procedure and its sensitivity, can be taken during the exposure period. These are analyzed by liquid scintillation counting if radiolabeled penetrants are used or by GLC/HPLC if unlabeled chemicals are used.

It is recommended that the concentration of the chemical remaining in the skin at the end of the experiment is determined. The distribution of the chemical in different skin layers can be evaluated by several methods, e.g., tape stripping, horizontal sectioning, or autoradiography.

The effects of decontaminating the skin after a defined period of exposure can be studied by washing the skin surface with saline and detergent solution.

9. RESULTS

The absorption profile should be characterized from immediately after application of a compound up to a minimum of 24 h. If the data allow the definition of lag times and calculation of absorption rates, these should be presented.

The slope of the regression line through the linear portion of the curve represents the amount of substance penetrated through the treatment area per time unit, dM/dt; the extrapolated intercept on the time axis represents the lag time L. From Fick's First Law of Diffusion a permeability coefficient P can be calculated:

$$P = \frac{dM / dt}{A \cdot C}$$

where

P = permeability coefficient in length/time
dM/dt = substance flux in mass units per time
A = surface area of skin exposed (length^2)
C = concentration of test substance in the donor solution in mass units per volume

From the lag time L, the diffusion coefficient D is obtained:

$$D = \frac{d2}{6L}$$

where

D = diffusion coefficient in length^2/time
d = thickness of membrane (horny layer) in length units
L = lag time

While the "infinite dose" technique has been of great value in elucidating the physico-chemical concepts of percutaneous absorption, this methodology is only of limited value for predicting skin absorption and systemic load *in vivo*. For this the "finite dose" technique was developed in which the skin surface can be exposed to solutions, ointments, powders, etc., similar to the exposure *in vivo*. Accumulated amounts penetrating a certain area of skin in a defined time can be directly obtained from cumulative amounts vs. time curves.

From these plots, a time-averaged substance absorption rate (flux *J*) can be derived according to:

$$J = \frac{M(o - f)}{A \cdot t}$$

where

$M(o - f)$ = cumulated amount absorbed within exposure time *t* in mass units
A = skin area exposed to test agent in cm[7]
t = exposure time *in vitro* (h)

From such experiments, the total *in vivo* body absorption may be estimated. An untested but possibly useful approach is to use the following equation, which takes account of different skin permeabilities in different regions of the human body:

$$E(o - t) = J(\textstyle\sum) \; i = n \; ai \cdot Pi$$

$$i = 1$$

where

$E(o - t)$ = total systemic exposure within an exposure time *t*
J = time averaged *in vitro* flux (exposure time *t*)
ai = area of exposure in region *i*
Pi = penetration index of region *i* relative to penetration index of skin site used in the *in vitro* experiment.

BIBLIOGRAPHY

Bracher, M., C. Faller and F. K. Noser, Evaluation of an *in vitro* percutaneous permeation model with two oxidative hair dyes, *International Journal of Cosmetic Science*, Vol. 9, p. 223, 1987.

ECETOC, Percutaneous absorption, *Monograph No. 20,* European Chemical Industry Ecology & Toxicology Center, Brussels, 1993.

Hotchkiss, S. A. M., P. Hewitt and J. Caldwell, Percutaneous absorption of 4,4'-methylene-bis(2-chloroaniline) and 4,4'-methylenedianiline through rat and human skin *in vitro, Toxicology In Vitro,* Vol. 7, No. 2, p. 141, 1993.

Hughes, M. F., S. P. Shrivastava, H. L. Fisher and L. L. Hall, Comparative *in vitro* percutaneous absorption of p-substituted phenols through rat skin using static and flow-through diffusion systems, *Toxicology In Vitro,* Vol. 7, No. 3, p. 221, 1993.

Moody, R. P. and B. Nadeau, An automated *in vitro* dermal absorption procedure: III. *In vivo* and *in vitro* comparison with the insect repellent N-N-diethyl-m-toluamide in mouse, rat, guinea pig, pig, human and tissue-cultured skin, *Toxicology In Vitro,* Vol. 7, No. 2, p. 167, 1993.

Moody, R. P. and P. A. Martineau, An automated *in vitro* dermal absorption procedure: I. Permeation of 14C-labeled N,N-diethyl-m-toluamide through human skin and effects of short-wave ultraviolet radiation on permeation, *In Vitro Toxicology,* Vol. 4, No. 3, p. 193, 1990.

Noser, F. K., C. Faller and M. Bracher, *In vitro* permeation with pig skin: Instrumentation and comparison of flow-through versus static-diffusion protocol, *Journal of Applied Cosmetology,* Vol. 6, No. 3, p. 111, 1988.

Wester, R. C., L. Sedik, J. Melendres, F. Logan, H. I. Maibach and I. Russell, Percutaneous absorption of diazinon in humans, *Food and Chemical Toxicology,* Vol. 31, No. 8, p. 569, 1993.

IN VITRO PHOTOMUTAGENICITY MAMMALIAN CYTOGENETIC TEST

1. METHOD

1.1 Introduction, 1.2 Definition, and 1.3 Reference Substances (to be defined)

1.4 Principle of the Test Method

The *in vitro* photomutagenicity cytogenic test is a short-term test for the detection of structural chromosomal aberrations induced by photoactive chemicals in cultured mammalian cells. Cultures of established cell line as well as primary cell cultures may be used. After exposure to test chemicals in the presence of UV light, cell cultures are treated with spindle inhibitors, such as colchicine, to accumulate cells in a metaphase-like stage of mitosis (c-metaphase). Cells are harvested at appropriate times and chromosome preparations are made.

Preparations are stained and metaphase cells are analyzed for chromosomal abnormalities.

1.5 Quality Criteria (to be defined)

1.6 Description of the Test Method
1.6.1 Preparations

Test chemicals are prepared in culture, in the dark, in triplicate, with solvent, and incubated at 37°C for at least 15 min prior to UV light exposure. Groups of flasks are exposed to a sunlamp (e.g., Osram Ultra-Vitalux) and the spectral radiation flux is calibrated before each experiment using a UV meter, both as unfiltered light and as light filtered through a sheet of 3 mm thick glass, which screened out almost all the UVB component. Both UVA and UVB measurements are recorded and doses calculated in mJ/cm2, using duration of exposure and dose rate.

1.6.2 Test Conditions
Number of Cultures

At least triplicate cultures are used for each experimental point.

Use of Negative and Positive Controls

A.C. solvent and untreated controls are used as negative controls. In each experiment a positive control is included.

Dose Level

At least three doses of test compounds and two doses of UVA/UVB irradiation are employed.

Culture Conditions

Appropriate culture medium, incubation conditions (e.g., temperature, culture vessels used, CO_2 concentration, and humidity) are used.

1.6.3 Procedure
Preparation of Cultures

Established Cell Line: Cells are generated from stock cultures (e.g., by trypsinization or by shaking off), seeded in culture vessels at appropriate density, and incubated at 37°C.

Treatment of the Cultures with the Test Substance

Cultures are treated in the dark, in triplicate with solvent and chemical in 25 cm² or, less frequently, 75 cm² flasks, and incubated at 37°C for at least 15 min prior to UV light exposure.

Following irradiation, and about 24 h after the addition of chemical, monolayers are rinsed with phosphate-buffered saline (PBS) and fresh medium added. Cultures are incubated for a further 18 h, the last two in the presence of 1 μg/ml colchicine.

Chromosome Preparations

Cells for chromosome aberration analysis (two or three flasks) are harvested by mitotic shakeoff. Those for mitotic index (MI) scoring (one or three flasks) are removed using 150 mM EDTA. Cells are swelled for 4 to 5 min, in 75 mM KCl and fixed with several changes of ice-cold methanol/glacial acetic acid (3:1 v/v).

Drop preparations are stained with 4% Gurrs Giemsa R66 at pH 6.8.

Analysis

At least 100 well-spread metaphase cultures are analyzed for chromosomal aberrations. Slides are coded before analysis.

In established cell lines, only metaphases containing ±2 centromeres of the modal number are analyzed.

2. DATA

Data are presented in a tabular form. Chromatid-type aberrations (gaps, breaks, interchanges), chromosome-type aberrations (gaps, breaks, minutes, rings, dicentris, polycentris) and the number of aberrant metaphases (including and excluding gaps) are listed separately for all treated and control cultures. The data are evaluated by appropriate statistical methods.

3. REPORTING
3.1 Test Report

The test report shall, if possible, include the following information:

- cells used;
- test conditions: composition of medium, CO_2 concentration, incubation temperature, incubation time, dose level, treatment time, UVA and UVB light doses, duration of treatment concentration of the spindle inhibitor used, type of liver enzyme activation mixture used, positive and negative controls;
- number of cell cultures;
- number of metaphases analyzed (data given separately for each culture);
- mitotic index;
- type and number of aberrations given separately for each treated and control culture, modal number of chromosomes in established cell line used;
- statistical evaluation;
- discussion of the results;
- interpretation of the results.

3.2 Evaluation and Interpretation
(to be defined)

4. ALTERNATIVE TO ANIMAL TEST

This method is used for the identification of photoclastogenic chemicals.

BIBLIOGRAPHY

Dean, S. W., R. H. Dunmore, S. P. Ruddock, J. C. Dean, C. N. Martin and D. J. Kirkland, Development of assays for the detection of photomutagenicity of chemicals during exposure to UV light, II. Results of testing three sunscreen ingredients, *Mutagenesis*, Vol. 7, No. 3, p. 179, 1992.

Dean, S. W., M. Lane, R. H. Dunmore, S. P. Ruddock, C. N. Martin, D. J. Kirkland and N. Loprieno, Development of assays for the detection of photomutagenicity of chemicals during exposure to UV light; I. Assay development, *Mutagenesis*, Vol. 6, No. 5, p. 335, 1991.

Loprieno, N., *In vitro* assay systems for testing photomutagenic chemicals, *Mutagenesis*, Vol. 6, No. 5, p. 331, 1991.

IN VITRO SISTER CHROMATID EXCHANGE ASSAY (SCE) (87/302/EEC DIR.)

1. METHOD

1.1 Introduction, 1.2 Definition, and 1.3 Reference Substances
None.

1.4 Principle of the Test Method
The Sister Chromatid Exchange (SCE) assay is a short-term test for detecting reciprocal exchanges of DNA between two sister chromatids of a duplicating chromosome. SCEs represent the interchange of DNA replication products at apparently homologous loci. The exchange process presumably involves DNA breakage and reunion, although little is known about its molecular basis. Detection of SCEs requires some means of differentially labeling sister chromatids and this can be achieved by incorporation of bromodeoxyuridine (BrdU) into chromosomal DNA for two cell cycles.

Mammalian cells *in vitro* are exposed to the test chemical with and without a mammalian exogenous metabolic activation system, if appropriate, and cultured for two rounds of replication in BrdU-containing medium. After treatment with a spindle inhibitor (e.g., colchicine) to accumulate cells in a metaphase-like stage of mitosis (c-metaphase), cells are harvested and chromosome preparations are made.

1.5 Quality Criteria
None.

1.6 Description of the Test Method
1.6.1 Preparations
Primary cultures, (human lymphocytes) or established cell lines (e.g., CHO) may be used in the assay. Cell lines should be checked for mycoplasma contamination.

Appropriate culture media and incubation conditions (e.g., temperature, culture vessels, CO_2 concentration, and humidity) should be used.

Test substances may be prepared in culture media or dissolved or suspended in appropriate vehicles prior to treatment of the cells. The final concentration of a vehicle in the culture system should not significantly affect cell viability or growth rate and effects on SCE frequency should be monitored by a solvent control.

Cells should be exposed to the test substance both in the presence and absence of an exogenous mammalian metabolic activation system. Alternatively, where cell types with intrinsic metabolic activity are used, the rate and nature of the activity should be appropriate to the chemical class being tested.

1.6.2 Test Conditions
Number of Cultures
At least duplicate cultures should be used for each experimental point.

Use of Negative and Positive Controls
Positive controls, using both a direct acting compound and a compound requiring metabolic activation, should be included in each experiment; a vehicle control should also be used.

The following are examples of substances that might be used as positive controls:

- direct acting compound
- ethylmethanesulfonate
- indirect acting compound
- cyclophosphamide

When appropriate, an additional positive control of the same chemical class as the chemical under test may be included.

Exposure Concentrations

At least three adequately spaced concentrations of the test substance should be used. The highest concentration should give rise to a significant toxic effect but must still allow adequate cell replication to occur. Relatively water-insoluble substances should be tested up to the limit of solubility using appropriate procedures. For freely water-soluble nontoxic substances the upper test substance concentration should be determined on a case-by-case basis.

1.6.3 Procedure
1.6.3.1 Preparation of Cultures

Established cell lines are generated from stock cultures (e.g., by trypsinization or by shaking off), seeded in culture vessels at appropriate density and incubated at 37°C. For monolayer cultures, the number of cells per culture vessel should be adjusted so that the cultures are not much more than 50% confluent at the time of harvest. Alternatively, cells may be used in suspension culture. Human lymphocyte cultures are set up from heparinized blood, using appropriate techniques, and incubated at 37°C.

1.6.3.2 Treatment of the Cultures with the Test Substance

Cells in an exponential stage of growth are exposed to the test substance for a suitable period of time; in most cases 1 to 2 h may be effective, but the treatment time may be extended up to two complete cell cycles in certain cases. Cells without sufficient intrinsic metabolic activity should be exposed to the test chemical in the presence and absence of an appropriate metabolic activation system. At the end of the exposure period, cells are washed free of test substance and cultured for two rounds of replication in the presence of BrdU. As an alternative procedure, cells may be exposed simultaneously to the test chemical and BrdU for the complete culture time of two cell cycles.

Human lymphocyte cultures are treated while they are in a semisynchronous condition. Cells are analyzed in their second posttreatment division, ensuring that the most sensitive cell cycle stages have been exposed to the chemical. All cultures to which BrdU is added should be handled in darkness or in dim light from incandescent lamps up to the harvesting of cells in order to minimize photolysis of BrdU-containing DNA.

Harvesting of Cells

Cell cultures are treated with a spindle inhibitor (e.g., colchicine) 1 to 4 h prior to harvesting. Each culture is harvested and processed separately for the preparation of chromosomes.

Chromosome Preparation and Staining

Chromosome preparations are made by standard cytogenetic techniques. Staining of slides to show SCEs can be performed by several techniques, (e.g., the fluorescence plus Giemsa method).

1.6.3.3 Analysis

The number of cells analyzed should be based on the spontaneous control frequency of SCE. Usually, at least 25 well-spread metaphases per culture are analyzed for SCEs. Slides are coded before analysis. In human lymphocytes only metaphases containing 46 centromeres are analyzed. In established cell lines only metaphases containing ±2 centromeres of the modal number are analyzed. It should be stated whether or not centromeric switch of label is scored as an SCE. The results should be confirmed in an independent experiment.

2. DATA

Data should be presented in tabular form. The number of SCEs for each metaphase and the number of SCEs per chromosome for each metaphase should be listed separately for all treated and control cultures.

The data should be evaluated using appropriate statistical methods.

3. REPORTING

3.1 Test Report

The test report shall, if possible, contain the following information:

- cells used, methods of maintenance of cell culture;
- test conditions: composition of media, CO_2 concentration, concentration of test substance, vehicle used, incubation temperature, treatment time, spindle inhibitor used, its concentration and the duration of treatment with it, type of mammalian activation system used, positive and negative controls;
- number of cell cultures per experimental point;
- details of the technique used for slide preparation;
- number of metaphases analyzed (data given separately for each culture);
- mean number of SCE per cell and per chromosome (data given separately for each culture);
- criteria for scoring SCE;
- rationale for dose selection;
- dose-response relationship, if applicable;
- statistical evaluation;
- discussion of results;
- interpretation of results.

3.2 Evaluation and Interpretation

There are several criteria for determining a positive result, one of which is a statistically significant dose-related increase in the mean number of SCEs per cell. Another criterion may be the detection of a reproducible and statistically significant positive response for at least one of the test points.

A test substance producing neither a statistically significant dose-related increase in the mean number of SCEs per cell nor a statistically significant and reproducible positive response at any one of the test points is considered not active in this system.

4. ALTERNATIVE TO ANIMAL TEST

This method may be used for the identification of DNA-damaging chemicals.

BIBLIOGRAPHY

Commission Directive 87/302/EEC, 18 November 1987, Adapting to technical progress for the ninth time Council Directive 67/548/EEC on the approximation of laws, regulations and administrative provisions relating to the classification, packaging and labelling of dangerous substances, *Official Journal of the European Communities,* No. L133, Vol. 31, p. 1, 1988.

Latt, S. A., J. W. Allen, S. E. Bloom, A. Carrano, E. Falke, D. Kram, E. Schneider, R. Schreck, R. Tice, B. Whitfield and S. Wolff, Sister chromatid exchanges, *Mutation Research,* Vol. 87, p. 17, 1981.

INHIBITION OF TUMOR CELL ATTACHMENT

1. METHOD

1.1 Introduction, 1.2 Definition, and 1.3 Reference Substances (to be defined)

1.4 Principle of the Test Method

Interactions between embryonic cells are generally thought to have a central role in the control of development. They are mediated by cell-to-cell or cell-to-extracellular matrix interactions involving carbohydrate to receptor binding. *In vitro* studies indicate that embryonic cell-to-cell interactions share several characteristics with cell attachment to lectin-coated surfaces. Both processes consist of two stages, the first being a passive ligand-receptor binding, and the second involving metabolic energy, cytoskeletal elements, and cell surface carbohydrates. These similarities suggest that the process involved in both systems may be similar and that *in vitro* cell to surface recognition system can be used for screening potential teratogens. Particularly, in this assay teratogens are identified by their ability to inhibit the attachment of tumor cells to a plastic surface coated with concanavalin A.

1.5 Quality Criteria (to be defined)

1.6 Description of the Test Method
1.6.1 Preparations
Solvent: DMSO (up to 0.3 M), ethanol.
Ascitic mouse ovarian tumor cells are used.

1.6.2 Test Conditions
Number of Cultures
Triplicate discs for each experimental point are used.

Use of Negative and Positive Controls
Triplicate bovine serum albumin-coated discs for each experimental point are used to evaluate background attachment.

Exposure Concentrations
The maximum concentration tested is limited by solubility of the drug in PBS or by its toxicity as judged by tripan blue exclusion.

Culture Conditions
In presence of chemicals requiring metabolic activation, the degree of inhibition can be affected by the duration of 37°C incubation (>30 min).

Metabolic Activation
When necessary, murine liver S9 mix is employed.

1.6.3 Procedure
1.6.3.1 Preparation of Cultures
Ascites mouse ovarian tumor cells are grown intraperitoneally in C3H/HeJ mice. The evening before use the mice are injected intraperitoneally with 0.2 mCi ($_1$Ci = 3.7×10^{10}

becquerels) of tritiated hymidine. The following morning the cells are harvested, washed three times in PBS, and resuspended at 10^8/ml in PBS. Concanavalin-A coated discs are made by floating 1.25 cm diameter polyethylene discs on a 0.1 mg/ml concanavalin A (Sigma), 2.5% glutaraldehyde, PBS solution, waiting 30 min and inverting the discs. Incubation is continued at room temperature with gentle oscillation overnight; the discs are washed in PBS and stored in 0.3 M glycine.

Bovine serum albumin-coated discs are made similarly.

1.6.3.2 Treatment of the Cultures with the Test Substance

Cells are incubated in PBS at 10^7 cells per ml (total volume, 1 ml) for 30 min at 37°C with various concentrations of the chemicals and, if necessary, with a microsomal activation system. Because attachment is sensitive to changes in pH, care is taken to titrate chemical solutions to pH 7.4 before use. The treated cell suspension is poured into a 35-mm bacterial plastic Petri dish (Falcon 1008), and three concavalin A-coated polyethylene discs introduced into the suspension. The cells are allowed to sediment onto the discs for 20 min; the discs are removed with fine forceps, washed in PBS, and the attached radioactivity counted in a scintillation counter.

Protocol Variations

To distinguish between drugs' effects on membrane function and the destruction of membrane structure, cells are incubated briefly with 0.4% trypan blue in PBS, and the fraction of cells excluding the dye is determined microscopically. Because dead cells do not attach to lectin-coated surfaces, only treatments that inhibit attachment but do not increase trypan permeability of the cells are considered to be inhibitory. Reduced attachment accompanied by trypan permeability is not considered to be true inhibition. In the case of chemicals found to be toxic, the use of FCS (5%) is found to protect cells from toxicity at chemical concentrations that inhibit attachment.

Chemicals that are not inhibitory or toxic at their solubility limit are reassayed at longer incubation intervals.

1.6.3.3 Analysis

Radioactivity attached to several concanavalin A-coated discs is averaged, background radioactivity (never exceeds 5% of maximal attachment) from bovine serum albumin-coated discs is subtracted, and the corrected value for attached cpm is plotted as a function of chemical concentration. The dose that decreases attachment by 50%, the ID_{50}, is a useful measure of the inhibitory potency of a drug.

2. DATA

3. REPORTING
3.1 Test Report
Animal strains must be mentioned.

3.2 Evaluation and Interpretation
(to be defined)

4. ALTERNATIVE TO ANIMAL TEST
This method may be used in the screening for potential teratogenic chemicals.

BIBLIOGRAPHY

Braun, A. G. and J. P. Dailey, Thalidomide metabolite inhibits tumor cell attachment to concanavalin A coated surfaces, *Biochemical Biophysical Research Communications*, Vol. 98, p. 1029, 1981.

Braun, A. G., C. A. Buckner, D. J. Emerson and B. B. Nichinson, Quantitative correspondence between the *in vivo* and *in vitro* activity of teratogenic agents, *Proceedings of the National Academy of Science*, Vol. 79, p. 2056, 1982.

Braun, A. G., D. J. Emerson and B. B. Nichinson, Teratogenic drugs inhibit tumour cell attachment to lectin-coated surfaces, *Nature*, Vol. 282, p. 507, 1979.

LDH RELEASE

1. METHOD

1.1 Introduction, 1.2 Definition, and 1.3 Reference Substances (to be defined)

1.4 Principle of the Test Method

The LDH (lactate dehydrogenase) release is a cytotoxic assay employing a biochemical marker. Test chemicals' effects, on both primary cultures and cell lines, are evaluated by the leakage to culture medium of LDH. The enzymatic activity is determined spectrophotometrically. LDH release, as earlier indicator of membrane damage, has been suggested to be applicable mainly to the study of the possible mechanisms of cytotoxicity rather than for screening purposes.

1.5 Quality Criteria (to be defined)

1.6 Description of the Test Method
1.6.1 Preparations

Primary cultures (isolated human lymphocytes; rabbit tracheal epithelium; rat hepatocytes), subcultures (human skin fibroblasts) and established cell line (HepG2; HEp-2, ATCC (CCL 23); FaO hepatoma; BALB 3T3) are used.

1.6.2 Test Conditions
Number of Cultures

From three to eight cultures for each experimental point and two to four separate experiments are used.

Use of Negative and Positive Controls
(to be defined)

Exposure Concentrations

For screening experiments chemicals are tested at half-interval dilutions starting at 2 mg/ml and 5% (v/v) for solid and liquid agents, respectively. Five concentrations in a twofold geometrical progression are used. Up to eight concentrations are used.

Culture Conditions

Appropriate culture medium, pretreatment time, dosing duration, and seeding density are used.

Metabolic Activation
(most chemicals require metabolic activation)

1.6.3 Procedure
1.6.3.1 Preparation of Cultures

1.6.3.2 Treatment of the Cultures with the Test Substance

LDH release is performed, after an appropriate culture treatment time, as follows: aliquots of supernatant are prepared and the activity of LDH determined. The activity of intracellular LDH is also performed after cell permeabilization. The released enzyme activity is expressed as a percentage of the total activity present in control cells. The activity of LDH is determined by measuring the decrease of absorbance, reflecting the oxidation of NADH at 340 nm.

1.6.3.3 Analysis

The toxic effect is expressed as the concentration of test chemical at which 50% of the LDH is released into the medium (LDHR$_{50}$), with respect to the total content (intracellular and extracellular).

2. DATA

3. REPORTING

3.1 Test Report

The test report shall, if possible, include the following information:

- test conditions: detailed description of treatment and sampling schedule, dose levels, toxicity data, negative and positive controls,
- dose/effect relationship when possible,
- statistical evaluation,
- discussion of the results,
- interpretation of the results.

3.2 Evaluation and Interpretation

(to be defined)

4. ALTERNATIVE TO ANIMAL TEST

This method may be used in the identification of cytotoxic chemicals.

BIBLIOGRAPHY

Blanquart, C., S. Romet, A. Baeza, C. Guennou and E. Marano, Primary cultures of tracheal epithelial cells for the evaluation of respiratory toxicity, *Toxicology In Vitro*, Vol. 5, No. 5/6, p. 499, 1991.

Commission of the European Communities, Collaborative study on the relationship between "*in vivo*" primary irritation and "*in vitro*" experimental models, Doc. CEC/V/E/3/Lux/157/188 Rev. 1, Brussels, 1989, p. 47.

Commission of the European Communities, Collaborative study on the evaluation of alternative methods to the eye irritation test — Part 1, Doc. XI/632/91 V/E/1/131/91, Brussels, 1991, p. 17.

Commission of the European Communities, Collaborative study on the evaluation of alternative methods to the eye irritation test — Part II, Doc. XI/632/91 V/E/1/131/91, Brussels 1991, p. 157.

Cornelis, M., C. Dupont and J. Wepierre, *In vitro* cytotoxicity tests on cultured human skin fibroblasts to predict the irritation potential of surfactants, *ATLA*, Vol. 19, p. 324, 1991.

Ekwall, B., I. Bondesson, J. V. Castell, M. J. Gomez-Lechon, S. Hellberg, J. Hogberg, R. Jover, X. Ponsoda, L. Romert, K. Stenberg and E. Walum, Cytotoxicity evaluation of the first ten MEIC chemicals: Acute lethal toxicity in man predicted by cytotoxicity in five cellular assays and by oral LD$_{50}$ tests in rodents, *ATLA*, Vol. 17, p. 83, 1989.

Fautrel, A., C. Chesné, A. Guillozo, G. De Sousa, R. Placidi, R. Rhamani, F. Braut, J. Pichon, H. Hoellinger, P. Vintezous, I. Diarte, C. Melcion, A. Cordier, G. Lorenzon, M. Benincourt, B. Vannier, R. Fournex, A. F. Peloux, N. Bichet, D. Gouy and J. P. Cano, A multicentre study of acute *in vitro* cytotoxicity in rat liver cells, *Toxicology In Vitro*, Vol. 5, No. 5/6, p. 543, 1991.

Mazziotti, I., A. L. Stammati and F. Zucco, *In vitro* cytotoxicity of 26 coded chemicals to HEp-2 cells: A validation study, *ATLA*, Vol. 17, p. 401, 1990.

Otoguro, K., K. Komiyama, S. Omura and C. A. Tyson, An *in vitro* cytotoxicity assay using rat hepatocytes and MTT and Coomassie Blue dye as indicators, *ATLA*, Vol. 19, p. 352, 1991.

Peloux, A.-F., C. Federici, N. Bichet, D. Gouy and J.-P. Cano, Hepatocytes in primary culture: An alternative to LD$_{50}$ testing? Validation of a predictive model by multivariate analysis, *ATLA*, Vol. 20, p. 8, 1992.

Schepers, G., C. Aschmann and S. Morchel, The use of primary cultured rat hepatocytes for the assessment of xenobiotic effects on biotransformation, *ATLA*, Vol. 19, p. 209, 1991.

Seibert, H., M. Gulden, M. Kolossa and G. Schepers, Evaluation of the relevance of selected *in vitro* toxicity test systems for acute systemic toxicity. *ATLA*, Vol. 20, p. 240, 1992.

Skaanild, M. T. and J. Clausen, Estimation of LC$_{50}$ values by assay of lactate dehydrogenase and DNA redistribution in human lymphocyte cultures. *ATLA*, Vol. 16, p. 293, 1989.

Zanetti, C., I. De Angelis, A. L. Stammati and F. Zucco, Evaluation of toxicity testing of 20 MEIC chemicals on HEp-2 cells using two viability endpoints, *ATLA*, Vol. 20, p. 120, 1992.

METHOD FOR *IN VITRO* CYTOTOXICITY TESTING

1. METHOD

1.1 Introduction, 1.2 Definition, and 1.3 Reference Substances (to be defined)

1.4 Principle of the Test Method

This *in vitro* assay has been performed in order to evaluate potential nephrotoxicity of chemicals, alone or in combination, by using proximal renal epithelium cell line. Cytotoxic evaluation is based on morphological (cellular detachment, cytoplasmatic vacuolation, and reduction in dome formation) and biochemical responses (LDH, ALP, GGT, AST, ALT, and ACP activities). Various doses and times of exposure are assessed.

1.5 Quality Criteria (to be defined)

1.6 Description of the Test Method
1.6.1 Preparations
Chemicals are dissolved in complete medium.
Cell lines (LLC-PK1) are used.

1.6.2 Test Conditions
Number of Cultures
Triplicate cultures are used.

Use of Negative and Positive Controls
Negative control is used.

Exposure Concentrations

Culture Conditions
The pH and osmolality of the chemical solutions are monitored to ensure they are within physiological range.

Metabolic Activation
(most chemicals require metabolic activation)

1.6.3 Procedure
1.6.3.1 Preparation of Cultures
Cell Lines: The LLC-PK1 (porcine kidney proximal tubule epithelium, passage 201) cell line, obtained from the American Type Culture Collection, is maintained in medium 199 with Hank's salt supplemented with 3% FBS and 20 mM-HEPES. Cells are seeded in 35-mm six-well culture plates (Corning) at 2×10^5 cells/culture.

1.6.3.2 Treatment of the Cultures with the Test Substance
Cell Lines: Cultures are treated approximately 24 h after seeding when they are 45 to 55% confluent. Cultures are placed in a humidified incubator at 37°C, 95% air/5% CO_2 and are replenished with freshly prepared dosing solutions on each study day. Cytotoxicity is assessed at days 3, 7, 10, and 14 using morphological and biochemical criteria. Cultures are observed for morphological alterations through an inverted phase-contrast microscope (cytoplasmic vacuolation, increased number of detached cells, and reduced dome formation). Biochemical assessment is made by removing the culture media and assaying for cell leakage of the following enzymes: lactate dehydrogenase (LDH), alkaline phosphatase (ALP), g-glutamyl transpeptidase (GGT), aspartate transaminase (AST), alanine transaminase (ALT), and acid phosphatase (ACP).

1.6.3.3 Analysis
The result of the biochemical analysis are subjected to statistical evaluation.

2. DATA

3. REPORTING
3.1 Test Report
Cell culture and treatment time conditions must be reported.

3.2 Evaluation and Interpretation
(to be defined)

4. ALTERNATIVE TO ANIMAL TEST
This method may be used in the screening for potential toxic chemicals.

BIBLIOGRAPHY
Bacon, J. A., R. J. Weaver and T. J. Raczniak, *In vitro* assessment of trospectomycin and gentamicin sulphate in the LLC-PK1 cell line, *Toxicology In Vitro*, Vol. 5, No. 5/6, p. 473, 1991.

METHOD FOR *IN VITRO* NEUROTOXICITY TEST

1. METHOD

1.1 Introduction, 1.2 Definition, and 1.3 Reference Substances (to be defined)

1.4 Principle of the Test Method
This *in vitro* assay, performed on neuroblastoma cell lines, is able to investigate the effects of sublethal doses of known neurotoxins on protein homeostasis. The intra/extracellular levels of cytoplasmatic proteins (LDH, lactate dehydrogenase, and NSE, neurone-specific enolase), measured by an automated bicinchoninic acid protein assay, are the parameters used. The evidences of deranged protein metabolism/cell death (altered intra/extracellular levels) may provide sensitive markers of neurotoxicity.

1.5 Quality Criteria (to be defined)

1.6 Description of the Test Method
1.6.1 Preparations
   Neuroblastoma cell lines (IMR 32) are used.

1.6.2 Test Conditions
Number of Cultures

Use of Negative and Positive Controls
   Negative control (medium) is used.

Exposure Concentrations
   (to be defined)

Culture Conditions
   (to be defined)
   Neuroblastoma cell lines must be differentiated by using bromodeoxyuridine.

Metabolic Activation
   (most chemicals require metabolic activation)

1.6.3 Procedure
1.6.3.1 Preparation of Cultures
Cell Lines: Human neuroblastoma IMR 32 cell line (Flow) is grown in modified Eagle's medium (MEM, Gibco) and differentiated with bromodeoxyuridine to induce the expression of neurone-specific enolase (NSE), a threefold increase.

1.6.3.2 Treatment of the Cultures with the Test Substance
Cell Lines: Differentiated IMR32 cells are exposed to test chemicals in 10 ml of complete medium; 1-ml samples of conditioned medium are removed at various times for analysis of NSE and LDH levels; the samples are replaced by 1 ml of the appropriate medium. At the end of the experiment (48 h) the cells are washed three times with PBS before freezing. Cells are resuspended in PBS (1 ml) and sonicated three times using a Dawes Ultrasonic Generator Type 7532B on half power for 15 sec. Protein concentration are measured using an automated bicinchoninic acid protein assay. NSE is measured using the coated bead "Prolifigen" NSE immunoradiometric assay (IRMA, Sangtec Medical): this is a two-site, monoclonal antibody radiometric assay; the antibodies recognizes different epitopes on the g-subunit of NSE. NSE activity in the sonicated cells is measured by the method outlined in the kit with the following change: the beads, coated with one antibody, are preincubated with 25 µl of standard diluted with 225 µl of fresh medium, or 250 µl of conditioned medium samples. The beads are then washed before incubating with the second antibody labeled with radiolabeled iodine (^{125}I). LDH activity is measured by automated fluorimetric and spectrophotometric methods (Sigma LDH Isoenzymes kit, No. 705-C).

1.6.3.3 Analysis
   Intra- and extracellular cytoplasmic protein levels are compared to distinguish between altered protein metabolism and cell death; a correlation analysis is performed.

2. DATA

3. REPORTING
3.1 Test Report
Cell culture and treatment time conditions must be reported.

3.2 Evaluation and Interpretation
(to be defined)

4. ALTERNATIVE TO ANIMAL TEST
This method may be used in the screening for potential neurotoxic chemicals.

BIBLIOGRAPHY

Thomas, S. M., C. L. Hartley and H. J. Mason, Effects of neurotoxins on neurone-specific enolase and lactate dehydrogenase activity and leakage in neuroblastoma cells, *Toxicology In Vitro,* Vol. 5, No. 5/6, p. 439, 1991.

METHODS OF ASSESSMENT OF THYROTOXICITY

1. METHOD

1.1 Introduction, 1.2 Definition, and 1.3 Reference Substances (to be defined)

1.4 Principle of the Test Method
This methodology has been performed in order to evaluate, by using primary culture of thyroid cells, the specific action of compounds on the different parts of thyroid biochemical pathways.
The parameters measured are:

- iodine uptake, by liquid scintillation counting;
- iodine organification, by liquid scintillation counting;
- release of the thyroid hormones T_3 (triiodothyronine) and T_4 (thyroxine), by radioimmunoassay;
- thyrocite viability, by MTT assay.

The use of an *in vitro* system may be useful to investigate direct effects of compounds on thyroid cells without the complication of metabolic influence that could be present in studies *in vivo*, namely the hypothalamic and pituitary influences and the hepatic clearance effects.

1.5 Quality Criteria (to be defined)

1.6 Description of the Test Method
1.6.1 Preparations
Test chemicals are dissolved in medium or in Earle's balanced salt solution (EBSS).
Primary cultures (canine thyrocytes) are used.

1.6.2 Test Conditions
Number of Cultures
From three to six cultures are used for each experimental point.

Use of Negative and Positive Controls
Control cultures are treated with DMSO or EBSS.

Exposure Concentrations
   (to be defined)

Culture Conditions
   (to be defined)

1.6.3 Procedure
1.6.3.1 Preparation of Cultures
   Primary Culture: For each experiment two whole thyroids, obtained from dogs post mortem, are used: tissue is minced and the cells disaggregated in 5 ml 0.25% (w/v) trypsin, 1.0% (w/v) collagenase, and 2% (w/v) bovine serum albumin for 60 min at 37°C with constant stirring. The suspension of cells and follicles is filtered through nylon mesh (150 µm) and pelleted by centrifugation at 1000 g for 10 min. The pellet of thyrocytes is then resuspended in Ham's F12 culture medium containing 5% (v/v) fetal calf serum, 100 IU penicillin/ml, 100 µg streptomycin/ml, 5 µg transferrin/ml, 100 ng somatostatin/ml, 200 ng glycyl-L-histidyl-L-lysine/ml, 10 mU TSH (thyroid stimulating hormone)/ml, 10 µg insulin/ml, 10^{-8} M-hydrocortisone, and 1.5 µg NaI/ml. Cells are established into culture at approximately 10^5 cells/well in standard 24-well tissue culture plates, precoated with 200 µl/well of 10 ng poly-L-lysine/ml. Cultures are maintained under standard conditions of 37°C and a humidified atmosphere of 95% air/5% CO_2.

1.6.3.2 Treatment of the Cultures with the Test Substance
Primary Culture
   Iodine uptake and organification: After an overnight incubation test chemicals, diluted in EBSS containing 2 µCi Na[125$_1$] radiolabel/ml and 150 µg Na[127$_1$] carrier/ml, are added to the culture plates. At the end of 4 h exposure period at 37°C, the medium is aspirated and the monolayer washed twice with 1 ml EBSS/well. Cells are then lysed with 1 M-NH4OH, 0.2% Triton X-100 (1 ml/well) for 10 min. Subsequently, 100-µl samples are taken and assessed for total iodine content by liquid scintillation counting (LSC). Further 500-µl samples are taken from each well and iodine-labeled protein content determined by trichloroacetic acid (10%, w/v) precipitation, collection of precipitate on 0.2-µm Millipore filters, and LSC of radioactivity content.

   Assessment of T_3T_4 release: After an overnight incubation, test chemicals are added to the culture plates. At the end of the 72-h exposure time, 100-µl (for T_3 assessment) and 25-µl (for T_4 assessment) samples are removed from the supernatant media. T_3 and T_4 contents are determined by radioimmunoassay (Coat-a-count total T_3 and T_4, Diagnostic Products Corporation).

   Thyrocyte viability: For both 4-h and 72-h experiments, duplicate cultures of compound-treated thyrocytes are maintained. At the end of the treatment time cells are tested for viability by MTT assay: 10% (v/v) of 5 mg MTT reagent/ml, in PBS, is added to each culture well. After incubation at 37°C for 60 min, acidified isopropanol (0.4 ml 1M-HCl in 10 ml isopropanol) is added. A quantitative assessment of viable thyrocytes is made by determination of optical density at 550 nm.

1.6.3.3 Analysis
   Percentage effect is taken as the difference between treated and control cultures, expressed as a percentage of control. For each test chemical, the values (mean ± SEM) are from replicates in one experiment on tissue from one animal.

2. DATA

3. REPORTING
3.1 Test Report
   Cell culture and treatment time conditions must be reported.

3.2 Evaluation and Interpretation
(to be defined)

4. ALTERNATIVE TO ANIMAL TEST
This method may be used in the screening for potential tyrotoxic chemicals.

BIBLIOGRAPHY

Duffy, P. A. and S. A. Yarnell, Use of primary canine thyroid monolayer cultures to investigate compounds that are thyrotoxic *in vivo, Toxicology In Vitro,* Vol. 5, No. 5/6, p. 373, 1991.

MICROMASS TERATOGEN TEST

1. METHOD

1.1 Introduction, 1.2 Definition, and 1.3 Reference Substances (to be defined)

1.4 Principle of the Test Method
The micromass assay is an *in vitro* test that gives an indication of potential teratogenic hazard of compounds. The technique is a method of culturing mammalian or avian embryo midbrain (CNS) or limb-bud (LB) cells so that many phases of cell differentiation related to normal embryogenesis are maintained *in vitro*. The assay measures the inhibition by test compounds of two phases of embryonic development: neurogenesis and chondrogenesis. Cytotoxicity also is measured to permit the comparison between cell differentiation and survival in order to determine whether an inhibitory effect is a result of specific inhibition of the process of cell differentiation or due to cytotoxicity. Cell differentiation, expressed as formation of small foci of neurons/chondrocytes, is revealed by staining with specific dyes; cytotoxicity, expressed as effect on cell proliferation, is revealed by staining with neutral red.

1.5 Quality Criteria (to be defined)

1.6 Description of the Test Method
1.6.1 Preparations
Test chemicals are diluted in DMSO or medium. When DMSO is used, the final concentration must be always <0.5% (v/v).
Rat and chick embryo limb-bud cells are used.

1.6.2 Test Conditions
Number of Cultures
Duplicate cultures are used.

Use of Negative and Positive Controls
A negative control (medium) is used.
Diphenylhydantoin can be used as positive control.

Exposure Concentrations
At least five concentrations of each chemicals are tested.

Culture Conditions
(to be defined)

Metabolic Activation

Metabolism can be modeled by the inclusion of rat liver homogenate plus cofactors (S9 mix).

1.6.3 Procedure

1.6.3.1 Preparation of Cultures

Limb-Bud Cells: Rats are killed on the morning of pregnancy day 13 (plug day = 1) and chicks are taken at 4 d of incubation. Rat embryos are at the 35- to 40-somite stage and forelimbs only are used. Chick embryos are at stage 23 and both fore- and hindlimbs are used. Limb buds are removed from embryos in Hanks' balanced salt solution, using watchmaker's forceps. About 100 to 200 limb buds are dissociated with 0.1% trypsin, followed by filtration through "Nytex" nylon mesh to form a single cell suspension. The cell density is adjusted to $1-2 \times 10^7$ cells/ml in Ham's F-12 medium (Imperial Laboratories) supplemented with 10% FCS or 5% FBS (Gibco). A 10-μl drop is placed in the center of each well of 24-well tissue culture plates (Flow) or to 35 mm Primaria dishes (for inhibition of cell differentiation assay) and to collagen coated 96-well plates (for cell survival assay). The culture plates are placed in a humidified CO_2 incubator at 37°C for 2 h, to allow for cell attachment.

Midbrain Cells: Rat embryo midbrain is dissected free and following enzymatic dissociation single cell suspensions are prepared in Ham's F12 culture medium plus 10% FCS to give 2.5 $\times 10^6$ CNS cells/ml. 10-μl drops are delivered to 35-mm Primaria dishes (for inhibition of cell differentiation assay) and to collagen-coated 96-well plates (for cell survival assay).

1.6.3.2 Treatment of the Cultures with the Test Substance

Limb-Bud Cells: The wells are then flooded with 1 ml of medium plus serum with test substance and eventually rat S9 mix. The cultures are incubated for 5 d, without change of the medium. Cultures then are washed and stained with either alcian blue (AB) or neutral red (NR). Bound dye is extracted and quantified spectrophotometrically to estimate the effect of the test compounds on the accumulation of cartilage proteoglycans and on cellular proliferation, respectively.

Midbrain Cells: After cell adherence, dishes and plates are supplemented with medium containing test chemicals and eventually rat S9 mix. The cells are cultured for 5 d at 37°C and 5% CO_2 in air. After fixation and staining, the number of foci of differentiated cells is determined with an automated colony counter. Cell survival is measured by neutral red uptake and elution of fixed cells.

1.6.3.3 Analysis

Data are expressed as a percentage of concomitant control, then pooled for the number of the separate experiments (n = 3). IC50 values and their standard errors are calculated from linear regression of the transformed data ($\log_{10}$ concentration vs. arcsin percentage).

Three criteria are used for the identification of teratogens *in vitro* using IC_{50} values:

1. the "<500 μg/ml rule" for either CNS or LB cultures (IC_{50} being the concentration that reduces the number of nodules formed by 50%);
2. the "<50 μg/ml rule" for either CNS or LB cultures (IC_{50} being the concentration that reduces the number of nodules formed by 50%);
3. the "twofold rule," which defines a positive response as: IC_{50} cytotoxicity/IC_{50} differentiation >2 (i.e., specific inhibition of cell differentiation).

2. DATA

3. REPORTING
3.1 Test Report
Animal species must be indicated; cell culture and treatment time conditions must be reported.

3.2 Evaluation and Interpretation
(to be defined)

4. ALTERNATIVE TO ANIMAL TEST
This method may be used in the screening for potential teratogenic chemicals.

BIBLIOGRAPHY

Brown, N. A. and R. Wiger, Comparison of rat and chick limb bud micromass cultures for developmental toxicity screening, *Toxicology In Vitro*, Vol. 6, No. 2, p. 101, 1991.

Parsons, J. F., J. Rockley and M. Richold, *In vitro* micromass teratogen test; interpretation of results from a blind trial of 25 compounds using three separate criteria, *Toxicology In Vitro*, Vol. 4, No. 4/5, p. 609, 1990.

MICRONUCLEUS TEST

1. METHOD

1.1 Introduction, 1.2 Definition, and 1.3 Reference Substances (to be defined)

1.4 Principle of the Test Method
The micronucleus test is a short-term test for the detection of chromosomal damage or damage of the mitotic apparatus of the cultured mammalian cells induced by chemicals. Cultures of established cell lines and also primary cell cultures may be used. After exposure to test chemicals with and without a liver enzyme activation mixture (a cofactor supplemented with postmitochondrial fraction), cell cultures are treated with cytochalasin B. Cells are harvested at appropriate times and analyzed for the presence of micronuclei.

1.5 Quality Criteria (to be defined)

1.6 Description of the Test Method
1.6.1 Preparations
Test chemicals are prepared in culture-medium or dissolved in appropriate vehicles (distilled water; DMSO, not more than 1%) prior to treatment of the cells.

Established cell lines or cultures of primary/secondary cells (human keratinocytes; human lymphocytes) are used.

1.6.2 Test Conditions
Number of Cultures
At least duplicate cultures are used for each experimental point.

Use of Negative and Positive Controls
Solvent (when the solvent is not the culture medium or water), liver enzyme activation mixture, liver enzyme activation mixture and solvent, and untreated controls are used as negative controls.

In each experiment, a positive control is included; when liver enzyme activation mixture is used to activate the test chemical, a compound known to require metabolic activation must be used as a positive control.

Exposure Concentrations

At least three doses of the test compound over at least a one-log dose range are employed, the highest dose producing some indication of cytotoxicity, expressed by a change in the ratio of binucleate cells to total cells (human lymphocytes).

Culture Conditions

Appropriate culture medium, incubation condition (e.g., temperature, culture vessels used, CO_2 concentration, and humidity) are used.

Metabolic Activation

Cells should be exposed to test substance both in the presence and absence of an appropriate mammalian liver enzyme activation mixture (a cofactor-supplemented postmitocondrial fraction) prepared from mice or rats.

1.6.3 Procedure

1.6.3.1 Preparation of Cultures

Primary Cultures: Heparinized whole human blood (0.3 ml) is added to 4.7 ml Ham's F10 culture medium supplemented with 10% fetal bovine serum, 100 IU penicillin/ml and 100 µg streptomycin/ml (all from Flow Laboratories, Irvine, Ayrshire, UK), and containing 1.5% phytohemagglutinin (PHA; Wellcome Diagnostics, Beckenham, Kent, UK). Cytochalasin B (3 µg/ml; Sigma Chemical Co., St. Louis, MO, USA) is added after 44 h of culture.

Secondary Cultures: Human epidermal cells are isolated and cultured. Murine 3T3 fibroblasts, treated with mitomycin C (Janssen Chimica, Tilburg, ND, 4 µg/ml for 2 h) to inhibit proliferation, are used as feeder layer cells.

Second passage human keratinocytes (1×10^5) are plated together with the 3T3 cells (2×10^5) in a 35 cm² culture dish. When metabolic activation is used, 4 d after plating the cells, the medium is changed with medium containing Aroclor 1254 (Monsanto, St. Louis, MO, USA, 10^{-5} M) to induce the biotransformation activity.

1.6.3.2 Treatment of the Cultures with the Test Substance

Primary Cultures: Chemicals are added to the test tubes after 24 h of culture. At the end of treatment time (either 48 h or 72 h) cells are harvested using the following steps: two passages in buffer (0.9 mM-NH_4CO_3 and 0.0132 mM-NH_4Cl) to lyse the red cells (each for 20 min at room temperature, followed by a centrifugation at 1200 g for 15 min); two passages in fresh fixative (methanol-acetic acid; 3:1, v/v) for 20 min at room temperature; preparation of slides by dropping the cell suspension. Slides then are stained with 4% Giemsa (E. Merck AG, Darmstadt, Germany) in distilled water and mounted in Eukitt.

Secondary Cultures: Chemical is added at the eighth day of culturing: after 24 h the mediun is removed and the cultures are rinsed with Hank's balanced salt solution (HBSS) and culture medium containing cytochalasin B (Janssen Chimica, Tilburg, ND, 5 µg/ml) is added. After either 48 h or 72 h the cells are harvested, fixed on slide, stained with May-Grunwald/Giemsa stain, and coverslipped.

1.6.3.3 Analysis

At least 500 binucleate cells are scored per slide: each data point is scored in duplicate (human keratinocytes).

For human lymphocytes, 2000 binucleate cells are scored, when possible, for each dose level; the ratio of binucleate cells to total cells is calculated by counting 2000 lymphocytes.

2. DATA
Data are presented in a tabular form.
Data are analyzed using Fisher's exact test.

3. REPORTING
3.1 Test Report
The test report shall, if possible, include the following information:

- test conditions: detailed description of treatment and sampling schedule, dose levels, toxicity data, negative and positive controls;
- criteria for scoring micronuclei;
- dose/effect relationship when possible;
- statistical evaluation;
- discussion of the results;
- interpretation of the results.

3.2 Evaluation and Interpretation
(to be defined)

4. ALTERNATIVE TO ANIMAL TEST
This test method may is used to identify clastogenic, aneuploidogenic, and mutagenic chemicals.

BIBLIOGRAPHY

Migliore, L. and M. Nieri, Evaluation of twelve potential aneuploidogenic chemicals by the *in vitro* human lymphocyte micronucleus assay, *Toxicology In Vitro*, Vol. 5, No. 4, p. 325, 1991.

Van Pelt, R. M. H. and P. J. J. M. Weterings, Micronucleus formation in cultured human keratinocytes: Involvement of intercellular bioactivation, *Toxicology In Vitro*, Vol. 5, No. 5/6, p. 515, 1991.

MICROTUBULE DISASSEMBLY

1. METHOD

1.1 Introduction, 1.2 Definition, and 1.3 Reference Substances (to be defined)

1.4 Principle of the Test Method
This *in vitro* assay has been performed in an attempt to identify chemicals that induce allergic contact dermatitis (ACD) *in vivo*. It is based on the evidence that chemicals (haptens) can conjugate with cellular proteins (carriers) to form hapten-protein complexes. Because cytoskeletal proteins may be good candidates for hapten/carrier conjugation, chemical-induced microtubule disassembly, qualitatively evaluated after indirect immunofluorescence, may be indicative of potential sensitizers.

1.5 Quality Criteria (to be defined)

1.6 Description of the Test Method
1.6.1 Preparations
Cell lines (3T3 murine fibroblast cell line; human skin fibroblasts cell line) are used.

1.6.2 Test Conditions
Number of Cultures

Use of Negative and Positive Controls
   A negative control is used.

Exposure Concentrations
   Cells are exposed to µM doses of halogenated nitrobenzene derivates.

Culture Conditions
   (to be defined)

Metabolic Activation
   (most chemicals require metabolic activation)

1.6.3 Procedure
1.6.3.1 Preparation of Cultures
   Cell Lines: Swiss 3T3 murine fibroblasts are maintained in Dulbecco's modified Eagle's medium (DMEM) containing 10% FBS (Sigma) and an antibiotic mixture of penicillin (250 U/ml) and streptomycin sulfate (250 µg/ml) in a humidified atmosphere of 7% CO_2. Quiescent cultures are obtained by plating $1.4–2.1 \times 10^3$ cells/cm² in DMEM containing 10% FBS and incubating for 24 h: glass coverslips (No. 1 thickness, 12×12 mm, Bradford Scientific) placed in culture dishes are utilized. Before use, coverslips are rinsed 10 times with deionized water purified through the Milli-Q Reagent Grade Water Systems (Millipore Corp.) and three times with 95% ethanol, and then stored in 95% ethanol. The coverslips are washed by dipping them into DMEM to remove residual ethanol and then placed in tissue culture dishes shortly before plating cells. The culture medium is replaced with DMEM containing 0.3% FBS for 48 h followed by fresh DMEM containing 0.3% FBS. Cells are used in experiments 48 to 72 h later.
   Normal diploid human foreskin fibroblasts (strain AG1522, obtained from the Coriel Institute for Medical Research, USA) are grown in Eagle's minimal essential medium supplemented with 10% FBS, D-glucose (0.9 g/l), sodium pyruvate (0.66 mg/l), penicillin (110 U/ml) and streptomycin sulfate (110 µg/ml). Cultures are incubated at 37°C in a humidified atmosphere of 95% air: 5% CO_2: glass coverslips (No. 1 thickness, 12×12 mm, Bradford Scientific) placed in culture dishes are utilized. Before use, coverslips are rinsed 10 times with deionized water purified through the Milli-Q Reagent Grade Water Systems (Millipore Corp.) and three times with 95% ethanol, and then stored in 95% ethanol. The coverslips are washed by dipping them into DMEM to remove residual ethanol and then placed in tissue culture dishes shortly before plating cells.

1.6.3.2 Treatment of the Cultures with the Test Substance
   Cell Lines: 3T3 cells and human foreskin fibroblasts are then incubated in medium-containing test chemicals for 3 h in the respective culture conditions.
   Immunofluorescent labeling procedure: after removal of the medium, cells on glass coverslips are rinsed once with PBS and incubated in an MT (microtubule) stabilizing buffer PM2G, pH 6.9 (100 mM-PIPES, 2 mM-EGTA, 1 mM-$MgSO_4$, 2 M-glycerol) for 1 min. The cells are fixed for 30 min in 3.7% formaldehyde (Aldrich) freshly diluted in PM2G, and then incubated in PBS for 5 min followed by incubation with 0.1 M-glycine in PBS, pH 7.4, for 5 min to quench residual formaldehyde. The cells are extracted for 10 min with 0.3% NP40 freshly prepared in PBS and washed three times with PBS. All steps are performed at room temperature and all reagents are warmed to room temperature before use. The extracted cells are stored at 4°C in PBS if they are not stained immediately for MT.

For MT visualization by indirect immunofluorescence, a polyclonal rabbit antitubulin antibody (Poly-sciences, Inc.) is used as the primary antibody and rhodamine conjugated sheep anti-rabbit IgG (Orga-non Teknika-Cappel) as the secondary antibody. The coverslips are drained, placed on a filter paper, overlaid with 20 μl of anti-tubulin antibody, and incubated at 37°C for 30 min in a moist chamber. The excess antibody is drained carefully using a paper towel and the coverslips are washed thoroughly by dipping five times in each of five beakers containing PBS. The coverslips are drained and overlaid with 20 μl of the secondary antibody, incubated in a moist chamber and washed with PBS as described above. The coverslips are washed once in deionized water before they are mounted on the slides using gelvatol (Monsanto). The slides are examined with a Nikon Optiphot microscope equipped with an epi-fluorescence attachment using the G-1A filter and Plan Apochromat 40 × oil objective. Photographs are taken using a UFX automatic exposure system (Nikon) with Kodak Tri-X pan film (ASA 400). The film is exposed at ASA 800 and push developed to an effective ASA 1600.

1.6.3.3 Analysis

MT disassembly is evaluated by qualitative analysis. The minimal dose of each chemical required to cause complete MT disassembly is determined.

2. DATA

3. REPORTING
3.1 Test Report
The test report shall, if possible, include the following information:

* test conditions: detailed description of treatment and sampling schedule, dose levels, toxicity data, negative and positive controls;
* dose/effect relationship when possible;
* statistical evaluation;
* discussion of the results;
* interpretation of the results.

3.2 Evaluation and Interpretation
(to be defined)

4. ALTERNATIVE TO ANIMAL TEST
This method may be used in the screening for potential skin sensitization chemicals.

BIBLIOGRAPHY

Leung, M. F., K. Geoghegan-Barek, G. B. Zamansky and I. N. Chou, Microtubule disassembly induced by sensitizing halogenated nitrobenzene derivatives, *Toxicology In Vitro*, Vol. 4, No. 4/5, p. 252, 1990,

MITOTIC RECOMBINATION TEST — *SACCHAROMYCES CEREVISIAE* (87/302/EEC DIR.)

1. METHOD

1.1 Introduction, 1.2 Definition, and 1.3 Reference Substances
None.

1.4 Principle of the Test Method

Mitotic recombination in *Saccharomyces cerevisiae* can be detected between genes (or more generally between a gene and its centromere) and within genes. The former event is called mitotic crossing-over and generates reciprocal products, whereas the latter event is most frequently nonreciprocal and is called gene conversion. Crossing-over generally is assayed by the production of recessive homozygous colonies or sectors produced in a heterozygous strain, whereas gene conversion is assayed by the production of prototrophic revertants produced in an auxotrophic heteroallelic strain carrying two different defective alleles of the same gene. The most commonly used strains for the detection of mitotic gene conversion are D4 (heteroallelic at ade 2 and trp 5) D7 (heteroallelic at trp 5) BZ34 (heteroallelic at arg 4) and JD1 (heteroallelic at his 4 and trp 5). Mitotic crossing-over producing red and pink homozygous sectors can be assayed in D5 or in D7 (which also measures mitotic gene conversion and reverse mutation at ilv 1–92) both strains being heteroallelic for complementing alleles of ade 2.

1.5 Quality Criteria

None.

1.6 Description of the Test Method

1.6.1 Preparations

Solutions of test chemicals and control or reference compounds should be prepared just prior to testing, using an appropriate vehicle. With organic compounds that are water insoluble not more than a 2% solution v/v of organic solvents such as ethanol, acetone or dimethylsulfoxide (DMSO) should be used. The final concentration of the vehicle should not significantly affect cell viability and growth characteristics.

Metabolic Activation

Cells should be exposed to test chemicals both in the presence and absence of an appropriate exogenous metabolic activation system. The system most commonly used is a cofactor-supplemented postmitochondrial fraction from the livers of rodents pre-treated with enzyme inducing agents. The use of other species, tissues, postmitochondrial fractions, or procedures also may be appropriate for metabolic activation.

1.6.2 Test Conditions

Tester Strains

The most frequently used strains are the diploids D4, D5, D7, and JD1. The use of other strains may be appropriate.

Media

Appropriate culture media are used for the determination of survival and the frequency of mitotic recombination.

Use of Negative and Positive Controls

Positive, untreated and solvent controls should be performed concurrently. Appropriate positive control chemicals should be used for each specific recombination endpoint.

Exposure Concentrations

At least five adequately spaced concentrations of the test substance should be used. Among the factors to be taken into consideration are cytotoxicity and solubility. The lowest concentration must have no effect on cell viability. For toxic chemicals, the highest concentration tested should not reduce survival below 5 to 10%. Relatively water-insoluble chemicals should be tested up to the limit of solubility using appropriate procedures. For freely water-soluble nontoxic substances, the upper concentration should be determined on a case-by-case basis.

Cells may be exposed to test chemicals in either the stationary phase or during growth for periods of up to 18 h. However, for long treatment times cultures should be microscopically inspected for spore formation, the presence of which invalidates the test.

Incubation Conditions

The plates are incubated in the dark for 4 to 7 d at 28 to 30°C. Plates used for the assay of red and pink homozygous sectors produced by mitotic crossing-over should be kept in a refrigerator (about 4°C) for a further 1 to 2 d before scoring to allow for the development of the appropriate pigmented colonies.

Spontaneous Mitotic Recombination Frequencies

Subcultures should be used with spontaneous mitotic recombination mutation frequencies within the accepted normal range.

Number of Replicates

A minimum of three replicate plates should be used per concentration for the assay of prototrophs produced by mitotic gene conversion and for viability. In the case of the assay of recessive homozygosis produced by mitotic crossing-over, the plate number should be increased to provide an adequate number of colonies.

1.6.3 Procedure

Treatment of *S. cerevisiae* strains is usually performed in a liquid test procedure involving either stationary or growing cells. Initial experiments should be done on growing cells. 1–5 × 10^7 cells/ml are exposed to the test chemical for up to 18 h at 28 to 37°C with shaking; an adequate amount of metabolic activation system is added during treatment when appropriate. At the end of the treatment, cells are centrifuged, washed, and seeded upon appropriate culture medium. After incubation, plates are scored for survival and the induction of mitotic recombination. If the first experiment is negative, then a second experiment should be carried out using stationary phase cells. If the first experiment is positive, it is confirmed in an independent experiment.

2. DATA

Data should be presented in tabular form indicating the number of colonies counted, the number of recombinants, survival, and the frequency of recombinants.

Results should be confirmed in an independent experiment.

The data should be evaluated using appropriate statistical methods.

3. REPORTING
3.1 Test Report

The test report shall, if possible, contain the following information:

- strain used;
- test conditions: stationary phase or growing cells, composition of media, incubation temperature and duration, metabolic activation system;
- treatment conditions: exposure concentration, procedure and duration of treatment, treatment temperature, positive and negative controls;

- number of colonies counted, number of recombinants; survival and recombination frequency, dose/response relationship if applicable, statistical evaluation of data;
- discussion of the results;
- interpretation of the results.

3.2 Evaluation and Interpretation

There are several criteria for determining a positive result, one of which is a statistically significant dose-related increase in the number of recombinants. Another criterion may be based upon the detection of a reproducible and statistically significant positive response for at least one of the test substance concentrations.

A test substance producing neither a statistically significant dose-related increase in the number of recombinants, nor a statistically significant and reproducible positive response at any one of the test substance concentrations is considered not to have produced DNA recombination in this test system.

Both biological and statistical significance should be considered together in this evaluation.

4. ALTERNATIVE TO ANIMAL TEST

This method is used for the identification of DNA damaging chemicals.

BIBLIOGRAPHY

Commission Directive 87/302/EEC, of 18 November 1987 Adapting to technical progress for the ninth time Council Directive 67/548/EEC on the approximation of laws, regulations and administrative provisions relating to the classification, packaging and labelling of dangerous substances, *Official Journal of the European Communities,* No. L133, Vol. 31, p.1, 1988.

Zimmermann, F. K., R. C. Von Borstel, E. S. Von Halle, J. M. Parry, D. Siebert, G. Zetterberg, R. Barale and N. Loprieno, Testing of chemicals for genetic activity with *Saccaromyces cerevisiae, Mutation Research,* Vol. 133, p. 199, 1984.

NEUTRAL RED RELEASE (NRR)

1. METHOD

1.1 Introduction, 1.2 Definition, and 1.3 Reference Substances (to be defined)

1.4 Principle of the Test Method

NRR assay is a cytotoxic assay used to measure cell damage expressed as loss of the vital dye neutral red (a weakly cationic dye) from confluent cell line culture preloaded with the dye, following exposure to relatively high concentrations of test chemicals for a short period of time. After extraction, the absorbance of the dye is spectrophotometrically determined.

1.5 Quality Criteria (to be defined)

1.6 Description of the Test Method
1.6.1 Preparations

Test chemicals are used neat or diluted in warm PBS. Insoluble substances are dissolved in vegetable oil. In the case of pipettable liquids, simple volume/volume dilutions are used. Viscous solutions are weighed and made up volumetrically. Samples not soluble in water are shaken with PBS to give a suspension.

Established cell lines (3T3-L1, ATCC (CCL 92.1), ATCC CCL 92.1) are used.

1.6.2 Test Conditions
Number of Cultures
Triplicate cultures on separate plates are used.

Use of Negative and Positive Controls
Untreated and negative control (solvent) are used.

Exposure Concentrations
Liquids are first tested at 50% and, depending on the approximate amount of neutral red released compared with the controls, then tested at higher or lower concentrations, so that almost total and minimal loss of neutral red can be detected.

Culture Conditions
(to be defined)

Metabolic Activation
(most chemicals require metabolic activation)

1.6.3 Procedure
1.6.3.1 Preparation of Cultures
Cell Lines: 3T3-L1 cells (mouse fibroblast-like cell line) are maintained in Dulbecco's modified Eagle's medium (DMEM), supplemented with 2 mM L-glutamine, 10% newborn calf serum, 100 μg/ml streptomycin sulfate, 100 IU/ml benzylpenicillin, and 2 μg/ml Fungizone. They are routinely grown on 80 cm^2 flasks, in a humidified 5% CO_2/95% air incubator, and passaged every 2 to 3 d.

For testing the culture, medium is decanted from the culture flask and the cell sheet monolayer washed with sterile PBS; 1 ml of 0.5% EDTA-trypsin solution is added and the flask gently agitated for a few minutes to loosen the cells and to provide a single-cell suspension; 30 to 50 ml of fresh medium is then added to terminate the proteolytic action of the trypsin. Cell counts are made and a suspension of $1-2 \times 10^4$ cells/ml is prepared.

Next, 150 μl of the cell suspension is added to 95 of the 96 wells of a flat-bottomed plate; 150 μl medium alone is added to the 96th well, which acts as a control blank. The plates are incubated at 37°C until confluency. This usually takes a period of 3 to 4 d. On the day of the test, the medium is aspirated and 100 μl of 50 μg/ml neutral red medium (made up from a filtered stock solution of 5 mg/ml neutral red in distilled water and preincubated overnight at 37°C) is added after spinning at 800 rpm for 5 min. The centrifugation step is important, since it removes any fine crystals of neutral red, which may interfere with the assay. The neutral red medium is left on the cells for 3 h before being replaced with fresh medium. If the cells are left in contact with the neutral red medium, they would continue to take up dye until they are eventually killed by the neutral red.

1.6.3.2 Treatment of the Cultures with the Test Substance
Cell Lines: The medium is aspirated (three wells at a time) and the cells washed with 200 μl warm PBS. The PBS is aspirated and 50 μl of the test sample added to wells. After 1 min, the test sample is removed by aspiration and the cells are again washed with 200 μl warm PBS. Precisely 100 μl neutral red destain solution (1% acetic acid, 50% ethanol, 49% distilled water) is then added, which fixes the cells and releases the remaining neutral red into a

solution. The plate is agitated on a microtiter plate shaker for a few minutes to disperse the released dye, then the optical density is read on a MicroELISA plate reader at 540 nm and a 404-nm reference filter. The plate reader is zeroed on the blank well, which contains no cell.

1.6.3.3 Analysis

From the optical density values obtained, the NRR concentrations of test chemicals that cause 50% loss of the neutral red dye are calculated with respect to the PBS-controls (NRR_{50}).

2. DATA

3. REPORTING

3.1 Test Report

The test report shall, if possible, include the following information:

- test conditions: detailed description of treatment and sampling schedule, dose levels, toxicity data, negative and positive controls;
- dose/effect relationship when possible;
- statistical evaluation;
- discussion of the results;
- interpretation of the results.

3.2 Evaluation and Interpretation

(to be defined)

4. ALTERNATIVE TO ANIMAL TEST

This method may be used in the screening for potential eye irritant chemicals.

BIBLIOGRAPHY

Commission of the European Communities, Collaborative study on the evaluation of alternative methods to the eye irritation test — Part 1, Doc. XI/632/91 V/E/1/131/91, Brussels, 1991, p. 13.

Commission of the European Communities, Collaborative study on the evaluation of alternative methods to the eye irritation test — Part II, Doc. XI/632/91 V/E/1/131/91, Brussels 1991, p. 152.

Gettings, S.D., J. J. Teal, D. M. Bagley, J. L. Demetrulias, L. C. Di Pasquale, K. L. Hintze, M. G. Rozen, S. L. Weise, M. Chudkowski, K. D. Marenus, W. J. W. Pape, M. Roddy, R. Schnetzinger, P. M. Silber, S. M. Glaza and P. J. Kurtz, The CTFA evaluation of alternatives program: An evaluation of *in vitro* alternatives to the Draize primary eye irritation test (Phase 1) Hydro-alcoholic formulations; (Part 2) Data analysis and biological significance, *In Vitro Toxicology*, Vol. 4, No. 4, p. 247, 1991.

INVITTOX **Protocol,** No. 54, July 1992.

Reader, S. J., V. Blackwell, R. O'Hara, R. H. Clothier, G. Griffin and M. Balls, A vital dye release method for assessing the short-term cytotoxic effects of chemicals and formulations, *ATLA*, Vol. 17, p. 28, 1989.

Shaw, A. J., R. H. Clothier and M. Balls, Loss of trans-epithelial impermeability of a confluent monolayer of Madin-Darby canine kidney (MDCK) cells as a determinant of ocular irritation potential, *ATLA*, Vol. 18, p. 145, 1990.

NEUTRAL RED UPTAKE (NRU)

1. METHOD

1.1 Introduction, 1.2 Definition, and 1.3 Reference Substances (to be defined)

1.4 Principle of the Test Method

The NRU assay is a cytotoxic assay used to identify reduction of cell proliferation/viability on both established cell lines and primary cultures exposed to test chemicals. It is based on the uptake of neutral red, a weakly cationic supravital dye (3-amino-7-dimethylamino-2-methylphenazine hydrochloride), and its accumulation in the lysosomes of viable uninjured cells. After extraction, the absorbance of the dye can be determined spectrophotometrically. This test has been suggested to be useful to screen chemicals for their irritative potential to eye.

1.5 Quality Criteria (to be defined)

1.6 Description of the Test Method
1.6.1 Preparations

Test chemicals are prepared in medium, or in distilled water or DMSO afterwards diluted in serum-free culture medium: final DMSO concentration must not exceed 1%. When present, DMSO is used at the same concentration for all chemical concentrations.

Other solvents are: various concentrations of ethanol (2%, 4%, 100%); methanol.

Hydro-alcoholic formulations are tested at a dilution of 0.1%.

Primary cultures (rabbit tracheal epithelial cells; freshly and cryopreserved rat, dog, and human hepatocytes), secondary cultures (human epidermal keratinocytes; human dermal fibroblast) and established cell lines (SIRC, ATCC CCL 60; BALB/3T3 clone A31, ATCC (CCL 163); 3T3-L1, ATCC (CCL 92.1); keratinocytes, Clonetics' EpiPack®; human fetal dermal fibroblasts, CCRL 1475; FaO rat hepatoma; L929 cell line) may be used in this assay.

1.6.2 Test Conditions
Number of Cultures

From two to eight cultures are tested for each experimental point.

Use of Negative and Positive Controls

Positive controls are made concurrently; negative control (medium) always is used. Positive controls are run only at the beginning of testing of new product categories and not on a routine basis.

Exposure Concentrations

For screening experiments chemicals are tested at half-interval dilutions starting at 2 mg/ml and 5% (v/v) for solid and liquid agents, respectively. Serial dilutions are adjusted to obtain a minimum of 7 to 10 data-points within a range of toxicity from 10 to 90%.

Culture Conditions

Appropriate culture media, seeding density, and incubation condition are used. To prevent evaporation of volatile test agents, plates are sealed with a CO_2-permeable plastic film that is unpermeable to volatile chemicals (permeable plastic film: Greiner, Germany, No. 676001).

Metabolic Activation

(most chemicals require metabolic activation)

1.6.3 Procedure
1.6.3.1 Preparation of Cultures
Primary Cultures: Tracheas are removed from rabbits and the epithelium is separated from the underlying cartilage and cut into 2 mm explants. The explants are grown on collagen matrix and covered with minimum essential medium (MEM).

Hepatocytes are isolated from rats by the two-step collagenase perfusion method. Cell viability, measured by the trypan blue exclusion test (final concentration of dye: 0.05% in phosphate buffered saline), is adequate if in excess of 85%. Cells are seeded at a density of 3×10^4 cells per well in 96-well plates (NUNC, Kamstrup, Denmark) in 100 μl nutrient medium. The medium consists of Williams' E medium (Flow, Les Ulis, France) containing 10% fetal calf serum (FCS, Boehringer, Mannheim, Germany), 0.1 IU bovine insulin/ml, 10 IU penicillin/ml, 10 μl streptomycin/ml and 2.5 mM-glutamine.

Human liver specimens are collected from multiorgan donors for transplantation. Human hepatocytes are obtained by a two-step collagenase perfusion and resuspended in Ham's F12 Coon's/Dulbecco's modified Eagle's medium (1:1, v/v) containing 10% FCS, and supplemented with penicillin, netilmicin, insulin, glucagon, thyroxine, sodium selenite, human transferrin and ethanolamine (Sigma). Cell viability is determined using erythrosin B exclusion test. Hepatocytes are seeded at a density of 30×10^3 cells/100 μl, in 96-multiwell plates and incubated in a humidified, 5% CO_2 atmosphere at 37°C. Media are renewed after 4 h of adhesion.

Human liver specimens are collected from multiorgan donors for transplantation. Human hepatocytes, obtained by a two-step collagenase perfusion method, are cryopreserved in Ham's F12 medium (Sigma) containing bovine serum albumin, polyvinylpyrrolidone (PVP), 10% DMSO, and 20% FCS, in vials (1.8 ml Nunc), and stored in liquid nitrogen. Cryopreserved cells are directly thawed by immersing the vials in a 37°C water-bath and then purified by Percoll density gradient. Seeding is performed as above.

Rat, dog, and human hepatocytes are isolated by the two-step collagenase perfusion method; cell viability is estimated by the trypan blue exclusion test. Then, isolated hepatocytes are suspended at a density of 4×10^6 cells per ml in Leibovitz (L-15) medium containing 20% FCS. An equal volume of L-15 medium, containing 20% FCS and DMSO (the cryoprotective agent) is then slowly introduced. DMSO is added at final concentrations of 16, 14, and 12% for rat, dog, and human hepatocytes, respectively. The cells are distributed in freezing vials in 1.6 ml of medium per vial, transferred at –20°C for 12 min then to a –80°C freezer for 1 h and plunged in liquid nitrogen. For recovery storage, vials are warmed in a water-bath at 37°C and cell suspensions are gently pipetted. Each cell sample is transferred in 15 ml of L-15 medium containing 0.6 or 0.8 M-glucose. Cell suspensions are centrifuged either directly or after being subjected to density gradient centrifugation on a Percoll 400 cushion to eliminate cell debris and dead cells. Freshly isolated and thawed hepatocytes are seeded at a density of 7×10^5 cells per 35 mm Petri dish in 2 ml culture medium and incubated at 37°C in a humidified atmosphere of 95% air/5% CO_2. The medium is a mixture of 75% minimum essential medium and 25% medium 199 supplemented with 0.1% bovine serum albumin, 5 μl bovine insulin/ml and 10% FCS.

Secondary Cultures: A secondary culture of proliferating normal human epidermal keratinocytes is harvested, when 50 to 80% confluent, by tripsinization (0.025% v/v) from a T-25 culture flask (Corning). The cells are centrifuged ($220 \times g$, 5 min), diluted in keratinocyte growth medium (KGM, Clonetics Corp., San Diego) and counted (1×10^4/ml). The cells are plated at 2500 cells/well in a 96-well tissue culture plate (Falcon). The plate is incubated for 3 d at 37°C in a 5% CO_2 humidified atmosphere.

Normal human fibroblasts, isolated from the dermis of freshly obtained neonatal foreskins, are propagated in complete DMEM (Dulbecco's modified Eagle's medium, Gibco) containing 10% fetal bovine serum (Hyclone), nonessential amino acids (Gibco), 2 mM-L-glutamine (Gibco), 1 mM-sodium pyruvate (Gibco), 100 IU penicillin G sodium/ml (Gibco), 100 μg streptomycin sulfate/ml (Gibco), and 0.25 μg/ml amphotericin B (Gibco); then they are seeded onto 8×8 cm nylon mesh, pretreated with acetic acid-fetal bovine serum, to obtain a three-dimensional substrate consisting of several layers of cells. When the cells become confluent (after 2 to 3 weeks), the sheets of nylon mesh are cut with a laser (Texcel) into 11×11 mm squares. Then these squares are placed into 24-well plates and treated.

Cell Lines: Microtiter plates are inoculated with 1.5×10^4 or 5×10^4 cells (SIRC, rabbit corneal cell line)/well in 0.2 ml culture medium using a multichannel pipette with the exception of the wells in the first row that will serve as blanks. The same suspension must be used to fill all microtiter plates. In the first case, the medium is composed of MEM supplemented with glutamine 2 mM, gentamycin 4 µg/ml, and fetal calf serum (10% for culture and 5% for treatment); in the second case, the medium is DMEM with 5% fetal calf serum (FCS) and 1% NEAA. In both cases, the cells are maintained in suspension with a magnetic shaker. About 10 ml are put in a reagent basin and distributed in wells. After each range, the cell suspension is shaken twice with a multichannel pipette. After inoculation, the microtiter plates are put on a microtiter shaker to obtain a good distribution of the cells in the wells. Microtiter plates are incubated for 24 h in humidified 5% CO_2 incubator at 37°C.

BALB c/3T3 (mouse embryonic lung fibroblasts, American Type Culture Collection) cells are maintained in DMEM, supplemented with 2 mM L-glutamine, 10% newborn calf serum or 2%/10% fetal bovine serum, 100 µg/ml streptomycin sulfate, 100 IU/ml benzylpenicillin and 1.25–2 µg/ml Fungizone (Squibb & Sons, Princeton, NJ). They are routinely grown on 80 cm² flasks in a humidified 5–7% CO_2 atmosphere at 37°C, and transferred every 2 to 3 d. The cells are then dissociated in a solution containing 0.5 g trypsin and 0.2 g ethylenediaminetetraacetic acid (EDTA) in 100 ml phosphate-buffered saline (PBS). Cells are plated in 0.2 ml of medium per well in 96-well tissue culture microtest plate at 1.6×10^4 or 4–5×10^4 cells/ml.

Keratinocytes (Clonetics' EpiPack®, grown in Clonetics' serum-free medium) and human fetal dermal fibroblasts (grown in DMEM with 10% fetal calf serum and penicillin/streptomycin) are plated in 96-well flat bottom plates and incubated for 24 h at 37°C, 5% CO_2.

FaO cells (subcloned from the hepatoma cell line H4IIEC3, isolated from the Reuber H35 hepatoma) are cultured in NCTC 135/Ham's F12 medium (v/v) supplemented with 5% FCS, 100 IU penicillin/ml and 100 µl streptomycin/ml: the medium is renewed every 2 d and the cells are transferred after about 10 d when they reached subconfluency using 0.5% trypsin. After five passages, the cells are stored in liquid nitrogen. For cytotoxicity studies, frozen FaO cells are thawed and put in culture; the functional capacity is controlled by measuring albumin secretion rates in media. After three passages, the cells are seeded in 96-well plates in Williams' E medium (Flow, Les Ulis, France) containing 10% fetal calf serum (FCS, Boehringer, Mannheim, Germany), 0.1 IU bovine insulin/ml, 10 IU penicillin/ml, 10 µl streptomycin/ml, and 2.5 mM-glutamine.

L929, a mouse fibroblast cell line, is grown as a monolayer in Eagle's Minimum Essential Medium (Biological Industries), supplemented with 10% fetal calf serum (Nordvacc), 50 µg gentamicin/ml (Nordvacc), 1% nonessential amino acids and 2 mM-L-glutamine (Biological Industries). The cells are subcultivated twice a week using 0.1% trypsin (Nordvacc) in phosphate-buffered saline without Ca^{2+} and Mg^{2+}, and maintained at 37°C in humidified air with 5% CO_2. Then the cells are taken from confluent cultures and inoculated into 96-well tissue culture plates (Greiner) at a density of 7000 cells/cm².

1.6.3.2 Treatment of the Cultures with the Test Substance
Primary Cultures

Chemicals are applied on day 7 (on cells that are near the end of the exponential growth phase) and NRU measurements are carried out after 24 h of treatments. The neutral red solution (Sigma) is diluted 1:40 in culture medium (500 µl per dish). After elimination of the supernatant culture, the dye is fixed with a solution containing 4% formol and 10% calcium chloride for 1 min, as a longer fixation is likely to damage cells. Neutral red extraction is performed with a mixture of 1% acetic acid in 50% ethanol for several minutes at room temperature and absorbance is determined at 540 nm.

Three hours after seeding, the medium is discarded and replaced by 100 µl FCS-free medium containing 10^{-6} M-hydrocortisone hemisuccinate (Roussel-Uclaf, Romainville, France) with the test compound. The cultures are incubated for 20 h at 37°C under a humidified atmosphere of 95% air-5% CO_2. At the end of the incubation period the cultures are examined under phase-contrast microscopy. Then the cells are preloaded with 100 µl neutral red solution (50 µg/ml) for 3 h at 37°C. Then this solution is discarded and replaced by 200 µl formol-calcium solution in distilled water. After 1 min the cells are washed with PBS before addition of an alcohol (50%)-acetic acid (1%) solution. Optical density is measured at 550 nm.

After 14 to 16 h, the media are discarded and test chemicals are added in serum-free medium, containing 10^{-6} M-dexamethasone. After 24 or 48 h of exposure neutral red assay is performed.

After 38 h, the media are discarded and test chemicals are added in serum-free medium (but containing 10^{-6} M-dexamethasone). After 20 h of exposure neutral red assay is performed.

After 4 h (rat and dog cells) or 24 h (human cells), the media are discarded and test chemicals are added in serum-free medium. After 24 h (rat and dog) or 48 h (human) of exposure, neutral red assay is performed.

Secondary Culture

Used KGM is removed from the wells by careful aspiration and 250 µl fresh KGM is added to control wells while 250 µl of various concentrations of test agents diluted in KGM are added to test wells. The plate is incubated for 2 d at 37°C. The spent medium/test agent solutions are removed and replaced with KGM supplemented with neutral red dye (Sigma) at a final concentration of 50 µg/ml to all wells except blanks; 250 µl of KGM without dye is added to the blanks. The plate is then incubated for 3 h at 37°C. Each well then receives 250 µl Wash/Fix Solution (an aqueous 1% formaldehyde/1% calcium chloride solution) for 1 min (room temperature). The Wash/Fix solution is decanted and each well receives 100 µl of a Solvent Solution (1% glacial acetic acid/50% ethanol) for 20 min at room temperature. Absorbances are measured at 540 nm in a microplate reader, after making the appropriate blank correction, and percentage of untreated control values calculated for each dilution of test agent.

Test chemicals are added in 2 ml of complete DMEM containing 2% fetal bovine serum (assay medium). After overnight incubation at 37°C in 5% CO_2, the used media are aspirated and replaced with 1 ml (per well) of assay medium containing 50 µg neutral red/ml (Sigma). The cultures are incubated for 3 h, washed twice with 1 ml PBS (Mediatech), and once for 1 min with 1 ml of an aqueous solution of 0.5% formaldehyde (Sigma) containing 1% calcium chloride (Sigma). NR taken up by viable cells is solvent-extract with 2 ml of 1% acetic acid (Sigma) in 50% aqueous ethanol (Quantum) on a shaker platform for 1 h. Aliquots (200 µl) of the extracted NR solutions are transferred to a 96-well plate and the optical density at 540 nm is determined spectrophotometrically using a VMAX microplate reader (Molecular Devices), making a blank correction to a pretreated nylon mesh (without cells) that has been similarly incubated with NR.

Cell Lines: On cell monolayers, prior to confluence (1.5×10^4 cells/well) and on confluent cell monolayers (5×10^4 cells/well), the medium is removed and replaced with medium supplemented with various concentrations of the test agent (8 wells/concentration, 0.2 ml/well). Two rows of culture (on both sides of the microtiter plate) receive normal medium and serve as controls. The microtiter plates are then incubated for 24 h in humidified 5% CO_2 incubator at 37°C. The cells are examined by a phase contrast microscope. The medium is removed and cells are washed in NaCl 0.9%; 0.2 ml of medium containing 0.05 mg NR/ml is added to each well with a multichannel pipette. The microtiter plates are incubated for 3 h in humidified 5% CO_2 incubator at 37°C. The medium is removed and the cell are rapidly (1 min) washed with 0.2 ml of fixative (formol-calcium). Then 0.2 ml of mixture of acetic acid-ethanol is used to extract the dye from the cells. After 15 min at room temperature and rapid agitation on a microtiter plate shaker, the plates are transferred to a microplate reader and the absorbance is measured at 540 nm with blank wells.

- NR (Neutral red solution): 4 mg/ml in distilled water (stability: 15 d) is diluted 1/80 in culture medium (5% serum); 24 h after solubilization or immediately prior to the test, a two-step centrifugation is made to remove fine precipitates of dye crystals.
- Formol-calcium solution: 1 ml formaldehyde 40% + 10 ml calcium chloride 10% + 89 ml distilled water.
- Acid-ethanol solution: 1 ml acetic acid + 99 ml ethanol 50%.

Cultures are treated 24 h after plating when cells are still in exponential growth: the medium is removed and the cells are re-fed with medium containing test agents. After a treatment time of either 18 to 24 h ($4–5 \times 10^4$ cells/well) or 72 h (1.6×10^4 cells/well) measurements of NRU are made as follows: a 50 mg/ml aqueous stock solution of neutral red is prepared and added to DMEM to give a final concentration of 50 µg/ml (designated as NR medium). This is preincubated overnight at 37°C and centrifuged before use to remove precipitated dye crystals, which may interfere with the assay. Three hours before termination of the experiment, the medium containing the test compound is removed and replaced with 0.2 ml NR medium. After 3 h (the lysosomes having taken up sufficient stain), the NR medium is removed and the cells rinsed with PBS (or with a mixture of 1% formaldehyde-1% $CaCl_2$) to remove excess unincorporated stain. Precisely 0.2 ml of NR destain solution (1% glacial acetic acid, 49% distilled water, 50% ethanol, by volume) is then added to each well, in order to both fix the cells and remove the neutral red into solution. The plates then are rapidly shaken for 1 to 2 h on an orbital shaker and the absorbance of the solution in each well read on a MicroELISA plate reader at 540 nm with a 404 nm reference filter. The well containing no cells is used as a blank and is set at 0.

Test agents are added to the wells in 200 µl of fresh medium and incubated for 24 to 48 h. Cultures are scanned with an inverted phase microscope and photodocumented. 24 h prior to the end of treatment time, neutral red solution is prepared by adding stock neutral red (Gibco neutral red stock, NR = 3 mg/ml) to complete medium, the final concentration being 50 µg/ml: it is incubated overnight at 37°C and the following day centrifuged 10 min at $1500 \times g$ to remove crystal dye precipitate. At the end of treatment time medium is replaced with 200 µl neutral red medium and cultures are incubated for 3 h at 37°C. Medium is again removed and cells are washed quickly with a solution of 1% formaldehyde and 1% $CaCl_2$. Medium then is aspirated and 200 µl of a solution of 1% acetic acid + 50% ethanol is added for 20 min. The plate then is shaken rapidly. Plates are read at 540 nm on an ELISA Plate Reader (Bio-Tek EL 309 Autoreader). Results are expressed as% OD of complete medium control.

At subconfluency (4 d after cell seeding), the medium is discarded and replaced by FCS-free medium containing 10^{-6} M-hydrocortisone hemisuccinate (Roussel-Uclaf, Romainville, France) with the test compound. The cultures are incubated for 20 h at 37°C under a humidified atmosphere of 95% air-5% CO_2. At the end of the incubation period the cultures are examined under phase-contrast microscopy. Then the cells are preloaded with 100 µl neutral red solution (50 µg/ml) for 3 h at 37°C. Then this solution is discarded and replaced by 200 µl formol-calcium solution in distilled water. After 1 min the cells are washed with PBS before addition of an alcohol (50%)-acetic acid (1%) solution. Optical density is measured at 550 nm.

The medium is removed 72 or 24 h after inoculation and test compounds are added at various concentrations. After a treatment time of 24 or 72 h, respectively, measurements of neutral red uptake are determined. The absorbance is measured with an automatic microtiter plate reader, Dynatech MR 700 (Billingshurst).

1.6.3.3 Analysis

Cell numbers (in terms of NRU absorbance readings) in treated cultures are compared to those in control cultures and the percentage inhibition of growth calculated: the NRU_{50} (the concentration producing 50% inhibition of growth) is determined using the linear regression analysis.

2. DATA

3. REPORTING
3.1 Test Report
The test report shall, if possible, include the following information:

- test conditions: detailed description of treatment and sampling schedule, dose levels, toxicity data, negative and positive controls;
- dose/effect relationship when possible;
- statistical evaluation;
- discussion of the results;
- interpretation of the results.

3.2 Evaluation and Interpretation
(to be defined)

4. ALTERNATIVE TO ANIMAL TEST
This test method may be used in the screening for potential eye irritant chemicals.

BIBLIOGRAPHY

Blanquart, C., S. Romet, A. Baeza, C. Guennou and E. Marano, Primary cultures of tracheal epithelial cells for the evaluation of respiratory toxicity, *Toxicology In Vitro,* Vol. 5, No. 5/6, p. 499, 1991.

Borenfreund, E., H. Babich and N. Martin-Alguacil, Comparisons of two *in vitro* cytotoxicity assays, the neutral red (NR) and tetrazolium MTT tests, *Toxicology In Vitro,* Vol. 2, No. 1, p. 1, 1988.

Chesné, C., C. Guyomard, L. Grislain, C. Clerc, A. Fautrel and Guillouzo, Use of cryopreserved animal and human hepatocytes for cytotoxicity studies, *Toxicology In Vitro,* Vol. 5, No. 5/6, p. 479, 1991.

Commission of the European Communities, Collaborative study on the evaluation of alternative methods to the eye irritation test — Part 1, Doc. XI/632/91 V/E/1/131/91, Brussels, 1991, p. 11.

Commission of the European Communities, Collaborative study on the evaluation of alternative methods to the eye irritation test — Part II, Doc. XI/632/91 V/E/1/131/91, Brussels 1991, p. 149.

De Sousa, G., M. Dou, D. Barbe, B. Lacarelle, M. Placidi and R. Rahmani, Freshly isolated or cryopreserved human hepatocytes in primary culture: Influence of drug metabolism on hepatotoxicity, *Toxicology In Vitro,* Vol 5, No. 5/6, p. 483, 1991.

Fautrel, A., C. Chesné, A. Guillozo, G. De Sousa, M. Placidi, R. Rhamani, F. Braut, J. Pichon, H. Hoellinger, P. Vintezous, I. Diarte, C. Melcion, A. Cordier, G. Lorenzon, M. Benincourt, B. Vannier, R. Fournex, A. F. Peloux, N. Bichet, D. Gouy and J. P. Cano, A multicentre study of acute *in vitro* cytotoxicity in rat liver cells, *Toxicology In Vitro,* Vol. 5, No. 5/6, p. 543, 1991.

Gettings, S. D., J. J. Teal, D. M. Bagley, J. L. Demetrulias, L. C. Di Pasquale, K. L. Hintze, M. G. Rozen, S. L. Weise, M. Chudkowski, K. D. Marenus, W. J. W. Pape, M. Roddy, R. Schnetzinger, P. M. Silber, S. M. Glaza and P. J. Kurtz, The CTFA evaluation of alternatives program: An evaluation of *in vitro* alternatives to the Draize primary eye irritation test (Phase 1) Hydro-alcoholic formulations; (Part 2) Data analysis and biological significance, *In Vitro Toxicology*, Vol. 4, No. 4, p. 247, 1991.

INVITTOX Protocol No. 3a, September 1990.

Nordin, M., A. Wieslander, E. Martinson and P. Kjellstrand, Effects of exposure period of acetylsalicylic acid, paracetamol and isopropanol on L929 cytotoxicity, *Toxicology In Vitro*, Vol. 5, No. 5/6, p. 449, 1991.

Spielmann, H., I. Gerner, S. Kalweit, R. Moog, T. Wirnsberger, K. Krauser, R. Kreiling, H. Kreuzer, N. P. Lüpke, H. G. Miltenburger, N. Muller, P. Murmann, W. Pape, B. Siegemund, J. Spengler, W. Steiling and F. J. Wiebel, Interlaboratory assessment of alternatives to the Draize eye irritation test in Germany, *Toxicology In Vitro*, Vol. 5, No. 5/6, p. 539, 1991.

Triglia, D., S. Sherard Braa, C. Yonan and G. K. Naughton, Cytotoxicity testing using neutral red and MTT assays on a three-dimensional human skin substrate, *Toxicology In Vitro*, Vol. 5, No. 5/6, p. 573, 1991.

PHOTOMUTAGENICITY BACTERIAL ASSAY

1. METHOD

1.1 Introduction, 1.2 Definition, and 1.3 Reference Substances (to be defined)

1.4 Principle of the Test Method

The bacterial photomutagenicity assay represents a microbial reverse mutation system that measures gene-mutations induced by photochemical products that can cause base changes in bacterial organism genoma. Bacteria are exposed concurrently to chemicals and UV light. After a suitable period of incubation on minimal medium, revertant colonies are counted and compared to the number of spontaneous revertants observed in an untreated and non-UV-exposed sample and/or solvent control culture.

1.5 Quality Criteria (to be defined)

1.6 Description of the Test Method

The following methods may be used to perform the assay: the direct incorporation method in which bacteria and test agent are mixed in overlay agar and poured over the surface of a selective agar plate; plates are exposed to various doses of unfiltered or glass-filtered UV light; plates are then incubated for 3 d at 37°C.

1.6.1 Preparations

Bacteria

Bacteria are grown at 37°C up to late exponential or early stationary phase of growth. Approximate cell density should be 10^8 to 10^9 cells per milliliter.

1.6.2 Test Conditions

Tester Strains

Salmonella typhimurium strain TA100 and *Escherichia coli* strains WP2 and WP2pKM101 should be used. Recognized methods of stock culture preparations and storage are to be used. The growth requirements and the genetic identity of strains, their sensitivity to UV radiation or mitomycin C and the resistance to ampicillin in strain WP2pKM101 has to be checked. The strains also should yield spontaneous revertants within the frequency ranges expected.

Medium

An appropriate medium for the expression and selection of mutants is used with an adequate overlay agar.

Use of Negative and Positive Controls

Concurrent untreated, unexposed to UV light and solvent controls have to be performed. Positive controls have to be conducted also for the following purposes:

- to confirm sensitivity of bacterial strains;
- 8-methoxypsoralen may be used as positive control for tests in presence of UV light;
- Methylmethanesulfonate may be used as positive control for tests in absence of UV light.

Amount of Test Substance per Plate

At least five different amounts of test chemical are tested with half-log intervals between plates. Substances are tested up to the limit of solubility or toxicity. Toxicity is evidenced by a reduction of the numbers of spontaneous revertants, a clearing of background lawn, or by degree of treated cultures survival. Nontoxic chemicals should be tested to 5 mg per plate before considering the test subsistance negative.

Irradiation Conditions

At least two different UVA/UVB radiation doses are used. Exposure of cultures to UV light is performed using a sun lamp, whose spectral radiation flux is calibrated before each experiment using a UV meter, both as unfiltered light and as light filtered through a sheet of 3 mm thick glass, which screened out almost all the UVB component. Both UVA and UVB measurements are recorded and doses calculated in mJ/cm_2, using duration of exposure and dose rate.

Incubation Conditions

A.C. plates are incubated for 72 h at 37°C.

1.6.3 Procedure

The chemical and 0.1 ml of a fresh bacterial culture A.C. are added to 2.0 ml of overlay agar, in a darkened laboratory. Once set, plates are exposed to various doses of unfiltered or glass-filtered UV light, and then incubated for 3 d at 37°C.

All plating is done at least in triplicate.

2. DATA

Numbers of per plate revertant colonies are reported for both control and treated series. Individual plate counts, per plate revertant colonies, mean number and standard deviation should be presented for tested chemicals under the exposed/unexposed conditions and controls.

All results are confirmed in an independent experiment.

Data should be evaluated using appropriate statistical methods.

3. REPORTING
3.1 Test Report

The test report shall, if possible, include the following information:

- bacteria, strain used;
- test conditions: dose level, UVA and UVB light doses, toxicity; composition of the media; treatment procedures; reference substances; negative controls;
- individual plate count, per plate revertant colonies mean number, standard deviation, dose/effect relationship (when possible);
- results interpretation.

3.2 Evaluation and Interpretation
(to be defined)

4. ALTERNATIVE TO ANIMAL TEST
This method is used for the identification of photomutagenic chemicals.

BIBLIOGRAPHY

Dean, S. W., R. H. Dunmore, S. P. Ruddock, J. C. Dean, C. N. Martin and D. J. Kirkland, Development of assays for the detection of photomutagenicity of chemicals during exposure to UV light. II. Results of testing three sunscreen ingredients, *Mutagenesis*, Vol. 7, No. 3, p. 179, 1992.

Dean, S. W., M. Lane, R. H. Dunmore, S. P. Ruddock, C. N. Martin, D. J. Kirkland and N. Loprieno, Development of assays for the detection of photomutagenicity of chemicals during exposure to UV light; I. Assay development, *Mutagenesis*, Vol. 6, No. 5, p. 335, 1991.

Loprieno, N., *In Vitro* assay systems for testing photomutagenic chemicals, *Mutagenesis*, Vol. 6, No. 5, p. 331, 1991.

PROTEIN SYNTHESIS INHIBITION

1. METHOD

1.1 Introduction, 1.2 Definition, and 1.3 Reference Substances (to be defined)

1.4 Principle of the Test Method
The test enables the measurement of protein synthesis within cultured cells, as determined by their ability to incorporate radiolabeled leucine into the cellular protein. Any detrimental effect of compounds upon the protein synthesis machinery can thus be determined.

1.4.1 Basic Procedure
Hel 30 cells are incubated in the presence of radiolabeled leucine with or without test chemical for a short period of time. Uptake of the radiolabeled leucine is terminated by the addition of unlabeled leucine. Cell protein is precipitated with trichloroacetic acid and harvested onto glass-fiber filters. Radioactivity of the samples is assessed by liquid scintillation counting.

1.4.2 Critical Assessment
A number of *in vitro* tests for cytotoxicity depend upon the fact that many chemicals affect the integrity of the plasma membrane, causing leakage of cell contents and eventually cell death. Loss of membrane integrity can thus be assessed by a nonspecific method, such as determination of LDH leakage, while the loss of cell protein from monolayers can be taken as a marker of cell death, which is accompanied by detachment of the previously adherent cells. However, chemicals that damage the plasma membrane could potentially affect other cytoplasmic lipid bilayers, such as the endoplasmic reticulum, where a less drastic degree of damage may nevertheless have consequences for protein synthesis.

Time course experiments using LDH leakage, total protein content, and *de novo* protein synthesis as parameters of cytotoxicity in cells exposed to surfactants showed the best dose-response relationship occurred after 2 h incubation with test concentrations in the range 1 to 500 g/ml. For both LDH leakage and total protein content, the plateau of the cytotoxic effect was at 300 to 500 ug/ml test substance, with the lower threshold being 50 μg/ml for cationic, and 100 g/ml for anionic compounds, while amphoteric and nonionic surfactants were active only at the highest concentrations used. Protein synthesis proved to be a more sensitive marker, with cationic substances producing profound inhibition at the lowest tested concentration (1 μg/ml), which had no effect on the other two parameters. The plateau of this effect was at 50 to 100 μg/ml.

Comparative toxicity followed the general order cationic > anionic > nonionic > amphoteric for all three parameters. However, some nonionic compounds were found to have a more pronounced effect on the anabolic function (protein synthesis) than on membrane integrity.

With respect to the choice of target cell, it has been found that many toxic substances show the same ranking, regardless of which cell type is used. The choice of the HEL 30 mouse epidermal cell line was therefore considered justified, and this was borne out by the good correlation achieved between *in vitro* results and reported *in vivo* irritation test data.

In summary, while loss of cell protein content and LDH leakage give valuable information about the relative potency of test compounds, protein synthesis provides a more sensitive indication of toxic effects at nonlethal concentrations that have no effect on the two former parameters. Further, although LDH leakage shows greater correlation with *in vivo* data, than does inhibition of protein synthesis, and therefore could be considered a more appropriate, even if less sensitive, parameter, it does not always indicate toxicity in other nonsurfactant classes of compound, whereas inhibition of protein synthesis appears to be an indicator of cytotoxicity over a broad spectrum of chemicals. Inhibition of protein synthesis is thus a sensitive and reproducible endpoint that may form a valuable part of an *in vitro* test battery designed not only to be an equivalent to the Draize test, but also to distinguish between substances giving an *in vivo* result judged to be of equal severity.

1.5 Quality Criteria (to be defined)

1.6 Description of the Test Method
1.6.1 Preparations
General Cell Maintenance
Storage of Frozen Cells

Cells may be grown to confluence in 100-mm dishes. The cells from each dish can then be harvested into 1.5 ml of storage medium and frozen until needed. When required an aliquot should be thawed out at 37°C and seeded into a 25 cm² flask containing 3 ml of culture medium (final volume 4.5 ml). After 24 h the medium should be removed, the cells rinsed once with 4 ml of room temperature PBS, and 3 ml fresh culture medium added. Cells should be rinsed and medium replaced every second day thereafter.

Continuation of the Cell Line

When cells are confluent in the flasks (after 4 d) trypsinize off:

- remove medium and add 2 ml of trypsin/EDTA (prewarmed to 37°C) to each flask and incubate for 5 min at 37°C;
- suspend the cells from each flask in 50 ml culture medium at room temperature and place 10 ml of this suspension into each of five 100-mm dishes;
- cells should be rinsed once (10 ml room temperature PBS/dish) and medium replaced every second day thereafter.

When the cells are confluent (after 4 d), trypsinize off:

- remove medium and add 2 ml of trypsin/EDTA to each dish and incubate for 5 min at 37°C;
- suspend the cells obtained from 5 dishes into 200 ml culture medium at room temperature;
- divide between two 100-mm dishes for continuation of the cell line and ninety 35-mm dishes (to be used for test purposes — see later).

1.6.2 Test Conditions
Number of Cultures
   Run triplicate dishes for each condition.

Use of Negative and Positive Controls
   (to be defined)

Exposure Concentrations
   (to be defined)

Culture Conditions
   (to be defined)

Metabolic Activation
   (most chemicals require metabolic activation)

1.6.3 Procedure
1.6.3.1 Preparation of Cultures
   Seed approximately 1×10^5 cells in 2 ml medium into each 35-mm dish. The cell suspension harvested above will provide this approximate concentration of cells. Incubate the cells at 37°C for 4 d until confluent. Cells should be rinsed once (2 ml room temperature PBS/dish) and medium replaced every 2 d thereafter.

1.6.3.2 Treatment of the Cultures with the Test Substance
   Once confluent, remove medium, rinse cells, and add:
   1 ml of fresh medium — blank
   1 ml of fresh medium containing 3H-leucine — control, or
   1 ml of fresh medium containing 3H-leucine and the test chemical — test
   Incubate for 2 h.
   Terminate the reaction by adding 10 µl of 0.1 M unlabeled leucine to each dish (final concentration — 0.1 M). Aspirate off the medium (this may be retained for analysis, e.g., LDH leakage, prostaglandin determination, etc.). Rinse the cell monolayer twice with 1 ml PBS (room temperature). Add 1 ml of 1N NaOH to each dish and store overnight at 4°C to ensure complete protein solubilization.

Protein Determination
   Remove 100 µl for protein determination by method of choice.

3H-Leucine Incorporation Determination
   Remove 500 µl and add to 500 µl of ice-cold 60% TCA to precipitate the protein. Store the samples on ice for 30 min. Filter the samples through glass-fiber filters. Place filters in vials and add 10 ml of scintillation fluid. Determine the quantity of leucine incorporated into the protein by liquid scintillation counting.

1.6.3.3 Analysis

Correct all readings with reference to the background reading, i.e., subtract blank values from test and control readings.

Calculate the cpm/mg protein for each sample (s) and control (c).

With the control cpm/mg value taken as 100, calculate the inhibition of leucine incorporation:

$$\% \text{ inhibition} = 100 - (s \times 100)/c$$

The PSI_{50} value for a given chemical is then obtained by performing a linear regression analysis on the data for different doses.

Note: Certain chemicals may cause an increase in protein synthesis.

2. DATA

3. REPORTING

3.1 Test Report

The test report shall, if possible, include the following information:

- test conditions: detailed description of treatment and sampling schedule, dose levels, toxicity data, negative and positive controls,
- dose/effect relationship when possible,
- statistical evaluation,
- discussion of the results,
- interpretation of the results.

3.2 Evaluation and Interpretation
(to be defined)

4. ALTERNATIVE TO ANIMAL TEST

This method may be used in screening for potential eye irritant chemicals.

BIBLIOGRAPHY

INVITTOX **Protocol**, No. 14, February 1993.

QSAR APPLIED TO THE DRAIZE EYE TEST 1

1. METHOD

The use of QSAR in toxicology consists of analysis of different quantitative parameters of a chemical that could be related to biological activities. The guideline's description for this method cannot conform, at present, to the format so far developed by OECD experts. This description is an attempt to organize the material in a way to allow analysis of the data according to a procedure used by some authors.

2.1 Description of the Test Method

In a QSAR quantitative analysis, biological activities are normally described as molar concentrations causing defined responses (e.g., LC_{50}, EC_{50}). The Draize eye irritation score is not, however, a conventional QSAR endpoint in terms of being a concentration producing a response, but is taken as the only quantitative description of overall eye irritation potentials suitable for QSAR modelling. The scores are adjusted for the molarity of the pure chemicals.

This will give a better description of the relative activity "per molecule". The molar adjusted eye irritation score then is calculated as follows:

1. The molarity of the solution (number of moles per liter) is obtained:

$$Molarity = (Density \times 1000)/Relative\ Molecular\ Mass$$

2. Density values are obtained from a standard source.
3. The molar adjusted eye irritation score is calculated as the original eye irritation score divided by the molarity of solution.

2.2 Eye Irritation Is Also Classified According to EEC Rules (1993) as: Nonirritant; R36-Irritant; R41-Severe Irritant

2.3 Physicochemical Descriptors of the Chemicals

A total of 23 physicochemical parameters describing three main chemical features (hydrophobicity, size and shape, and electronic characteristics) of each molecule are calculated.

Hydrophobicity is modeled using a calculated estimate of the logarithm of the octanol-water partition coefficient (ClogP) obtained from the MEDCHEM software. The estimate is based on the fragmental approach, with appropriate correction factors. The square of the partition coefficient is used to describe the possible parabolic relationship between eye irritation and hydrophobicity.

Shape and size are modeled by molecular connectivities and calculated molar refractivity. Molecular connectivities are calculated from a knowledge of the interatom structure and connectivity within a molecule. As such they are thought to describe the size or bulk of a molecule. Kappa indices are calculated in a similar manner, but are thought to measure more sutble effects such as molecular shape, symmetry, and flexibility. In addition to molecular weight, therefore, the following molecular connectivities are calculated using the MOLCONN-X software: zero- to third-order simple and valence-corrected path molecular connectivities; zero- to third-order Kappa alpha, and first- to third-order Kappa indices.

Electronic Parameters are calculated estimates of the compound's reactivity and stability, obtained from molecular modeling techniques and molecular orbital calculations. Each molecule is modeled using the QUANTA software and the molecular geometry partially minimized. Full geometry optimization is performed using the AM1 Hamiltonian in MOPAC6. On this optimized structure, AM1 molecular orbital calculations are performed to obtain the dipole moment, heat of formation and the energies of the highest occupied and lowest unoccupied molecular orbitals (HOMO and LUMO, respectively). HOMO and LUMO are thought to be good approximations of the electron donating and accepting capabilities, respectively, of the molecules.

2.4 Statistical Analysis

Relationships between the molar adjusted eye irritation score and the physicochemical parameters are investigated using forward stepwise regression analysis in the MINITAB statistical software. Stepwise regression is initially performed on the complete set of compounds and then on individual classes. Regression analysis is not a suitable technique for analyzing categorical data such as information as to whether a chemical is an eye irritant; other multivariate statistical methods are required. Stepwise linear discriminant analysis is applied to the dataset using the BMDP program P7M. This attempts to establish physicochemical parameters that will linearly separate the two groups of compounds (i.e., the eye irritants from nonirritants). Such techniques have been found to be successful for discriminating between mutagens and nonmutagens, and for other toxicological endpoints. The resulting model may not only provide a predictive technique for assessing compounds of unknown irritant potential, but also may shed some light on the underlying mechanism of toxic action. To distinguish parameters able to discriminate significantly between the two classifications, the default F-to-enter value of 4 is retained in the discriminant analysis. A reduction in this to facilitate the entry of parameters is not considered because it is felt that this would jeopardize the validity of any resulting linear discriminant function. Principal component analysis is also applied to the physicochemical data set using MINITAB statistical software. This proceeds by the formation of new orthogonal (i.e., uncorrelated) variables from the original data matrix. These new principal components contain as much of the variance of the data as possible and are seen as a valuable method of understanding the information contained in a physicochemical data set. Each new variable is made up of a linear combination of all the physicochemical parameters such that with reference to the original data, interpretation can be made of the principal components. For each chemical, a score can be calculated for each of the significant principal components. These then are utilized in simple plots as an unsupervised (i.e., without prior knowledge of the biological activity) pattern recognition technique.

2.5 List of the Chemicals
Acetates

1. Methyl trimethyl acetate
2. Ethyl trimethyl acetate
3. n-Butyl acetate
4. Ethyl acetate
5. Cellosolve acetate
6. Ethyl-2-methylacetoacetate
7. Methyl acetate
8. Triacetine

Acids

9. 2,2,-Dimethylbutanoic acid

Alcohols

10. Propylene glycol
11. Glycerol
12. Isopropanol
13. 2-Ethyl-1-hexanol
14. Isobutanol
15. n-Butanol
16. Hexanol
17. Butyl cellosolve
18. Cyclohexanol
19. 2-Propenol
20. 2-Methoxyethanol
21. 1-Octanol
22. 2(2-Ethoxyethoxy)ethanol

Aromatics

23. 4,4,-Methylene bis(2,6-di-tert-butyl) phenol
24. 4-Bromophenetole
25. 3-Chloro-4-fluoronitrobenzene
26. 1,3-Diisopropylbenzene
27. 1-Methylpropylbenzene
28. 3-Ethyltoluene
29. 2,4-Difluoronitrobenzene
30. Styrene
31. Toluene
32. Xylene
33. 2,6-Dichlorobenzoyl chloride
34. 4-Carboxybenzaldehyde
35. 4-Fluoroaniline

Hydrocarbons

36. 3-Methylhexane
37. 2-Methylhexane
38. 1,9-Decadiene
39. Dodecane
40. 1,5-Dimethylcyclooctadiene
41. cis-Cyclooctene
42. Methylcyclopentane
43. 1,5-Hexadiene
44. Methyl isobutyl ketone
45. Methyl amyl ketone
46. Methyl ethyl ketone
47. Acetone

Miscellaneous

48. Chloroform
49. Skolelal
50. Dimethylsulfoxide
51. Diethyl amine
52. Formamide
53. Methyl formamide

2.6 QSAR Analysis of Maximum Draize Eye Score

Stepwise regression analysis of the eye irritation scores for all the compounds in the dataset against the 23 physicochemical parameters reveals the following three QSARs:

$$\text{Molar Eye Score} = -0.118(\text{ClogP})^2 + 3.33$$

$n = 38$, $r^2 = 0.16$, $s = 2.56$, $F = 8.2$

where:

Molar Eye Score = Draize eye irritation score adjusted for molarity of solution

$(ClogP)^2$ = square of the calculated logarithm of the octanol-water partition coefficient
n = number of observations
r^2 = coefficient of determination adjusted for degrees of freedom
s = standard error of the estimate
F = F statistic

$$\text{Molar Eye Score} = -0.125(ClogP)^2 + 0.713 \text{ LUMO} + 2.33$$

n = 38, r^2 = 0.27, s = 2.40, F = 7.7
where:
LUMO = energy of the lowest unoccupied molecular orbital

$$\text{Molar Eye Score} = -0.156(ClogP)^2 + 1.13 \text{ LUMO} + 0.397 \text{ kalpha0} - 0.44$$

n = 38, r^2 = 0.35, s = 2.26, F = 7.6
where:
kalpha0 = zero order kappa alpha index
In QSAR much reliance is placed on the statistical analysis of the relationship to assess its validity and quality. An excellent relationship might be defined as having an r^2 greater than 0.9, with a low standard error and a highly significant F statistic. As the statistics for a QSAR become less significant, the QSAR's value as a predictive tool for comprehension of the mechanism of action decreases. It must, however, be noted that a QSAR can only be as good as the original data. All biological data will contain error that will be transferred to the goodness-of-fit of an equation. For the above equations for all the compounds in the dataset, no statistically significant QSARs are obtained, suggesting that it is not possible to model the eye irritation responses of such a chemically heterogeneous set of compounds. When, however, certain subgroups of the dataset are studied, improvements in the quality of the QSARs are observed.

For the alcohols, stepwise regression with the 23 physicochemical parameters gives the following two QSARs:

$$\text{Molar Eye Score} = 2.06 \text{ ClogP} + 4.13$$

n = 9, r^2 = 0.72, s = 1.89, F = 21.3
where:
ClogP = calculated logarithm of the octanol-water partition coefficient

$$\text{Molar Eye Score} = 1.72 \text{ ClogP} + 9.04 \text{ HOMO} + 102$$

n = 9, r^2 = 0.80, s = 1.58, F = 17.3
where:
HOMO = energy of the highest occupied molecular orbital
Both equations are highly significant, revealing that more than 80% of the variance of the biological activity can be explained by parameters describing hydrophobicity and the electron-donating capabilities of the molecule. This suggests that for the alcohols, transport of the molecule as described by ClogP is the most important feature governing eye irritation; and to a lesser extent, electronic reactivity as described by HOMO.

For the acetates, a somewhat different QSAR is obtained:

$$\text{Molar Eye Score} = -1.37 \text{ ClogP} + 2.97$$

n = 7, r^2 = 0.74, s = 0.52, F = 18.2

Again, ClogP is the best correlated single parameter to eye irritation score. In this equation, however, a negative slope is obtained with hydrophobicity, suggesting that the more hydrophobic acetates are weaker eye irritants. This may be a result of such compounds being retained more readily in lipid tissue and not reaching the active site, or may possibly be the downslope of a parabolic relationship between eye irritation and ClogP. No statistically significant two-parameter equation is obtained for the acetates from stepwise regression. Such an equation would have to be treated with caution as it would break the QSAR "rule of thumb" stating that in a regression equation there should be a greater than five to one ratio of number of observations to physicochemical parameters. For the other subgroups of chemicals studied, no QSARs can be formed, owing to lack of data for strong eye irritants. For instance, the hydrocarbons in the dataset show a small range of activity, but this is much too insignificant to be used in a meaningful QSAR analysis.

2.7 QSAR Analysis of Categorical Data

Stepwise linear discriminant analysis on the expanded eye irritation dataset with 23 physiochemical parameters has found no significant variables that can discriminate between the eye irritants and nonirritants. This suggests that there is no linear distribution of the irritants with any of the variables considered.

BIBLIOGRAPHY

Cronin, M. T. D., D. A. Basketter and M. York, A quantitative structure-activity relationship (QSAR) investigation of a Draize eye irritation database, *Toxicology In Vitro*, Vol. 8, No. 1, p. 21, 1994.

QSAR APPLIED TO THE DRAIZE EYE TEST 2
(MULTI-CASE METHODOLOGY)

1. METHOD

The use of QSAR in toxicology consists of the analysis of different quantitative parameters of a chemical that could be related to biological activities. The guideline's description for this method cannot conform, at present, to the format so far developed by OECD experts. This description is an attempt to organize the material in a way to allow analysis of the data according to a procedure used by some authors.

2.1 Description of the Test Method

The Multiple Computer Automated Structure Evaluation (Multi-CASE) methodology is an artificial intelligence system capable of analyzing a set of chemicals with defined biological activity. It is a computer-assisted expert system that correlates the structural and physico-chemical parameters of organic chemicals with a specified pattern of their activity in biological systems. When being trained, the system analyzes the experimental data and creates an expert dictionary of structural and physicochemical descriptors found relevant to activity. This dictionary can be used to predict the activity of novel compounds. The input required to train the Multi-CASE system for toxicity predictions includes chemical structures and their experimental toxicity values. Chemical structures can be entered through the computer terminal graphically or by using the Klopman Line Notation code. Multi-CASE automatically breaks up each molecule of the training set into all possible linear fragments of 2 to 20 heavy atoms with attached hydrogens. The relevance of each individual fragment to toxicity is determined by its distribution between toxic and nontoxic molecules. The fragments that occur randomly in both toxic and nontoxic molecules are assumed to be irrelevant to observed toxicity. Each fragment exhibiting statistically significant deviation from such random distribution, and encountered predominantly in either toxic or nontoxic molecules, is believed to contribute toxicity (biophore) or lake of toxicity (biophobe), respectively. The presence of a biophore in a molecule is assumed to be a prerequisite for toxicity. Initially, Multi-CASE uses the whole database to identify a fragment that can account uniquely for the toxicity of the largest number of chemicals in the database. All the compounds whose activities can be explained on the basis of the same biophore are removed from the set. The remainder of the data are searched for the next most significant attribute. Once that attribute is found, the data set is reduced again. The procedure is repeated until the toxicity (or lack of such) for every compound has been explained or no additional biophores or biophobes can be identified. Local QSAR analysis then is performed on each subset of congeneric molecules containing the same biophore. During the analysis, the relevance of physicochemical properties is established. Biophores, biophobes, and pertinent physicochemical parameters constitute the expert dictionary. New data then can be submitted to the program for *a priori* predictions of toxicity. On receiving a query structure, Multi-CASE uses the expert dictionary to identify the presence of relevant attributes in a molecule to make a prediction. To train the system, the experimental toxicity can be entered as the actual numerical values whenever such data are available. Predictions then are given in the same units as entered for the training set. In cases when only qualitative or semiquantitative data are available, Multi-CASE uses internal activity units ranging from 10 to 99.

Multi-CASE Index	Index Interpretation
10–19	Nontoxic
20–19	Marginally toxic
30–39	Toxic
40–49	Very toxic
50–99	Extremely toxic

In this study, the Multi-CASE methodology is used to develop a predictive model of ocular irritation based on an evaluation of the significance of chemical structure in the induction of eye irritation. The Multi-CASE program is trained with a noncongeneric database of 186 compounds, previously evaluated in a modified Draize test for their ability to cause eye irritation *in vivo*. Multi-CASE analysis creates an expert dictionary of structural attributes pertaining to eye irritation. These attributes are used by the Multi-CASE program to predict a priori the eye irritation potential of test chemicals. The "challenge" set of test materials consists of 21 individual chemicals, chemical mixtures, and polymers. The irritation potential of chemical mixtures is determined on the basis of the structures of the major constituents under the assumption of accumulative effects of eye irritation properties. Irritation potential of polymers is assessed on the basis of the structure of the repeat units. In the eye irritation tests, the measure of toxicity is a Draize score. The reproducibility of the numerical Draize scores is too low to be used directly in the Multi-CASE analysis. Therefore, the data are grouped into six categories based on six eye irritation judgments (EIJs) to make it more consistent. The EIJs are determined by both the maximum Draize score and the number of days it takes the eye to return to its normal appearance. EIJs are verbal descriptors; thus, the analysis is semiquantitative. For such an analysis, it is convenient to enter the Multi-CASE internal units of activity directly on input, choosing them in such a way as to adequately present the toxicity of molecules to the program. Five activity indices are used. Each index corresponds to a certain EIJ. Predictions are also made in Multi-CASE units and can be translated easily into EIJ values. The database (learning set) consists in 186 compounds originated from three sources. Each source uses a different scale, making it necessary to establish equivalency between them. Avon Products Inc. provides *in vivo* results for 66 of the compounds from their historical database. Eye irritation potential has been scored on the 110-point Draize scale and classified using the Kay & Calandra scale. Three to six rabbits per chemical are used. Animals are adult New Zealand White rabbits of either sex, weighing 1.6 to 2 kg. Anesthesia is used when appropriate. Observations of ocular changes are made on the first, second, third, fourth, and seventh days after instillation. Each observation yields a numerical Draize score based on changes in the cornea, iris, and conjunctivae. The maximum daily score then is selected to represent the eye irritation potential of the chemical. Based on the Draize score and recovery time, six irritation judgments (nonirritating, minimal, mild, moderate, severe, and extreme) are used to characterize the degree of chemical injury. All nonirritating and minimally irritating chemicals are assigned a Multi-CASE index of 10, and both groups are therefore treated as nontoxic. Mild irritants fall into the category of marginally active (Multi-CASE index = 25). Moderate, severe, and extreme irritants form the active group. Most of the remaining 120 compounds are tested according to a somewhat different protocol, described by Carpenter & Smyth. One of the major differences is that a 10-point rather than a 110-point rating scale is used. The Draize irritation judgment is the most suitable yardstick for establishing equivalency between the results of Avon Products Inc. and those of Carpenter & Smyth. Indeed, a 10-point scale can be conveniently broken into five regions of two points each. The number of such regions equals the number of Multi-CASE activity indices assigned to Avon chemicals based on their irritation judgments.

Avon EIJ	Carpenter 10-Point Scale	Multi-CASE Index
Non/minimal	1–2	10
Mild	3–4	25
Moderate	5–6	35
Severe	7–8	45
Extreme	9–10	55

Using the total (combined) data set and the standard Multi-CASE program, 37 substructures are found to be relevant to the eye irritation potential of organic chemicals.

No.	Activity	Substructure
1.	active	$N=CH-$
2.	active	NH_2-CH_2-
3.	active	$Cl-CH-$
4.	inactive	$=C-O-$
5.	active	$CO-OH-$
6.	active	SO_2-O-
7.	active	$N-CH_2-CH_3$
8.	active	$NH-CH-CH_3$
9.	active	$NH-CH_2-CH_2-$
10.	active	$OH-C=C-$
11.	active	$OH-CH_2-C=$
12.	active	$OH-CO-CH_2-$
13.	active	$Cl-Si-Cl$
14.	active	$CO-O-CO-$
15.	active	$SO_2-O^\wedge Na+$
16.	active	$CH=C(-C)-CH=$
17.	active	$CH=C(-Cl)-CH=$
18.	active	$CH_3-CH(-NH_2)-CH_2-$
19.	active	$Cl-CH(-COH)-CH_2-$
20.	active	$C=CH-C=C-$
21.	inactive	$CH=C-CH_2-CH-$

22.	active	$O-CH=CH-CH=$
23.	active	$O^-CH-CH-O^\wedge$
24.	inactive	$O-CO-CH_2-N-$
25.	active	$OH-CH_2-CH-NH_2$
26.	active	$OH-CH_2-CH_2-N-$
27.	active	$Cl-CO-CH-Cl$
28.	active	$CH_2-O-CH(-CH_2)-CH_2-$
29.	active	$CH_2-CH_2-N-CH_2-CH_2-$
30.	active	$OH-CH-CH_2-CH-CH_2-$
31.	active	$OH-CH_2-CH-CH_2-CH_3$
32.	active	$Na^\wedge+\cdot-^\wedge O-CO-CH_2-CH_2-$
33.	active	$CO-O-CH_2-CH_2-Cl$
34.	active	$COH-CH_2-CH-CH_2-COH$
35.	active	$OH-CH_2-CH_2-O-CH_2-CH-$
36.	active	$Br-CH_2-CH=CH-CH_2-Br$
37.	inactive	$CH_3-CH_2-CH_2-CH_2-CH_2-CH_2-CH_2-CH_2-CH=$

Note: $O^\wedge$ = epoxide oxygen.
– open valence indicates a bond to a nonhydrogen, nonoxygen atom.

3. PROCEDURES

Local QSAR analyses are performed for groups of compounds containing specific biophores. Within each group, the program provides successful retrofits of the experimental eye irritation data.

3.1 Local QSAR Result for Biophores CO–OH, CO–Cl, and SO₂–O⁻
Equation:

$$EIJ = -32.45[CH=C-CH_2-CH-]-24.42[CH=C-CH=C-]$$

$$- 21.25[CH=CH-C(CO)=CH-CH=]-29.94[O-CH_2-CH_3]$$

$$- 0.82[LOG\ P]-5.63[HO-CO-CH_2] + 10.53[SO_2-\ OH] + 58.13$$

$F(7, 17, 0.05) = 26.06$, n = 25, $R^2 = 0.92$

3.2 Local QSAR Result for Biophore C=CH–C=C–
Equation:

$$EIJ = -10.09[NH2-C=]-9.77[CO-OH] + 8.77[HO-C=CH-C=]$$

$$+ 0.47[LOG\ P] + 9.27[O-\ CH-] + 44.70$$

$F(5, 3, 0.05) =126.79$, n= 9, $R^2 = 0.99$

3.3 Local QSAR Result for Biophore –CO–O–CO–
Equation:

$$EIJ = -7.01[CO-CH_2]-56.01$$

$F(1, 2, 0.05) = 20.79$, n = 4, $R^2 = 0.91$

3.4 Local QSAR Result for Biophore CH₂–O–CH–CH₂–
Equation:

EIJ = 25.77[CH$_2$–CH$_2$–CH–CH$_2$] + 32.63[O^–CH–CH–O^] + 3.06[LOG P] + 23.06

$F(3, 6, 0.05) = 100.6$, n = 10, $R^2 = 0.98$

A test set of 21 chemicals, with experimentally determined eye irritation potential, is taken randomly from the initial data and submitted for evaluation by the Multi-CASE program. None of these 21 chemicals are included in the learning set. Importantly, any structural bias is avoided intentionally during the selection of the test set. Indeed, the model is intended to make predictions for structurally diverse novel molecules from different chemical classes that may or may not overlap with the chemical space of the learning set. There is an extended agreement between the eye irritation potentials predicted by Multi-CASE and those determined *in vivo*.

BIBLIOGRAPHY

Klopman, G., D. Ptchelintsev, M. Frierson, S. Pennisi, K. Renskers and M. Dickens, Multiple Computer Automated Structure Evaluation methodology as an alternative to *in vivo* eye irritation testing, *ATLA*, Vol. 21, p. 14, 1993.

QSAR APPLIED TO THE DRAIZE EYE TEST 3

1. METHOD

The use of QSAR in toxicology consists of analysis of different quantitative parameters of a chemical that could be related to biological activities. The guideline's description for this method cannot conform, at present, to the format so far developed by OECD experts. This description is an attempt to organize the material in a way to allow analysis of the data according to a procedure used by some authors.

2.1 Description of the Test Method

The method proposed permits the measurement of pH and acidic/alkaline reserve of all types of chemicals, under conditions that reproduce possible hydrolysis, in order to identify chemicals severely irritant to the eye. Under these conditions, the pH and the acidic/alkaline reserve of 166 chemicals from different chemical classes are measured. According to EEC classification criteria, 90 chemicals are considered to be nonirritant, 22 irritant, and 54 severely irritant to the eye. These physicochemical parameters, individually or in combination, are then correlated with the results from ocular irritation tests.

After 10 g of the test substance (liquid or solid) is added to 100 ml of distilled water in a 250-ml beaker, the solution or suspension is maintained for 4 h with agitation at 37°C. Directly in the solution, or in the aqueous phase of suspensions (after decantation or centrifugation), the pH is measured and titrated with diluted sodium hydroxide or hydrochloric acid until neutrality (pH 7 to 8) is obtained. The acidic or alkaline reserve (R) is expressed as the number of grams of pure acid or base necessary to neutralize 100 g of product (%).

The physicochemical index is defined as a weighting of the pH by the decimal logarithm of the acidic/alkaline reserve:

Index = pH + log R for pH ≥ 7
Index = (14-pH) + log R for pH <7.

For three parameters — pH, acidic/alkaline reserve, and physicochemical index — the sensitivity, the specificity and the predictive value are determined. The physicochemical index has the greatest sensitivity (83% of the SI products correctly identified) and predictive value of noncorrosive potential (91% of the products with index <9 are not severely irritant). The pH value has the best specificity (98% of the NI/I products has pH >2.5 or 9.5) and predictive value of corrosiveness (94% of the products having pH ≤2.5 or ≥9.5 are severely irritant). The best equivalence (88%) between the *in vitro* and *in vivo* results is obtained the decimal logarithm of the acidic/alkaline reserve. Finally, all chemicals that meet at least two of the following three criteria are considered as potentially severely irritant:

pH ≤ 2.5 or pH ≤ 9.5

log R ≥ 0

I ≥ 9

Under these conditions, it is possible to identify 74% of the SI products with a predictive value of 93%, and 97% of the NI/I products with a predictive value of 88%.

BIBLIOGRAPHY

Regnier, J. F. and C. Imbert, Contributions of physicochemical properties to the evaluation of ocular irritation, *ATLA*, Vol. 20, p. 457, 1992.

SALMONELLA TYPHIMURIUM — REVERSE MUTATION ASSAY (92/69/EEC DIR.)

1. METHOD

1.1 Introduction, 1.2 Definition, and 1.3. Reference Substances
None.

1.4 Principle of the Test Method
The *Salmonella typhimurium* histidine (his) reversion system is a microbial assay that measures his⁻-his⁺ reversion by chemicals which cause base substitutions or frameshift mutations in the genome of this organism.

Bacteria are exposed to test chemicals with and without metabolic activation and plated on minimal medium. After a suitable period of incubation, revertant colonies are counted and compared to the number of spontaneous revertants in an untreated and/or solvent control culture.

1.5 Quality Criteria
None.

1.6 Description of the Test Method
1.6.1 Preparations
1.6.1.1 Bacteria
Fresh cultures of bacteria are grown at 37°C until late exponential or early stationary phase of growth. Approximate cell density should be 10^8 to 10^9 cells per milliliter.

1.6.1.2 Metabolic Activation
Bacteria should be exposed to the test substance both in the presence and absence of an appropriate mammalian liver enzyme activation mixture (a cofactor supplemented postmitochondrial fraction) prepared from mice or rats pretreated with enzyme inducing agents.

1.6.2 Test Conditions
Tester Strains
At least four strains (TA 1535, TA 1537 or TA 97, TA 98, and TA 100) are to be used; other strains, such as TA 1538 and TA 102, may be used in addition. Recognized methods of stock culture preparation and storage are to be used. The growth requirements and the genetic identity of the strains, their sensitivity to UV radiation and crystal violet, and their resistance to ampicillin

must be checked. The strains also should yield spontaneous revertants within the frequency ranges expected.

Media

An appropriate selective medium is used with an adequate overlay agar.

Use of Negative and Positive Controls

Concurrent untreated and solvent controls have to be performed. Positive controls have to be conducted also for two purposes:

1. To confirm the sensitivity of the bacterial strains. The following compounds may be used for tests without metabolic activations:

    Strains revert with
    *   TA 1535, TA 100 Sodium azide
    *   TA 1538, TA 98 TA 97 2-nitrofluorene
    *   TA 1537 9-aminoacridine
    *   TA 102 cumene hydroperoxide

2. To ensure the activity of the appropriate metabolizing system. A positive control for the activity of one metabolizing system for all strains is 2-aminoanthracene. When available a positive control of the same chemical class as the chemical under test should be used.

Amount of Test Substance per Plate

At least five different amounts of test chemical are tested, with half-log intervals between plates. Substances are tested up to the limit of solubility or toxicity. Toxicity is evidenced by a reduction in the number of spontaneous revertants, a clearing of the background lawn, or by degree of survival of treated cultures. Nontoxic chemicals should be tested to 5 mg per plate before considering the test substance negative.

Incubation Conditions

Plates are incubated for 48 to 72 h at 37°C.

1.6.3 Procedure

For the direct plate incorporation method without enzyme activation, the test chemical and 0.1 ml of fresh bacterial culture are added to 2.0 ml of overlay agar. For tests with metabolic activation, 0.5 ml of liver enzyme activation mixture containing an adequate amount of postmitochondrial fraction is added to the agar overlay after the addition of the test chemical and bacteria. The contents of each tube are mixed and poured over the surface of a selective agar plate. Overlay agar is allowed to solidify and plates are incubated at 37°C for 48 to 72 h. At the end of the incubation period, revertant colonies per plate are counted. For the preincubation method, a mixture of the test chemical, 0.1 ml of fresh bacterial culture and an adequate amount of liver enzyme activation mixture or the same amount of buffer is preincubated before adding 2.0 ml of overlay agar. All other procedures are the same as for the direct plate incorporation method.

All plating for both methods is done at least in triplicate.

2. DATA

The number of revertant colonies per plate are reported for both control and treated series.

Individual plate counts, the mean number of revertant colonies per plate and standard deviation should be presented for the tested chemical and the controls.

All results are confirmed in an independent experiment.

Data should be evaluated using appropriate statistical methods.

At least two independent experiments are conducted. It is not necessary to perform the second one in an identical way to the initial experiment. Indeed, it may be preferable to alter certain test conditions in order to obtain more useful data.

3. REPORTING
3.1 Test Report
The test report shall, if possible, include the following information:

- bacteria, strain used;
- test conditions: dose levels, toxicity, composition of media, treatment procedures (preincubation, incubation) liver enzyme activation mixture, reference substances, negative controls;
- individual plate count, the mean number of revertant colonies per plate, standard deviation, dose/effect relationship when possible;
- discussion of the results;
- interpretation of the results.

3.2 Evaluation and Interpretation
There are several criteria for determining a positive result, one of which is a statistically significant dose-related increase in the number of revertants. Another criterion may be the detection of a reproducible and statistically significant positive response for at least one of the test points. A test substance producing neither a statistically significant dose-related increase in the number of revertants nor a statistically significant and reproducible positive response at any one of the test points is considered non-mutagenic in this system. Positive results from the *S. typhimurium* reverse mutation assay indicate that a substance induces point mutations by base changes or frameshifts in the genome of this organism. Negative results indicate that under the test conditions the test substance is not mutagenic in *S. thyphimurium*.

4. ALTERNATIVE TO ANIMAL TEST
This method is used for the identification of mutagenic chemicals.

BIBLIOGRAPHY

Annex to Commission Directive 92/69/EEC, 31 July 1992, Adapting to technical progress for the seventeenth time Council Directive 67/548/EEC on the approximation of laws, regulations and administrative provisions relating to the classification, packaging and labelling of dangerous substances, *Official Journal of the European Communities,* No. L383A, Vol. 35, p. 160, 1992.

Ames B., J. McCann and E. Yamasaki, Methods for detecting carcinogens and mutagens with the *Salmonella/* mammalian microsome mutagenicity test, *Mutation Research,* Vol. 31, p. 347, 1975.

Note: The *Salmonella typhimurium* and *Escherichia coli* reverse mutation assays are being combined at present by OECD experts in one single guideline.

SEX-LINKED RECESSIVE LETHAL TEST IN *DROSOPHILA MELANOGASTER* (87/302/EEC DIR.)

1. METHOD

1.1. Introduction, 1.2. Definition, and 1.3. Reference Substances
None.

1.4. Principles of the Test Method

The sex-linked recessive lethal (SLRL) test using *Drosophila melanogaster* detects the occurrence of mutations, both point mutations and small deletions, in the germ line of the insect. This test is a forward mutation assay capable of screening for mutations at about 800 loci of the X-chromosome; this represents about 80% of all X-chromosomal loci. The X-chromosome represents approximately one fifth of the entire haploid genome. Mutations in the X-chromosome of *D. melanogaster* are expressed phenotypically in males carrying the mutant gene. When the mutation is lethal in the hemizygous condition, its presence is inferred from the absence of one class of male offspring out of the two that normally are produced by a heterozygous female. The SLRL test takes advantage of these facts by means of specially marked and arranged chromosomes.

1.5 Quality Criteria
None.

1.6 Description of the Test Method
16.61 Preparations
Stocks

Males of a well-defined wild-type stock and females of the Muller-5 stock may be used. Other appropriately marked female stocks with multiple inverted X-chromosomes also may be used.

Test Substance

The test substance should be dissolved in water. Substances which are insoluble in water may be dissolved or suspended in appropriate vehicles (e.g., a mixture of ethanol and Tween-60 or 80), then diluted in water or saline prior to administration. Dimethylsulfoxide (DMSO) should be avoided as a vehicle.

Number of Animals

The test should be designed with a predetermined sensitivity and power. The spontaneous mutant frequency observed in the appropriate control will influence strongly the number of treated chromosomes that must be analyzed.

Route of Administration

Exposure may be oral, by injection, or by exposure to gases or vapors. Feeding of the test may be done in sugar solution. When necessary, substances may be dissolved in a 0.7% NaCl solution into the thorax or abdomen.

Exposure Levels

Three exposure levels should be used. For a preliminary assessment, one exposure level of the test substance may be used, that exposure level being either the maximum tolerated concentration or that producing some indication of toxicity. For nontoxic substances, exposure to the maximum practicable concentration should be used.

Procedure

Wild-type males (3 to 5 d old) are treated with the test substance and mated individually to an excess of virgin females from the Muller-5 stock or from another appropriately marked (with multiple inverted X-chromosomes) stock. The females are replaced with fresh virgins every two to three days to cover the entire germ cell-cycle. The offspring of these females are scored for lethal effects corresponding to the effects on mature sperm, mid or late-stage spermatids, early spermatids, spermatocytes, and spermatogonia at the time of treatment. Heterozygous F1 females from the above crosses are allowed to mate individually (i.e., one female per vial) with their brothers. In the F2 generation, each culture is scored for the absence of wild-type males. If a culture appears to have arisen from an F1 female carrying a lethal in the parental X-chromosome (i.e., no males with the treated chromosome are observed) daughters of that female with the same genotype should be tested to ascertain whether the lethality is repeated in the next generation.

2. DATA

Data should be tabulated to show the number of X-chromosomes tested, the number of nonfertile males and the number of lethal chromosomes at each exposure concentration and for each mating period for each male treated. Numbers of clusters of different sizes per male should be reported. These results should be confirmed in a separate experiment. Appropriate statistical methods should be used in evaluation of sex-linked lethal tests. Clustering of recessive lethals originating from one male should be considered and evaluated in an appropriate statistical manner.

3. REPORTING
3.1 Test Report

The test report shall, if possible, contain the following information:

- stock: Drosophila stocks or strains used, age of insects, number of males treated, number of sterile males, number of F2 culture established, number of F2 cultures without progeny, number of chromosomes carrying a lethal detected at each germ cell stage;
- criteria for establishing the size of treated groups;
- test conditions: detailed description of treatment and sampling schedule, exposure levels, toxicity data, negative (solvent) and positive controls, if appropriate;
- criteria for establishing the size of treated groups;
- exposure/effect relationship where possible;
- evaluation of data;
- discussion of results;
- interpretation of results.

3.2 Evaluation and Interpretation

There are several criteria for determining a positive response, one of which is a statistically significant dose-related increase in the frequency of sex-linked recessive lethal.

Positive results from the SLRL-test in *Drosophila* indicate that a substance induces mutations in the germ line of the insect. Negative results indicate that, under the test conditions the test substance does not induce mutations in the germ line of the insect.

BIBLIOGRAPHY

Commission Directive 87/302/EEC, 18 November 1987, Adapting to technical progress for the ninth time Council Directive 67/548/EEC on the approximation of laws, regulations and administrative provisions relating to the classification, packaging and labelling of dangerous substances, *Official Journal of the European Communities*, No. L133, Vol. 31, p. 71, 1988.

TETRAHYMENA THERMOPHYLA MOTILITY ASSAY

1. METHOD

1.1 Introduction, 1.2 Definition, and 1.3 Reference Substances (to be defined)

1.4 Principle of the Test Method

The *Tetrahymena* motility assay is used to identify cytotoxic chemicals (water soluble or water miscible substances). The endpoint is the dilution of test material that inhibits by 10% of the normal motility.

1.5 Quality Criteria (to be defined)

1.6 Description of the Test Method

1.6.1 Preparations

Chemical dilutions are prepared just before they are ready to be tested.
Tetrahymena thermophila, ATCC 30377.

1.6.2 Test Conditions

Number of Cultures

The test is performed in triplicate.

Use of Negative and Positive Controls

The negative control culture is *Tetrahymena* suspension in 0.4% NaCl.

The positive control culture is 1% sodium hydroxide diluted at 1:50, 1:55, and 1:60 (historic control values).

Exposure Concentrations

(to be defined)

Culture Conditions

(to be defined)

1.6.3 Procedure

1.6.3.1 Preparation of Cultures

Tetrahymena thermophila is grown in 15-ml, screw-top glass test tubes, in MM2 medium composed by liver powder 0.1%, *Saccharomyces cerevisiae* 0.1%, soy lecithin 0.001%, and distilled water to 100 ml for 48 h at 21°C. Cultures are not synchronized as to the stage of the cell cycle or the number of organisms present.

1.6.3.2 Treatment of the Cultures with the Test Substance

First, 50 µl of the diluted chemicals and 50 µl of *Tetrahymena* suspension are mixed in a test tube for 2 to 3 sec on a low-speed vortex action mixer. Just prior to the 2-min exposure time after the mixing of the test sample and the *Tetrahymena*, a bacteriological loopful of this suspension is placed on a microscope coverslip. The coverslip is inverted onto a microscope depression slide and the mixture examined at 40 or 100 magnifications, at the 2-min exposure time, using low-light illumination. The motility of the cell, excluding speed of movement, is evaluated.

1.6.3.3 Analysis

The highest tolerated dose is the dilution of test chemical that allowed 90% cell motility. The reciprocals of the highest tolerated doses are averaged.

2. DATA

3. REPORTING

3.1 Test Report

The test report shall, if possible, include the following information:

- test conditions: detailed description of treatment and sampling schedule, dose levels, toxicity data, negative and positive controls;
- dose/effect relationship when possible;
- statistical evaluation;
- discussion of the results;
- interpretation of the results.

3.2 Evaluation and Interpretation
(to be defined)

4. ALTERNATIVE TO ANIMAL TEST
This method may be used in the identification of cytotoxic chemicals.

BIBLIOGRAPHY

Gettings, S.D., J. J. Teal, D. M. Bagley, J. L. Demetrulias, L. C. Di Pasquale, K. L. Hintze, M. G. Rozen, S. L. Weise, M. Chudkowski, K. D. Marenus, W. J. W. Pape, M. Roddy, R. Schnetzinger, P. M. Silber, S. M. Glaza and P. J. Kurtz, The CTFA evaluation of alternatives program: An evaluation of *in vitro* alternatives to the Draize primary eye irritation test (Phase 1) Hydro-alcoholic formulations; (Part 2) Data analysis and biological significance, *In Vitro Toxicology*, Vol. 4, No. 4, p. 247, 1991.

INVITTOX Protocol No. 22, June 1991.

TETRAZOLIUM SALT ASSAY (MTT)

1. METHOD

1.1 Introduction, 1.2 Definition, and 1.3 Reference Substances (to be defined)

1.4 Principle of the Test Method
The MTT assay is a cytotoxic assay used to identify reduction of cell viability and alteration of cell metabolism on both established cell lines and primary cultures exposed to test chemicals. MTT (3-[4,5-dimethylthiazol-2-yl]-2,5-dephenyl tetrazolium bromide) is a soluble pale yellow salt that is reduced by mitochondrial succinate dehydrogenase of living cells to form an insoluble dark blue formazan product. After solubilization and extraction of the formazan, the absorbance is determined spectrophotometrically.

1.5 Quality Criteria (to be defined)

1.6 Description of the Test Method
1.6.1 Preparations
Test chemicals are prepared in medium, or in distilled water or DMSO, then diluted in serum-free culture medium: final DMSO concentration must not exceed 1%. When present, DMSO is used at the same concentration for all chemical concentrations.

Other solvent: methanol.

Hydro-alcoholic formulations are assayed at 0.1% v/v dilution.

Primary cultures (rabbit tracheal epithelium; freshly and cryopreserved rat, dog, and human hepatocytes), secondary cultures (human dermal fibroblasts) or established cell lines (keratinocytes, Clonetics' EpiPack®; human fetal dermal fibroblasts, CCRL 1475; FaO hepatoma; BALB 3T3 fibroblast cell line; L929 cell line) are used.

1.6.2 Test Conditions
Number of Cultures
From two to eight cultures are used for each experimental point.

Use of Negative and Positive Controls
Negative control (medium) is used.

Exposure Concentrations
For screening experiments, chemicals are tested at half-interval dilutions starting at 2 mg/ml and 5% (v/v) for solid and liquid agents, respectively.

Culture Conditions
Appropriate culture medium, pretreatment time, dosing duration are used.

Metabolic Activation
(most chemicals require metabolic activation)

1.6.3 Procedure
1.6.3.1 Preparation of Cultures
Primary Cultures: Tracheas are removed from rabbits and the epithelium is separated from the underlying cartilage and cut into 2 mm explants. The explants are grown on collagen matrix and covered with minimum essential medium (MEM).

Hepatocytes are isolated from rats by the two-step collagenase perfusion method. Cell viability, measured by the trypan blue exclusion test (final concentration of dye: 0.05% in phosphate-buffered saline), is good if in excess of 85%. Cells are seeded at a density of 3×10^4 cells per well in 96-well plates (NUNC, Kamstrup, Denmark) in 100 µl nutrient medium. The medium consists of Williams' E medium (Flow, Les Ulis, France) containing 10% fetal calf serum (FCS, Boehringer, Mannheim, Germany), 0.1 IU bovine insulin/ml, 10 IU penicillin/ml, 10 µl streptomycin/ml and 2.5 mM-glutamine.

Human liver specimens are collected from multiorgan donors for transplantation. Human hepatocytes are obtained by a two-step collagenase perfusion and resuspended in Ham's F12 Coon's/Dulbecco's modified Eagle's medium (1:1, v/v) containing 10% FCS, and supplemented with penicillin, netilmicin, insulin, glucagon, thyroxine, sodium selenite, human transferrin, and ethanolamine (Sigma). Cell viability is determined using erythrosin B exclusion test. Hepatocytes are seeded at a density of 30×10^3 cells/100 µl, in 96-multiwell plates and incubated in a humidified, 5% CO_2 atmosphere at 37°C. Media are renewed after 4 h of adhesion.

Human liver specimens are collected from multiorgan donors for transplantation. Human hepatocytes, obtained by a two-step collagenase perfusion, are cryopreserved in Ham's F12 medium (Sigma) containing bovine serum albumin, polyvinylpyrrolidone PVP, 10% DMSO, and 20% FCS, in vials (1.8 ml Nunc), and stored in liquid nitrogen. Cryopreserved cells are directly thawed by immersing the vials in a 37°C water-bath and then purified by Percoll density gradient. Seeding is performed as above.

Rat, dog, and human hepatocytes are isolated by the two-step collagenase perfusion method; cell viability is estimated by the trypan blue exclusion test. Then, isolated hepatocytes are suspended at a density of 4×10^6 cells per ml in Leibovitz (L-15) medium containing 20% FCS. An equal volume of L-15 medium, containing 20% FCS and DMSO (the cryoprotective agent) is then slowly introduced. DMSO is added at a final concentration of 16, 14, and 12% for rat, dog, and human hepatocytes, respectively. The cells are distributed in freezing vials in 1.6 ml of medium per vial, then transferred at −20°C for 12 min to a −80°C freezer for 1 h and plunged in liquid nitrogen. For recovery storage, vials are warmed in a water-bath at 37°C and cell suspensions are gently pipetted. Each cell sample is transferred in 15 ml L-15 medium containing 0.6 or 0.8 M-glucose. Cell suspensions are centrifuged either directly or after being subjected to density gradient centrifugation on a Percoll 400 cushion to eliminate cell debris and dead cells. Freshly isolated and thawed hepatocytes are seeded at a density of 7×10^5 cells per 35-mm Petri dish in 2 ml culture medium and incubated at 37°C in a humidified atmosphere of 95% air/5% CO_2. The medium is a mixture of 75% minimum essential medium and 25% medium 199 supplemented with 0.1% bovine serum albumin, 5 µl bovine insulin/ml and 10% FCS.

Secondary Cultures: Normal human fibroblasts, isolated from the dermis of freshly obtained neonatal foreskins, are propagated in complete DMEM (Dulbecco's modified Eagle's medium, Gibco) containing 10% fetal bovine serum (Hyclone), nonessential amino acids (Gibco), 2 mM-L-glutamine (Gibco), 1 mM-sodium pyruvate (Gibco), 100 U penicillin G sodium/ml (Gibco), 100 µg streptomycin sulfate/ml (Gibco) and 0.25 µg/ml amphotericin B (Gibco); then they are seeded onto 8×8 cm nylon mesh, pretreated with acetic acid-fetal bovine serum, to obtain a three-dimensional substrate consisting of several layers of cells. When the cells become confluent (after 2 to 3 weeks), the sheets of nylon mesh are cut with a laser (Texcel) into 11×11 mm squares. Then these squares are placed into 24-well plates and treated.

Cell Lines: Keratinocytes (Clonetics' EpiPack®, grown in Clonetics' serum-free medium) and human fetal dermal fibroblasts (grown in DMEM with 10% fetal calf serum and penicillin/streptomycin), are plated in 96-well flat bottom plates and incubated for 24 h at 37°C, 5% CO_2.

FaO cells (subcloned from the hepatoma cell line H4IIEC3, isolated from the Reuber H35 hepatoma) are cultured in NCTC 135/Ham's F12 medium (v/v) supplemented with 5% FCS, 100 IU penicillin/ml, and 100 µl streptomycin/ml. The medium is renewed every 2 d and the cells are passaged after about 10 d when they reached subconfluency using 0.5% trypsin. After five transfers, the cells are stored in liquid nitrogen. For cytotoxicity studies, frozen FaO cells are thawed and put in culture; the functional capacity is controlled by measuring albumin secretion rates in media. After three passages, the cells are seeded in 96-well plates in Williams' E medium (Flow, Les Ulis, France) containing 10% fetal calf serum (FCS, Boehringer, Mannheim, Germany), 0.1 IU bovine insulin/ml, 10 IU penicillin/ml, 10 µl streptomycin/ml, and 2.5 mM-glutamine.

BALB c/3T3 (mouse embryonic lung fibroblasts, American Type Culture Collection) cells are maintained in DMEM, supplemented with 10% fetal bovine serum, 100 µg/ml streptomycin, 100 IU/ml penicillin G and 1.25 µg/ml Fungizone (Squibb & Sons, Princeton, NJ). They are grown in a humidified 5.5% CO_2 atmosphere at 37°C. The cells then are dissociated in a solution containing 0.5 g trypsin and 0.2 g ethylenediaminetetraacetic acid (EDTA) in 100 ml phosphate-buffered saline (PBS). Cells are plated in 0.2 ml of medium per well (in a 96-well tissue-culture microtiter plate) at $4–5 \times 10^4$ cells/ml.

L929, a mouse fibroblast cell line, is grown as a monolayer in Eagle's Minimum Essential Medium (Biological Industries), supplemented with 10% fetal calf serum (Nordvacc), 50 µg gentamicin/ml (Nordvacc), 1% nonessential amino acids and 2 mM-L-glutamine (Biological Industries). The cells are subcultivated twice a week using 0.1% trypsin (Nordvacc) in phosphate-buffered saline without Ca^{2+} and Mg^{2+}, and maintained at 37°C in humidified air with 5% CO_2. Then the cells are taken from confluent cultures and inoculated into 96-well tissue culture plates (Greiner) at a density of 7,000 cells/cm².

1.6.3.2 Treatment of the Cultures with the Test Substance

Primary Cultures: Chemicals are applied on day 7 (on cells that are near the end of the exponential growth phase) and MTT measurements are carried out after 24 h of treatments. 500 μl MTT solution (0.5 mg/ml, Sigma) is directly added to cell cultures *in situ*. Cell cultures are then incubated for 2 h at 37°C. Collagenase (Boehringer, Mannheim, Germany), 0.35% in culture medium, is used to separate cells from collagen matrix for 20 min at 37°C. A viability measurement using trypan blue (Fluka Buchs, Switzerland) is made on cell cultures after preliminary exposure to the enzyme. After dye extraction with DMSO, absorbance at 560 nm is measured with an SP8-100 Pye Unicam ultraviolet spectrophotometer.

Three hours after seeding, the medium is discarded and replaced by 100 μl FCS-free medium containing 10^{-6} M-hydrocortisone hemisuccinate (Roussel-Uclaf, Romainville, France) with the test compound. The cultures are incubated for 20 h at 37°C under a humidified atmosphere of 95% air-5% CO_2. At the end of the incubation period, the cultures are examined under phase-contrast microscopy. The cells are washed once before adding 100 μl FCS-free medium containing 0.05% MTT in each well. After 2 h of incubation at 37°C, the medium is discarded and the formazan blue formed into the cells is released by adding 100 μl DMSO and stirring for 15 min. Optical density is measured at 550 nm.

After 14 to 16 h, the media are discarded and test chemicals are added in serum-free medium (but containing 10^{-6} M-dexamethasone). After 24 or 48 h of exposure, MTT assay is performed.

After 38 h, the media are discarded and test chemicals are added in serum-free medium (but containing 10^{-6} M-dexamethasone). After 20 h of exposure, MTT assay is performed.

After 4 h (rat and dog cells) or 24 h (human cells), the media are discarded and test chemicals are added in serum-free medium. After 24 h (rat and dog) or 48 h (human) of exposure, MTT assay is performed.

Secondary Cultures: Test chemicals are added in 2 ml of complete DMEM containing 2% fetal bovine serum (assay medium). After overnight incubation at 37°C in 5% CO_2, the used media are aspirated and replaced with 1 ml (per well) of assay medium containing 500 μg MTT/ml (Sigma). The cultures are incubated for 2 h, then washed twice with 1 ml PBS (Mediatech). Isopropanol (Sigma) is used as the solvent to extract the formazan from the mitochondria of the viable cells. Aliquots (200 μl) of used bluish solvent are transferred to a 96-well plate and the optical density at 540 nm is determined spectrophotometrically using a VMAX microplate reader (Molecular Devices), making a blank correction to a pretreated nylon mesh (without cells) that has been similarly incubated with MTT.

Cell Lines: 24 h before treatment, MTT reagent is prepared adding 10 ml PBS ph 7.4 to 50 mg MTT and mixing well, overnight, to dissolve the MTT dye; the solution is stored at 4°C and sterile filtered prior to use. All test agents are added to the wells in 200 μl of fresh medium and incubated for 24 to 48 h. At the end of the exposure period, the incubation medium is aspirated and cells rinsed once with PBS; 10% MTT reagent in complete medium (without phenol indicator) is added (100 μl) to the wells for 4 h at 37°C and mixed with gentle agitation. Isopropanol solution containing 0.04 N HCl is then added (100 μl) to each well and mixed thoroughly by repeated pipetting. Plates are read (540 nm) within 1 h in an ELISA Plate Reader (Bio-Tek EL 309 Autoreader).

At subconfluency (4 d after cell seeding), the medium is discarded and replaced by FCS-free medium containing 10^{-6} M-hydrocortisone hemisuccinate (Roussel-Uclaf, Romainville, France) with the test compound. The cultures are incubated for 20 h at 37°C under a humidified atmosphere of 95% air-5% CO_2. At the end of the incubation period the cultures are examined under phase-contrast microscopy. The cells are washed once before adding 100 μl FCS-free medium containing 0.05% MTT in each well. After 2 h of incubation at 37°C, the medium is discarded and the formazan blue formed into the cells is released by adding 100 μl DMSO and stirring for 15 min. Optical density is measured at 550 nm.

Cultures are treated 24 h after plating when cells are still in exponential growth; the medium is removed and the cells are re-fed with medium containing test agents. After a treatment time of 24 h, the plates are prepared for MTT assay. MTT tetrazolium salt is prepared as a stock solution of 5 mg/ml in PBS, stored in the dark at 4°C and filter-sterilized; before use it is diluted 1:10 into DMEM containing 1% fetal calf serum but no phenol red. 100 μl MTT-containing medium is added to each well, then the plates are covered with foil and incubated at 37°C for 3 h. Thereafter, the supernatants are removed by inverting the plates and 100 μl of a solution of 1 N HCl-isopropanol (1:24, v/v) is added. After 10 min at room temperature and a brief agitation on a microtiter plate shaker, the plates are transferred to a microplate reader and the optical density of each well is measured using a 550 nm test wavelength and a 700 nm reference wavelength.

The medium is removed 72 or 24 h after inoculation and test compounds are added at various concentrations. After a treatment time of 24 or 72 h, respectively, measurements of MTT are determined. The absorbance is measured with an automatic microtitre plate reader, Dynatech MR 700 (Billingshurst).

1.6.3.3 Analysis

Data is expressed as: (1) percentage difference in chromophore formation compared to untreated controls and assigned a toxicity rating; (2) IC$_{50}$, i.e., the concentration that inhibits cell viability (expressed in terms of absorbance readings) by 50%: linear regression analysis is used to compute the concentration.

2. DATA

3. REPORTING
3.1 Test Report
The test report shall, if possible, include the following information:

- test conditions: detailed description of treatment and sampling schedule, dose levels, toxicity data, negative and positive controls;
- dose/effect relationship when possible;
- statistical evaluation;
- discussion of the results;
- interpretation of the results.

3.2 Evaluation and Interpretation
(to be defined)

4. ALTERNATIVE TO ANIMAL TEST
This method may be used in screening for potential respiratory tract, eye irritant, and other toxic chemicals.

BIBLIOGRAPHY
Arnould, J. Dubois, F. Abikhalil, A. Libert, G. Ghanem, G. Atassi, M. Hanocq and F. J. Lejeune, Comparative sensitivity of two mouse lymphoid tumor cell lines (P388 and P388D1) to five anticancer drugs *in vitro, ATLA*, Vol. 18, No. 3, p. 225, 1990.

Blanquart, C., S. Romet, A. Baeza, C. Guennou and E. Marano, Primary cultures of tracheal epithelial cells for the evaluation of respiratory toxicity, *Toxicology In Vitro*, Vol. 5, No. 5/6, p. 499, 1991.

Borenfreund, E., H. Babich and N. Martin-Alguacil, Comparisons of two *in vitro* cytotoxicity assays, the neutral red (NR) and tetrazolium MTT tests, *Toxicology In Vitro*, Vol. 2, No. 1, p. 1, 1988.

Chesné, C., C. Guyomard, L. Grislain, C. Clerc, A. Fautrel and A. Guillouzo, Use of cryopreserved animal and human hepatocytes for cytotoxicity studies, *Toxicology In Vitro*, Vol. 5, No. 5/6, p. 479, 1991.

Cornelis, M., C. Dupont and J. Wepierre, *In vitro* cytotoxicity tests on cultured human skin fibroblasts to predict the irritation potential of surfactants, *ATLA*, Vol. 19, p. 324, 1991.

Cornelis, M., C. Dupont and J. Wepierre, Prediction of eye irritancy potential of surfactants by cytotoxicity test *in vitro* on cultures of human skin fibroblasts and keratinocytes, *Toxicology In Vitro*, Vol. 6, No. 2, p. 119, 1992.

De Sousa, G, M. Dou, D. Barbe, B. Lacarelle, M. Placidi and R. Rhamani, Freshly isolated or cryopreserved human hepatocytes in primary culture: Influence of drug metabolism on hepatotoxicity, *Toxicology In Vitro*, Vol. 5, No. 5/6, p. 483, 1991.

Fautrel, A., C. Chesné, A. Guillouzo, G. De Sousa, M. Placidi, R. Rhamani, F. Braut, J. Pichon, H. Hoellinger, P. Vintezous, I. Diarte, C. Melcion, A. Cordier, G. Lorenzon, M. Benincourt, B. Vannier, R. Fournex, A. F. Peloux, N. Bichet, D. Gouy and J. P. Cano, A multicentre study of acute *in vitro* cytotoxicity in rat liver cells, *In Toxicology In Vitro*, Vol. 5, No. 5/6, p. 543, 1991.

Gettings, S. D., J. J. Teal, D. M. Bagley, J. L. Demetrulias, L. C. Di Pasquale, K. L. Hintze, M. G. Rozen, S. L. Weise, M. Chudkowski, K. D. Marenus, W. J. W. Pape, M. Roddy, R. Schnetzinger, P. M. Silber, S. M. Glaza and P. J. Kurtz, The CTFA evaluation of alternatives program: An evaluation of *in vitro* alternatives to the Draize primary eye irritation test (Phase 1) Hydro-alcoholic formulations; (Part 2) Data analysis and biological significance, *In Vitro Toxicology*, Vol. 4, No. 4, p. 247, 1991.

INVITTOX Protocol No. 17, April 1990.

Jover, R., X. Ponsoda, J. V. Castell and M. J. Gomez-Lechon, Evaluation of the cytotoxicity of ten chemicals on human cultured hepatocytes: Predictability of human toxicity and comparison with rodent cell culture systems, *Toxicology In Vitro*, Vol. 6, No. 1, p. 47, 1992.

Nordin, M., A. Wieslander, E. Martinson and P. Kjellstrand, Effects of LDH exposure period of acetylsalicylic acid, paracetamol and isopropanol on L929 cytotoxicity, *Toxicology In Vitro*, Vol. 5, No. 5/6, p. 449, 1991.

Otoguro, K. Komiyama, S. Omura and C. A. Tyson, An *in vitro* cytotoxicity assay using rat hepatocytes and MTT and Coomassie Blue dye as indicator, *ATLA*, Vol. 19, p. 352, 1991.

Peloux, A. F., C. Federici, N. Bichet, D. Gouy and J. P. Cano, Hepatocytes in primary culture: An alternative to LD$_{50}$ testing? Validation of a predictive model by multivariate analysis, *ATLA*, Vol. 20, p. 8, 1992.

Triglia, D., S. Sherard Braa, C. Yonan and G. K. Naughton, Cytotoxicity testing using neutral red and MTT assays on a three-dimensional human skin substrate, *Toxicology In Vitro*, Vol. 5, No. 5/6, p. 573, 1991.

THE POLLEN TUBE TEST

1. METHOD

1.1 Introduction, 1.2 Definition, and 1.3 Reference Substances (to be defined)

1.4 Principle of the Test Method

The *in vitro* culture of pollen can provide a sensitive indication of toxicity at cellular level, because germination and growth of pollen tubes are inhibited in the presence of toxic substances. Since the main metabolic activity of the growing pollen tube is the production of tube wall material, such a quantification may be achieved by measuring the amount of tube wall material present, either directly after sonication or by determining the binding of Alcian blue, which has an affinity for water-insoluble polysaccharides, a major component of plant walls.

1.5 Quality Criteria (to be defined)

1.6 Description of the Test Method
1.6.1 Preparations
Pollen tubes from tobacco plants (Nicotiana sylvestris) are used. For this test system, it is necessary to dissolve test substances in the aqueous culture medium. For compounds of low solubility in water, it is possible to use DMSO as the initial solvent. DMSO is shown to have no effect on pollen germination and tube growth when present in the culture medium at a concentration not exceeding 1%.

1.6.2 Test Conditions
Number of Cultures
The assay is carried out in duplicate for each experimental point, in quadruplicate for medium and solvent control, and repeated on at least five separate occasions in order to obtain at least five dose-response curves.

Use of Negative and Positive Controls
Negative controls (aqueous, solvent and zero-time) are used.

Exposure Concentrations
Under normal circumstances, a range-finding experiment should be performed first: seven different final concentrations between 10 and 10^5 mM should be employed in order to estimate the critical range of tube-growth inhibition. This may be detected with the naked eye by checking the turbidity of test suspensions against that of the control, to which only an equivalent quantity of water has been added.

A narrower range of concentrations, chosen as a result of the range-finding experiment, is used. In practice, increasing test compound concentrations by a factor of two has proved very useful.

Culture Conditions
(to be defined)

1.6.3 Procedure
1.6.3.1 Preparation of Cultures
Mature anthers are harvested prior to their dehiscence from open flowers. They are spread in a petri dish and kept at room temperature in a dry place until they have all opened, which should not take longer than 2 d. The pollen is separated from the anthers using a sieve and small brush; then it is divided into small portions and frozen until required. Pollen culture medium (pH 5.G — adjusted with KOH): water containing 5% sucrose (w/v), 0.01% boric acid, 3 mM $Ca(NO_3)_2$, 10 mM 2-[N-morpholino]ethanesulfonic acid (MES).

A suspension of 1 mg pollen per 1 ml culture medium is prepared in the following manner: pollen is placed into a test tube, a trace of culture medium is added and then it is mixed with a glass rod until a homogenous pulp is obtained. The pulp is diluted with the rest of the culture medium; 900-μl aliquots of the pollen suspension are placed into 50-ml screw-capped Erlenmeyer flasks (the suspension should be constantly stirred while the aliquots are being taken).

1.6.3.2 Treatment of the Cultures with the Test Substance
The flasks are set up in the following manner:

- aqueous control: 100 μl water
- solvent control: 100 μl 10% DMSO in water

- zero-time control: 100 µl absolute ethanol*
- test condition (aqueous): 100 µl test compound stock solution
- test condition (gaseous): using a syringe, inject various quantities of gas through the septum of the flask

* ethanol is used at a final concentration of 10%, which is sufficient to reduce pollen tube growth to zero.

The flasks are incubated for 18 h at 25°C in the dark.

Determination of Pollen Tube Production
   At the end of the 18-h incubation:

Alcian Blue Method: Contents of each flask are transferred separately into centrifuge tubes; flasks are washed out two times with 4 ml water to ensure that no pollen remains in the flasks, and the washings are added to their respective centrifuge tubes; then the tubes are centrifuged at 1000 g for 1 min. After aspiration of the supernatant, the pellet is resuspended in 2 ml 0.05% Alcian blue for 30 min (aqueous Alcian blue solution is freshly prepared by diluting a 0.5% ethanolic Alcian blue stock solution, which is made by dissolving 0.5 g Alcian blue in 100 ml absolute ethanol); 7 ml water is added to the tubes, and then they are centrifuged at 1000 g for 1 min. After aspiration of the supernatant, the pellet is resuspended in 9 ml distilled water. The centrifugation and wash are repeated. After the second wash, each pellet is resuspended in 2 ml 40% citric acid for 10 min to redissolve the bound dye. The tubes are centrifuged and the extinction of the supernatant is determined at 607 nm.

Turbidity Method: Contents of each flask are suspended separately in 9 ml water in a centrifuge tube. Sonication is performed for 20 sec on setting No. 4. The tubes are centrifuged for 1 min at 1000 g. After aspiration of the supernatant, the pellet is resuspended in 3 ml water. The tubes are whirled up and turbidity is measured at 500 nm without delay.
   Because the photometer readings are unstable, it is necessary to integrate over the first 30 sec. Alternatively, take five readings in 30 sec and calculate the mean value.

1.6.3.3 Analysis
Generation of Dose-Response Curve: Extinction values of zero-time control are subtracted from those of test and control cultures. Corrected values are used to calculate percentage growth inhibition. A plot of these percentage values vs. the ϵ of test concentrations will produce a dose-response curve. Graphic presentations can be obtained with the aid of graphics software.

Calculation of POL$_{50}$: From at least five dose-response curves, the POL$_{50}$ (i.e., the concentration of test substance that reduces pollen tube growth to 50% of the control) for each curve is estimated by interpolation from the data of the two concentrations confining the POL$_{50}$. The mean and standard deviation may be calculated.

2. DATA

3. REPORTING
3.1 Test Report
   The test report shall, if possible, include the following information:

- test conditions: detailed description of treatment and sampling schedule, dose levels, toxicity data, negative and positive controls;
- dose/effect relationship when possible;

- statistical evaluation;
- discussion of the results;
- interpretation of the results.

3.2 Evaluation and Interpretation
(to be defined)

4. ALTERNATIVE TO ANIMAL TEST
This method may be used in screening for potential eye irritant chemicals.

BIBLIOGRAPHY

Gettings, S.D., J. J. Teal, D. M. Bagley, J. L. Demetrulias, L. C. Di Pasquale, K. L. Hintze, M. G. Rozen, S. L. Weise, M. Chudkowski, K. D. Marenus, W. J. W. Pape, M. Roddy, R. Schnetzinger, P. M. Silber, S. M. Glaza and P. J. Kurtz, The CTFA evaluation of alternatives program: An evaluation of *in vitro* alternatives to the Draize primary eye irritation test (Phase 1) Hydro-alcoholic formulations; (Part 2) Data analysis and biological significance, *In Vitro Toxicology*, Vol. 4, No. 4, p. 247, 1991.

INVITTOX **Protocol,** No. 55, February 1993.

TOTAL PROTEIN CONTENT (BIO-RAD ASSAY)

1. METHOD

1.1 Introduction, 1.2 Definition, and 1.3 Reference Substances (to be defined)

1.4 Principle of the Test Method
The total protein content is a cytotoxic assay used to identify a reduction of cell viability both on primary cultures and established cell lines. The reduction of cell number, determined by the test chemicals, is reflected by the measurement of total cell protein content. Bio-Rad assay is a dye-binding method with Coomassie Brilliant Blue, in which the amount of dye found is proportional to protein content. Total protein content has been suggested to be useful to screen chemicals for their irritative potential to eye.

1.5 Quality Criteria (to be defined)

1.6 Description of the Test Method
1.6.1 Preparations
Test chemicals are prepared in medium or in DMSO, afterwards diluted in serum-free culture medium: final DMSO concentration must not exceed 1%. When present, DMSO is used at the same concentration for all chemical concentrations.

Hydro-alcoholic formulations are tested at a dilution of 0.1% v/v.

Primary cultures (rat hepatocytes) and established cell lines [keratinocytes, Clonetics' Epi-Pack® human fetal dermal fibroblasts, CCRL 1475; HEp-2, ATCC (CCL 23); BALB 3T3, ATCC (CCL 163); FaO hepatoma; L929 cell line] are used.

1.6.2 Test Conditions
Number of Cultures
From four to five cultures are used for each experimental point.

Use of Negative and Positive Controls
Positive (known toxicant) as well as negative controls (complete medium only) are included.

Exposure Concentrations

Serial dilutions of chemicals are adjusted to obtain a minimum of ten data points within a range of toxicity from 10 to 90% of control values.

For screening experiments, chemicals are tested at half-interval dilutions starting at 2 mg/ml and 5% (v/v) for solid and liquid agents, respectively.

Culture Conditions

Appropriate culture medium, seeding density, pretreatment time and dosing duration are used.

Metabolic Activation

(most chemicals require metabolic activation)

1.6.3 Procedure

1.6.3.1 Preparation of Cultures

Primary Cultures: Hepatocytes are isolated from rats by the two-step collagenase perfusion method. Cell viability, measured by the trypan blue exclusion test (final concentration of dye: 0.05% in phosphate-buffered saline, PBS), is adequate if in excess of 85%. Cells are seeded at a density of 3×10^4 cells per well in 96-well plates (NUNC, Kamstrup, Denmark) in 100 µl nutrient medium. The medium consists of Williams' E medium (Flow, Les Ulis, France) containing 10% fetal calf serum (FCS, Boehringer, Mannheim, Germany), 0.1 IU bovine insulin/ml, 10 IU penicillin/ml, 10 µl streptomycin/ml, and 2.5 mM-glutamine.

Cell Lines: HEp-2 cells derived from a human carcinoma of the larynx are routinely cultured in monolayers at 37°C in disposable plastic flasks containing minimum essential medium (MEM), supplemented with Earle salts, 5% FCS, 2 mM glutamine, 0.14% sodium bicarbonate, 100 UI penicillin, and 100 µg/ml streptomycin. Cells are seeded in 35-mm dishes at a density of about 1×10^5 cells/dish.

Keratinocytes (Clonetics' EpiPack®, grown in Clonetics' serum-free medium) and human fetal dermal fibroblasts (grown in Dulbecco's modified Eagle medium, DMEM, with 10% fetal calf serum and penicillin/streptomycin) are plated in 96-well flat bottom plates and incubated for 24 h at 37°C, 5% CO_2.

BALB 3T3 cells (mouse embryonic lung fibroblasts) are maintained in a humidified, 37°C incubator at 7% CO_2 in DMEM supplemented with either 2% or 10% fetal bovine serum, 100 units/ml penicillin G, 100 µg/ml streptomycin, and 1.25 µg/ml Fungizone. Cells are plated at 3×10^3 cells in 200 µl of medium into a 96-well tissue culture test plate.

FaO cells (subcloned from the hepatoma cell line H4IIEC3, isolated from the Reuber H35 hepatoma) are cultured in NCTC 135/Ham's F12 medium (v/v) supplemented with 5% FCS, 100 IU penicillin/ml, and 100 µl streptomycin/ml. The medium is renewed every 2 d and the cells are transferred after about 10 d when they reach subconfluency using 0.5% trypsin. After five passages, the cells are stored in liquid nitrogen. For cytotoxicity studies, frozen FaO cells are thawed and put in culture; the functional capacity is controlled by measuring albumin secretion rates in media. After three passages, the cells are seeded in 96-well plates in Williams' E medium (Flow, Les Ulis, France) containing 10% fetal calf serum (FCS, Boehringer, Mannheim, Germany), 0.1 IU bovine insulin/ml, 10 IU penicillin/ml, 10 µl streptomycin/ml, and 2.5 mM-glutamine.

L929, a mouse fibroblast cell line, is grown as a monolayer in Eagle's MEM (Biological Industries), supplemented with 10% fetal calf serum (Nordvacc), 50 µg gentamicin/ml (Nordvacc), 1% nonessential amino acids, and 2 mM-L-glutamine (Biological Industries). The cells are subcultivated twice a week using 0.1% trypsin (Nordvacc) in PBS without Ca^{2+} and Mg^{2+}, and maintained at 37°C in humidified air with 5% CO_2. Then the cells are taken from confluent cultures and inoculated into 96-well tissue culture plates (Greiner) at a density of 7000 cells/cm^2.

1.6.3.2 Treatment of the Cultures with the Test Substance

Primary Cultures: 3 h after seeding, the medium is discarded and replaced by 100 µl FCS-free medium containing 10^{-6} M-hydrocortisone hemisuccinate (Roussel-Uclaf, Romainville, France) with the test compound. The cultures are incubated for 20 h at 37°C under a humidified atmosphere of 95% air-5% CO$_2$. At the end of the incubation period, the cultures are examined under phase-contrast microscopy. The cells are washed twice with PBS, then 50 µl 0.2 N-NaOH is added to each well. After a 15 to 20 min incubation at 37°C, 200 µl Coomassie Blue solution (2:5 in distilled water) is added to each well. Plates are stirred until staining appears homogenous and are then kept at room temperature for 30 min. Optical density is measured at 410 and 620 nm.

Cell Lines: At confluence, the culture supernatant is removed and fresh medium containing the test substance is added. After a treatment time of 24 h, protein total content is determined. The cell monolayer is washed three times with 1 ml cold PBS; 0.9 ml bi-distilled water is added; cells are disrupted by sonication before addition of 100 µl Triton X-100 and the suspensions centrifuged at 1930 g for 15 min. A 0.1 ml sample of supernatant is used for protein determination using the Bio-rad protein assay. The spectrophotometer is equipped with a 595-nm filter.

All test agents are added to the wells in 200 µl of fresh medium and incubated for 24 to 48 h. Cultures are scanned with an inverted phase microscope and photodocumented. After completion of neutral red assay, the same cells are assessed for protein content as follows: the cells are washed once with PBS, washed a second time with distilled water, then lysed in 40 ml 0.1 N NaOH for 2 h at 37°C; 200 µl of a 1:6 dilution of Bio-Rad Coomassie Blue is then added and incubated for 30 min at room temperature. The ODs are then read using 405 nm as a reference and 650 nm for the samples. A serial dilution of BSA (20 to 200 mg/well) in 0.1 N NaOH is used for protein standards. Results are expressed as %OD of complete medium control.

At 24 h after plating, medium is removed from the cells with gentle aspiration and replaced with 200 µl of fresh medium (for control wells), or with medium containing test agents at various concentrations. Then, 24 h after addition of test media, plates are scanned by phase microscopy to visually assess toxicity. Media are removed and cells are washed twice with Tris-buffered saline (135 mM NaCl, 5.4 mM KCl, 0.8 mM MgSO$_4$, 0.14 mM CaSO$_4$; 20 mM Tris, ph 7.4), care being taken to fill the wells completely with wash fluid. Media and washes are removed by inverting the plates and shaking them. After the second wash is removed, a standard curve is prepared in 8 empty wells so that they contained a range of 0 to 10 µg of protein in 0.1 N NaOH and a final volume of 50 µl. Each of the remaining wells received 50 µl 0.1 N NaOH. Cell plates are incubated for at least 15 min at 37°C and then 200 µl of diluted dye reagent Coomassie Blue (1 part Bio-Rad dye reagent, 3 parts distilled water) is added to each well. The plate is agitated on a shaker after dye addition. After 30 min of incubation at room temperature, the plate is scanned in a microplate reader using a 405-nm filter for the reference wavelength and a 630-nm filter for the absorption wavelength. The curve obtained with the standards is used to calculate micrograms of cell protein per well in the experimental samples. A dose-dependent curve is prepared from this data and an EC$_{50}$ determined (concentration of chemical causing a 50% reduction in protein level relative to controls).

At subconfluency (4 d after cell seeding), the medium is discarded and replaced by FCS-free medium containing 10^{-6} M-hydrocortisone hemisuccinate (Roussel-Uclaf, Romainville, France) with the test compound. The cultures are incubated for 20 h at 37°C under a humidified atmosphere of 95% air-5% CO$_2$. At the end of the incubation period, the cultures are examined under phase-contrast microscopy.

The cells are washed twice with PBS, then 50 μl 0.2 N-NaOH is added to each well. After a 15 to 20 min incubation at 37°C, 200 μl Coomassie Blue solution (2:5 in distilled water) is added to each well. Plates are stirred until staining appears homogenous, and are then kept at room temperature for 30 min. Optical density is measured at 410 and 620 nm.

The medium is removed 72 or 24 h after inoculation and test compounds are added at various concentrations. After a treatment time of 24 or 72 h, respectively, measurements of total protein content are determined. The absorbance is measured with an automatic microtiter plate reader, Dynatech MR 700 (Billingshurst).

1.6.3.3 Analysis

The results are expressed in percentages compared to control cultures. The relative toxicity of the test compounds is established by determination of the ID_{50}: (concentration of test compound required to induce a 50% reduction in total protein content).

2. DATA

3. REPORTING
3.1 Test Report
The test report shall, if possible, include the following information:

- test conditions: detailed description of treatment and sampling schedule, dose levels, toxicity data, negative and positive controls;
- dose/effect relationship when possible;
- statistical evaluation;
- discussion of the results;
- interpretation of the results.

3.2 Evaluation and Interpretation
(to be defined)

4. ALTERNATIVE TO ANIMAL TEST
This method may be used in the screening for potential eye irritant chemicals.

BIBLIOGRAPHY

Commission of the European Communities, Collaborative study on the evaluation of alternative methods to the eye irritation test — Part 1, Doc. XI/632/91 V/E/1/131/91, Brussels, 1991, p. 17.

Commission of the European Communities, Collaborative study on the evaluation of alternative methods to the eye irritation test — Part II, Doc. XI/632/91 V/E/1/131/91, Brussels 1991, p.157.

Fautrel, A., C. Chesné, A. Guillozo, G. De Sousa, M. Placidi, R. Rhamani, F. Braut, J. Pichon, H. Hoellinger, P. Vintezous, I. Diarte, C. Melcion, A. Cordier, G. Lorenzon, M. Benincourt, B. Vannier, R. Fournex, A. F. Peloux, N. Bichet, D. Gouy and J. P. Cano, A multicentre study of acute *in vitro* cytotoxicity in rat liver cells, *Toxicology In Vitro,* Vol. 5, No. 5/6, p. 543, 1991.

Gettings, S. D., J. J. Teal, D. M. Bagley, J. L. Demetrulias, L. C. Di Pasquale, K. L. Hintze, M. G. Rozen, S. L. Weise, M. Chudkowski, K. D. Marenus, W. J. W. Pape, M. Roddy, R. Schnetzinger, P. M. Silber, S. M. Glaza and P. J. Kurtz, The CTFA evaluation of alternatives program: An evaluation of *in vitro* alternatives to the Draize primary eye irritation test (Phase 1) Hydro-alcoholic formulations; (Part 2) Data analysis and biological significance, *In Vitro Toxicology,* Vol. 4, No. 4, p. 247, 1991.

Mazziotti, T., A. L. Stammati and F. Zucco, *In vitro* cytotoxicity of 26 coded chemicals to HEp-2 cells: A validation study, *ATLA,* Vol. 17, p. 401, 1990.

Nordin, M., A. Wieslander, E. Martinson and P. Kjellstrand, Effects of exposure period of acetylsalicylic acid, paracetamol and isopropanol on L929 cytotoxicity, *Toxicology In Vitro,* Vol. 5, No. 5/6, p. 449, 1991.

Otoguro, K. , K. Komiyama, S. Omura and C. A. Tyson, An *in vitro* cytotoxicity assay using rat hepatocytes and MTT and Coomassie Blue Dye as indicator, *ATLA,* Vol. 19, p. 352, 1991.

Peloux, A. F., C. Federici, N. Bichet, D. Gouy and J.-P. Cano, Hepatocytes in primary culture: An alternative to LD50 testing? Validation of a predictive model by multivariate analysis, *ATLA,* Vol. 20, p. 8, 1992.

Rougier, A., M. Cottin, O. De Silva, R. Roguet, P. Catroux, A. Toufic and K. G. Dossou, *In vitro* methods: Their relevance and complementarity in ocular safety assessment, *Lens and Eye Toxicity Research,* Vol. 9, No. 3–4, p. 229, 1992.

Zanetti, C., I. De Angelis, A. L. Stammati and F. Zucco, Evaluation of toxicity testing of 20 MEIC chemicals on HEp-2 cells using two viability endpoints, *ATLA,* Vol. 20, p. 120, 1992.

TOTAL PROTEIN CONTENT (KENACID BLUE METHOD, KB)

1. METHOD

1.1 Introduction, 1.2 Definition, and 1.3 Reference Substances (to be defined)

1.4 Principle of the Test Method
The total protein content is a cytotoxic assay used to identify an inhibition of cell proliferation on established cell lines. The reduction of cell number, determined by the test chemicals, is reflected by the measurement of total cell protein content obtained by staining with KB followed by a spectrophotometric determination. This test has been suggested to be useful to screen chemicals for their irritative potential to the eye.

1.5 Quality Criteria (to be defined)

1.6 Description of the Test Method
1.6.1 Preparations
Test chemicals are dissolved initially in medium, ethanol, or dimethyl sulfoxide to give a final concentration of solvent of 1% (v/v) in the culture medium; in the case of pipettable liquids, simple volume/volume dilutions are used while viscous solutions are weighed and made up volumetrically; weight/volume dilutions are used for solid material.
Established cell lines (3T3-L1, ATCC CCL 92.1 BALB/3T3, ATCC (CCL 163)) are used.

1.6.2 Test Conditions
Number of Cultures
The assay is carried out in triplicate for each experimental point, including medium and solvent control, and repeated on three separate occasions.

Use of Negative and Positive Controls
Negative controls (medium and solvent) are used.

Exposure Concentrations
(to be defined)

Culture Conditions
Different seeding density and treatment times are used.

Metabolic Activation
(most chemicals require metabolic activation)

1.6.3 Procedure
1.6.3.1 Preparation of Cultures
Cell Lines: 3T3-L1 cells (mouse fibroblast-like cell line) are maintained in Dulbecco's modified Eagle's medium (DMEM), supplemented with 2 mM L-glutamine, 10% newborn calf serum, 100 µg/ml streptomycin sulfate, 100 IU/ml benzylpenicillin, and 2 µg/ml Fungizone. They are routinely grown on 80 cm^2 flasks in a humidified 5% CO_2/95% air incubator, and passaged every 2 to 3 d. The 3T3-L1 cells are plated in 0.2 ml of medium per well in 95 out of 96 wells in a 96 multi-well tissue culture plate, either at 4–5 × 10^4 cells/ml or at 1.6 × 10^4 cells/ml.

1.6.3.2 Treatment of the Cultures with the Test Substance
Cell Lines: Cultures are treated 24 h after plating when cells are still in exponential growth. After a treatment time of either 18 to 24 h (4–5 × 10^4 cells/ml) or 72 h (1.6 × 10^4 cells/ml), the KB assay is performed on fixed cells by NR destain solution (1% acetic acid, 50% ethanol, 49% distilled water). Following removal of fixative, the cells are rinsed with PBS and then stained with KB stain (prepared immediately before use by adding 12 ml glacial acetic acid to 88 ml of a stock solution made by dissolving 0.4 g KB R in 250 ml ethanol and 630 ml distilled water). The plates then are shaken for 20 min. The stain is removed and the cells rinsed with washing solution (10% ethanol, 5% glacial acetic acid, 85% distilled water, by volume) to remove unbound stain. The plates are agitated for 5 min, and a fresh washing solution is added. After the final washing, exactly 0.2 ml of desorbing solution (1 M potassium acetate in 70% ethanol) is added to each well. The plates are agitated for a further 1 to 2 h and absorbance are read at 577 nm on a Kontron SLT-210 plate reader with a 404-nm reference filter, against the blank well containing no cells.

1.6.3.3 Analysis
Cell protein contents (in terms of KB absorbance readings) in treated cultures are compared to those in control cultures and the percentage inhibition of growth calculated: the ID$_{50}$ for protein content concentrations (the concentration producing 50% inhibition of growth) is determined.

2. DATA

3. REPORTING
3.1 Test Report
The test report shall, if possible, include the following information:

- test conditions: detailed description of treatment and sampling schedule, dose levels, toxicity data, negative and positive controls;
- dose/effect relationship when possible;
- statistical evaluation;
- discussion of the results;
- interpretation of the results.

3.2 Evaluation and Interpretation
(to be defined)

4. ALTERNATIVE TO ANIMAL TEST
This method may be used in the screening for potential eye irritant chemicals.

BIBLIOGRAPHY

Atkinson, K., L. Hulme, R. H. Clothier and M. Balls, *In vitro* cytotoxicity of 24 chemicals to mouse teratocarcinoma cells, *ATLA*, Vol. 17, p. 34, 1989.

Clothier, R. H., L. Hulme, A. B. Ahmed, H. L. Reeves, M. Smith and M. Balls, *In vitro* cytotoxicity of 150 chemicals to 3T3-L1 cells, assessed by the FRAME kenacid blue method, *ATLA*, Vol. 16, p. 84, 1988.

Commission of the European Communities, Collaborative study on the evaluation of alternative methods to the eye irritation test — Part 1, Doc. XI/632/91 V/E/1/131/91, Brussels, 1991, p. 18.

Commission of the European Communities, Collaborative study on the evaluation of alternative methods to the eye irritation test — Part II, Doc. XI/632/91 V/E/1/131/91, Brussels 1991, p. 159.

Garle, M., A. H. Hammond and J. R. Fry, The cytotoxicity of 27 chemicals to V79 Chinese hamster cells, *ATLA*, Vol. 15, p. 30, 1987.

Gettings, S. D., J. J. Teal, D. M. Bagley, J. L. Demetrulias, L. C. Di Pasquale, K. L. Hintze, M. G. Rozen, S. L. Weise, M. Chudkowski, K. D. Marenus, W. J. W. Pape, M. Roddy, R. Schnetzinger, P. M. Silber, S. M. Glaza and P. J. Kurtz, The CTFA evaluation of alternatives program: An evaluation of *in vitro* alternatives to the Draize primary eye irritation test (Phase 1) Hydro-alcoholic formulations; (Part 2) Data analysis and biological significance, *In Vitro Toxicology*, Vol. 4, No. 4, p. 247, 1991.

Knox, P., P. F. Uphill, J. R. Fry, J. Benford and M. Balls, The FRAME multicentre project on *in vitro* cytotoxicology, *Food and Chemical Toxicology*, Vol. 24, No. 6/7, p. 457, 1986.

Riddell, R. J., D. S. Panacer, S. M. Wilde, R. H. Clothier and M. Balls, The importance of exposure period and cell type in *in vitro* cytotoxicity tests, *ATLA*, Vol. 14, p. 86, 1986.

Smith, L. M., R. H. Clothier, S. Hillidge and M. Balls, Modification of the FRAME Kenacid Blue method for citotoxicity tests on volatile materials, *ATLA*, Vol. 20, p. 230, 1992.

TOTAL PROTEIN CONTENT (LOWRY METHOD)

1. METHOD

1.1 Introduction, 1.2 Definition, and 1.3 Reference Substances (to be defined)

1.4 Principle of the Test Method
The total protein content is a cytotoxic assay used to identify a reduction of cell viability on established cell lines. The reduction of cell number, determined by the test chemicals, is reflected by the measurement of total cell protein content. This test has been suggested to be useful to screen chemicals for their irritative potential to the eye.

1.5 Quality Criteria (to be defined)

1.6 Description of the Test Method
1.6.1 Preparations
Test chemicals are prepared in complete medium.
Cell lines (SIRC, ATCC CCL 60) are used.

1.6.2 Test Conditions
Number of Cultures
   (to be defined)

Use of Negative and Positive Controls
   Negative control (fresh complete medium) is used.

Exposure Concentrations
   (to be defined)

Culture Conditions
   (to be defined)

Metabolic Activation
   (most chemicals require metabolic activation)

1.6.3 Procedure
1.6.3.1 Preparation of Cultures
   Cell Lines: SIRC cells (rabbit corneal cell line) are plated into the 24 wells of a multidish with 1 ml complete medium per well and incubated at 37°C in a 5% CO_2 atmosphere: the medium is composed by Dulbecco's modified Eagle's medium (DMEM) supplemented with 5% fetal calf serum (FCS), 1% nonessential amino acids (NEAA), 100 units/ml penicillin, and 100 µg/ml streptomycin.

1.6.3.2 Treatment of the Cultures with the Test Substance
Cell Lines: After 24 h, the medium is removed from the wells containing confluent cultures. Test cultures are treated with 1 ml aliquots of different concentrations of freshly prepared chemicals. The cultures are incubated at 37°C for 24 h. After 24 h, the cells are washed three times with 1 ml HBSS per well; 1 ml Lowry solution A per well is added. After 15 min at 37°C, 200 ml of this solution is mixed with 500 ml solution C; 15 min thereafter, 100 ml 50% Folin Ciocalteu reagent is added. The extinction is read at 500 nm after 30 min.
   Solution A: 2% Na_2CO_3 in NaOH 1 N; Solution C: 35 ml solution A + 500 µl 1% $CuSO_4 \cdot 5H_2O$ + 500 µl 2% potassium sodium tartrate.

1.6.3.3 Analysis
   The results are expressed in percentage compared to control cultures. The relative toxicity of the test compounds is established by determination of the ID_{50} (concentration of test compound required to induce a 50% reduction in total protein content).

2. DATA

3. REPORTING
3.1 Test Report
   The test report shall, if possible, include the following information:

* test conditions: detailed description of treatment and sampling schedule, dose levels, toxicity data, negative and positive controls;
* dose/effect relationship when possible;
* statistical evaluation;
* discussion of the results;
* interpretation of the results.

3.2 Evaluation and Interpretation
   (to be defined)

4. ALTERNATIVE TO ANIMAL TEST
   This test may be used in the screening for potential eye irritant chemicals.

BIBLIOGRAPHY

Commission of the European Communities, Collaborative study on the evaluation of alternative methods to the eye irritation test — Part 1, Doc. XI/632/91 V/E/1/131/91, Brussels, 1991, p. 15.

Commission of the European Communities, Collaborative study on the evaluation of alternative methods to the eye irritation test — Part II, Doc. XI/632/91 V/E/1/131/91, Brussels 1991, p. 155.

Cornelis, M., C. Dupont and J. Wepierre, *In vitro* cytotoxicity tests on cultured human skin fibroblasts to predict the irritation potential of surfactants, *ATLA*, Vol. 19, p. 324, 1991.

Dierickx, P. J., Cytotoxicity testing of 114 compounds by the determination of the protein content in HEP G2 cell cultures, *Toxicology In Vitro*, Vol. 3, No. 3, p. 189, 1989.

Dierickx, P. J. and B. Ekwall, Long-term cytotoxicity testing of the first twenty MEIC chemicals by the determination of the protein content in human embryonic lung cells, *ATLA*, Vol. 20, p. 285, 1992.

Ekwall, B., I. Bondesson, J. V. Castell, M. J. Gomez-Lechon, S. Hellberg, J. Hogberg, R. Jover, X. Ponsoda, L. Romert, K. Stenberg and E. Walum, Cytotoxicity evaluation of the first ten MEIC chemicals: Acute lethal toxicity in man predicted by cytotoxicity in five cellular assays and by oral LD_{50} tests in rodents, *ATLA*, Vol. 17, p. 83, 1989.

Schepers, G., C. Aschmann and S. Morchel, The use of primary cultured rat hepatocytes for the assessment of xenobiotic effects on biotransformation, *ATLA*, Vol. 19, p. 209, 1991.

Seibert, H., M. Gulden, M. Kolossa and G. Schepers, Evaluation of the relevance of selected *in vitro* toxicity test systems for acute systemic toxicity, *ATLA*, Vol. 20, p. 240, 1992.

UNSCHEDULED DNA SYNTHESIS (87/302/EEC DIR. MODIFIED)

1. METHOD

1.1 Introduction, 1.2 Definition, and 1.3 Reference Substances
None.

1.4 Principle of the Test Method
The unscheduled DNA synthesis (UDS) test measures the DNA repair after excision and removal of a stretch of DNA containing the region of damage induced by chemical and physical agents. The test is based on the incorporation of tritium labeled thymidine (^{3}H-TdR) into the DNA of mammalian cells which are not in the S phase of the cell cycle. The uptake of ^{3}H-TdR may be determined by autoradiography or by liquid scintillation counting (LSC) of DNA extracted from the treated cells. Mammalian cells in culture, unless primary rat hepatocytes are used, are treated with the test agent with and without an exogenous metabolic activation system.

1.5 Quality Criteria
None.

1.6 Description of the Test Method
1.6.1 Preparations
Test chemicals and control or reference substances should be prepared in growth medium or dissolved or suspended in appropriate vehicles and then further diluted in growth medium for use in the assay. The final concentration of the vehicle should not affect cell viability.

Primary cultures (rat hepatocytes; human lymphocytes; rat tracheal epithelial cells; hamster tracheal epithelial cells), tertiary cultures (human keratinocytes), or established cell lines (e.g., human diploid fibroblasts) may be used in the assay. Cells should be exposed to the test chemical both in the presence and absence of an appropriate metabolic activation system.

1.6.2 Test Conditions
Number of Cultures
At least two cell cultures for autoradiography and six cultures (or less if scientifically justified) for liquid scintillation counting (LSC) UDS determinations are necessary for each experimental point.

Use of Negative and Positive Controls
Concurrent positive and negative (untreated and/or vehicle) controls with and without metabolic activation should be included in each experiment. Examples of positive controls for the rat hepatocyte assay include 7,12-dimethylbenzanthracene (7,12-DMBA) or 2-acetylaminofluorene (2-AAF). In the case of established cell lines 4-nitroquinoline-N-oxide (4-NQO) is an example of a positive control for both the autoradiographic and LSC assays performed without metabolic activation; N-dimethylnitrosamine is an example of a positive control compound when metabolic activation systems are used.

Exposure Concentrations
Multiple concentrations of the test substance over a range adequate to define the response should be used. The highest concentration should elicit some cytotoxic effects. Relatively water-insoluble compounds should be tested up to the limit of solubility. For freely water-soluble nontoxic chemicals, the upper test chemical concentration should be determined on a case-by-case basis.

Culture Conditions
Appropriate growth media, CO_2 concentration, temperature and humidity should be used in maintaining cultures. Established cell lines should be periodically checked for mycoplasma contamination.

Metabolic Activation
A metabolic activation system is not used with primary hepatocyte cultures. Established cell lines and lymphocytes are exposed to test substance both in the presence and absence of an appropriate metabolic activation system.

1.6.3 Procedure
1.6.3.1 Preparation of Cultures
Primary Cultures: Short-term cultures of rat hepatocytes are established by allowing freshly dissociated hepatocytes in an appropriate medium to attach themselves to the growing surface.

Human lymphocyte cultures are set up using appropriate techniques.

Both rat and hamster tracheal epithelial cells are isolated with protease type XIV at 4°C for 16 h and then flushed with 20 ml cold Dulbecco's minimum essential medium (DMEM, Gibco) containing 10% fetal calf serum (FCS, Gibco). Cells are harvested by washing twice in culture medium (Ham's F12 supplemented with 50 IU penicillin/ml, 50 µg streptomycin/ml, 100 µg kanamycin/ml, 10 mM-glutamine, 5 mM-pyruvate, 5 µg transferrin/ml, 5 µg insulin/ml, 10 µg epidermal growth factor/ml, and 0.1% FCS, all purchased from Gibco) and centrifuged (50 g for 5 min). Cells isolated from four animals are then pooled and plated out onto collagen-coated glass coverslips at a cell density of 2×10^5 cells/ml in 1 ml culture medium per well of a 24-well multiwell plate (Gibco). Cells are incubated for 24 h to allow them to attach, in an atmosphere of 5% CO_2/95% O_2 at 37°C.

Tertiary Cultures: Skin samples (taken from patients undergoing mastectomy but resulting macroscopically normal) are incubated overnight at 4°C in Type XIV protease (10 mg/ml) in serum-free DMEM. The epidermis is peeled away from the dermis and then floated on a solution of 0.05% trypsin plus 0.01% EDTA in phosphate-buffered saline (PBS). After a 20 min incubation at 37°C, medium is added and complete dispersion of epidermal cells is achieved by repeated pipetting. Confluent layers of mouse 3T3 fibroblasts (Flow Labs, Irvine, UK) are mitotically arrested by treatment with mitomycin C (4.0 µg/ml) for 4 h.

Tertiary cultures of human keratinocytes are seeded at 5×10^4 cells/well in the presence of a 3T3 feeder layer (5×10^4 cells/well) onto 13-mm glass coverslips in 24-well tissue culture plates (Gibco Europe Ltd., Paisley, UK). Triplicate wells are prepared for each treatment group and cultures are grown for 3 to 5 d to allow the cells to reach 50% confluence.

Cell Lines: Established cell lines are generated from stock cultures (e.g., by trypsinization or by shaking off), seeded in culture vessels at appropriate density, and incubated at 37°C.

1.6.3.2 Treatment of the Cultures with the Test Substance

Primary Cultures: Freshly isolated rat hepatocytes are treated with the test substance in a medium containing ³H-TdR for an appropriate length of time. At the end of the treatment period, medium should be drained off the cells, which then are rinsed, fixed, and dried. Slides should be dipped in autoradiographic emulsion (alternative stripping film may be used), exposed, developed, stained, and counted.

Culture medium is removed, the cell layer is washed with prewarmed PBS, and culture medium is replaced by culture medium containing appropriate concentrations of the test compound; [³H]thymidine (µCi/ml final concentration) is added to each well after 8 h. After a total incubation time of 24 h, the medium is removed, and the cell layer is washed and incubated for further 6 h with medium containing 0.25 mM-thymidine. The cells are finally washed three or four times with PBS (37°C), fixed for 30 min with 3:1 (v/v) mixture of absolute alcohol and glacial acetic acid, washed twice with distilled water, air-dried, and mounted cell-surface-uppermost onto glass slides. Slides are left overnight to dry before processing for autoradiography. The autoradiography is performed using fresh Ilford K2 emulsion, Kodak D19 developer and Ilford fixer following established procedures for liquid emulsion techniques. The slides each are covered carefully with the emulsion mixture, dried, and transferred into exposure boxes containing anhydrous silica. Sealed boxes are stored for the appropriate exposure period (10 d at 4°C or 21 d at –20°C), after which slides are developed and stained with hematoxylin and eosin. Slides are observed using ×100 objective under oil immersion and grains counted using an AMS 40-10 Image Analyzer (Analytical Measuring Systems, Cambridge, UK).

Tertiary Cultures: Cultures are exposed to test chemicals in serum-free culture medium containing 10 µCi [³H-methyl]thymidine (Amersham International, Bucks, UK). After an overnight incubation cells are washed twice in PBS and then incubated in culture medium containing unlabeled thymidine (0.25 mM) for 24 h. Cultures are examined microscopically for evidence of toxicity and then washed in PBS, followed by 0.02% EDTA to remove any remaining 3T3 cells and a final wash in PBS. Cells then are fixed and autoradiographed. Slides are examined with an oil immersion objective (×100) and analyzed with an AMS 40-10 image analyzer.

Cell Lines and Human Lymphocyte Cultures

Autoradiographic techniques: Cell cultures are exposed to the test substance for appropriate durations followed by treatment with ³H-TdR. The times will be governed by the nature of the substance, the activity of metabolizing systems and the type of cells. To detect the peak of UDS, ³H-TdR should be added either simultaneously with the test substance or within a few minutes after exposure to test substance. The choice between these two procedures will be influenced by possible interactions between test substance and ^{3}H-TdR. In order to discriminate between UDS and semiconservative DNA replication, the latter can be inhibited, for example, by the use of an arginine-deficient medium, low serum content, or addition of hydroxyurea in the culture medium.

LSC measurements of UDS: Prior to treatment with test substance, entry of cells into S-phase should be blocked as described above; cells should then be exposed to test chemical as described for autoradiography. At the end of the incubation period, DNA should be extracted from the cells and the total DNA content, and the extent of 3H-TdR incorporation determined.

It should be noted that, when human lymphocytes are used in the above techniques, the suppression of semiconservative DNA replication is unnecessary in unstimulated cultures.

1.6.3.3 Analysis

Autoradiographic determinations: In determining UDS in cells in culture, S-phase nuclei are not counted. At least 50 cells per concentration should be counted. Slides should be coded before counting. Several widely separated random fields should be counted on each slide. The amount of ^{3}H-TdR incorporation in the cytoplasm should be determined by counting three nucleus-sized areas in the cytoplasm of each cell counted.

LSC determinations: An adequate number of cultures should be used at each concentration and in the controls in LSC UDS determinations.

All results should be confirmed in an independent experiment.

2. DATA

Data should be presented in tabular form.

Autoradiographic determinations: The extent of ^{3}H-TdR incorporation in the cytoplasm and the number of grains found over the cell nucleus should be recorded separately. Mean, median, and mode may be used to describe the distribution of the extent of ^{3}H-TdR incorporation in the cytoplasm and the number of grains per nucleus.

LSC determinations: For LSC determinations, ^{3}H-TdR incorporation should be reported as dpm/µg DNA. The mean dpm/µg DNA with standard deviation may be used to describe the distribution of incorporation.

Data should be evaluated using appropriate statistical methods.

3. REPORTING
3.1 Test Report

The test report shall, if possible, contain the following information:

- cells used, density and passage number at time of treatment, number of cell cultures;
- methods used for maintenance of cell cultures including medium, temperature, and CO_2 concentration;
- test substance, vehicle, concentrations, and rationale for selection of concentrations used in the assay;
- details of metabolic activation systems;
- treatment schedule;
- positive and negative controls;
- autoradiographic technique used;
- procedures used to block entry of cells into S-phase;
- procedures used for DNA extraction and determination of total DNA content in LSC determination;
- dose/response relationship, where possible;

- statistical evaluation;
- discussion of results;
- interpretation of results.

3.2 Evaluation and Interpretation

There are several criteria for determining a positive result, one of which is a statistically significant dose-related increase in radiolabel incorporation (expressed either as grains per nucleus or as dpm/μg DNA). Another criterion may be the detection of a reproducible and statistically significant positive response for at least one of the test points.

A test substance producing neither a statistically significant dose-related increase in radiolabel incorporation (expressed either in grains per nucleus or as dpm/μg DNA) nor a statistically significant and reproducible positive response at any one of the test points is considered not active in this system.

4. ALTERNATIVE TO ANIMAL TEST

This test method is used to identify genotoxic chemicals.

BIBLIOGRAPHY

Lawrence, J. N. and D. J. Benford, Detection of chemical-induced unscheduled DNA synthesis in cultures of normal adult human keratinocytes, *Toxicology In Vitro,* Vol. 5, No. 5/6, p. 377, 1991.

Kuper, A. and D. J. Benford, Unscheduled DNA synthesis in tracheal epithelial cell cultures, *Toxicology In Vitro,* Vol. 5, No. 5/6, p. 511, 1991.

Commission Directive 87/302/EEC, 18 November 1987, Adapting to technical progress for the ninth time Council Directive 67/548/EEC on the approximation of laws, regulations and administrative provisions relating to the classification, packaging and labelling of dangerous substances, *Official Journal of the European Communities,* No. L133, Vol. 31, p. 64, 1988.

Chapter 6

FUTURE DEVELOPMENTS

Every year, a small percentage of the population shows negative health reactions deriving from the use of cosmetic products. Although this does not represent a general risk, it is crucial for cosmetic products put on the market to contain chemical ingredients in accordance with the provisions of Council Directive 76/768/EEC,[1] in which Article 2 states that:

"A cosmetic product put on the market within the Community must not cause damage to human health when applied under normal or reasonably foreseeable conditions of use, taking into account, in particular, the product's presentation, its labeling, any instructions for its use and disposal, as well as any other indication or information provided by the manufacturer or his authorized agent or by any other person responsible for placing the product on the Community market."

Moreover, according to the EC legislation, it is not permissible to market cosmetic products containing more than 400 cosmetic ingredients defined as dangerous for human health. For roughly an equal number of ingredients, EC legislation also provides limits of concentration, beyond which cosmetic products containing them may cause damages to consumers' health.

Since 1976, the prohibition and limitation of use of approximately 1000 cosmetic ingredients has been made possible, thanks to toxicological studies carried out by industries and research laboratories, aiming at the identification of effects negative to human health. Such research has mainly used models of study based on the utilization of animals, according to analytic biological methodologies defined by the international scientific community, and regulated in Europe by Directives 87/302/EEC[7] and 92/69/EEC.[8]

According to EC regulations, certain types of cosmetic ingredients (coloring agents, preservatives, sunscreens, and hair dyes), as recommended by the SCC, are submitted to a series of studies before their introduction on the market. This approach is the same followed and approved in the rest of the world by the scientific community, especially in the U.S. and Japan. Such an approach enables the identification of undesirable effects prior to consumers' exposure.

In 1986, Council Directive 86/609/EEC, on the approximation of laws, regulations, and administrative provisions of the Member States regarding the protection of animals used for experimental and other scientific purposes,[10] pointed out a series of actions to be put into operation by all countries, with the intent of:

• reducing pain deriving to animals utilized in tests and scientific studies;
• reducing to a minimum the number of animals used for these reasons;
• prohibiting the carrying out of a test based on the use of animals whenever another method is available, if scientifically valid and geared to reach the same significance, etc.

The approval of this Directive partially satisfies those public opinion groups that in the past decade have promoted the safety and life of animals utilized for scientific purposes in educational programs and in those of toxicological analysis of chemical substances.

The administrative authorities of the Commission have therefore taken special care in the use of animals in toxicity testing. The possible reduction of the number of animals used in "safety testing" programs should be discussed at the scientific level, together, if possible, with the problem of the full replacement of animal studies with alternative methodologies able to meet the objective of defining health risks deriving from chemical substances used in cosmetic products.

6.1 ALTERNATIVE METHODOLOGIES: STATE OF THE ART

An alternative methodology means any modification of the official guidelines on conducting toxicological studies for the assessment of toxic potentiality affecting human health and exerted by chemical substances in general, including cosmetic ingredients, as integral parts of the cosmetic product being marketed. Taking into account such a definition, we should consider "alternative" any methodology based on the "three R" principle, i.e., being able to:

1. Replace the use of animals,
2. Reduce the number of animals used, or
3. Refine existing procedures so that animals are subject to less pain and suffering.[57]

However, in another widely accepted definition, alternative methodologies means any analytic biological methodologies that avoid using animals.

Instead of animals, these alternative methodologies use as study objects simpler biological systems, represented by bacterial cell cultures and different mammalians or human cultures, or tissues and particular animal organs, or abiotic artificial systems, or computerized analysis programs.

In this book, exclusive emphasis has been given to these types of methodologies, because they better represent the goals of the animal rights movement, and meet the needs of legislative bodies for a different regulation of toxicological studies.

The basis of "risk assessment" or "safety evaluation" of a chemical ingredient is represented by the necessity for assessing its capability to produce any kind of damage to an organism, to such an extent as to affect its health, life, and progeny. In technical terms this is represented by the phase of "hazard identification." Hazard identification therefore includes all those studies that will identify not only terminal toxic effects produced by chemical ingredients, but also all those modifications necessary to cells, tissues, and organs, bringing as a consequence such terminal toxic effects (for example, all the knowledge that will enable us to understand the mechanism of toxic action accomplished by the chemical substance, including the existing relationships between dose administered and exposure, and the entity of the biological damages provoked).

Scientific studies have identified systems of cells and organs, by means of which it is possible to develop research aimed at explaining the aforesaid needs of knowledge. By using the systems described above and analytical procedures, toxicity tests for many chemical substances have been developed, and a few dozen *in vitro* methodologies have been demonstrated, capable of defining toxic effects for distinct toxicological studies. One of the attempts to systemize these *in vitro* tests, was carried out by Frazier et al.[46]

Examples referred to the possibility of identifying chemical agents recognized as potential eye irritants, based on different toxic effects or endpoints are represented by methods reported in Table 6.1.

6.2 METHODOLOGIES STANDARDIZATION

At present, every methodology described in the scientific literature and those quoted in this book are influenced by the personal experience of the researchers who have developed and implemented them. Other experiences, developed through the same methodology in other laboratories, allow the identification of the differences in the procedures that may prove decisive in the quantitative production of the effect under study. For each of these methodologies utilizing cell cultures, it is necessary to define experimentally a series of technical parameters, such as:

TABLE 6.1

Examples of Toxic Effects or Endpoints[93] in Cell Cultures

Cytotoxicity

Balb/c 3T3 Cells / Morphological Assays (HTD)	(1984)
BHK Cells / Colony Formation Efficiency	(1985)
BHK Cells / Growth Inhibition	(1985)
BHK Cells / Cell Detachment	(1985)
SIRC Cells / Colony Forming Assay	(1982)
Balb/c 3T3 Cells / Total Protein	(1985)
BCL-D1 Cells / Total Protein	(1985)
LS Cells / Dual Dye Staining	(1982)
Thymocytes / Dual Fluorescent Dye Staining	(1986)
LS Cells / Dual Dye Staining	(1985)
L 929 Cells / Cell Viability	(1981)
RCE - SIRC - P 815 - YAC - 1 / 51Cr Release	(1985)
Bovine Red Blood Cell / Hemolysis	(1987)
LS Cells / ATP Assay	(1984)
Balb/c 3T3 Cells	(1984)
Balb/c 3T3 Cells / Neutral Red Uptake	(1984)
HeLa Cells / Metabolic Inhibition Test (MIT-24)	(1985)

Release of Inflammatory Mediators

Normal human epidermal keratinocytes neutral red uptake	(1989)
Normal human epidermal keratinocytes cellular metabolism	(1989)
L 929 Cells / Agarose diffusion assay	(1987)
Chorioallantoic Membrane (CAM)	(1985)
HET-CAM	(1985)
Bovine Corneal Cup Model / Leukocyte Chemotactic Factors	(1987)
Rat Peritoneal Cells / Histamine Release	(1985)
Rat Peritoneal Mast Cells / Serotonin Release	(1979)
Rat Vaginal Explant / Prostaglandin Release	(1985)

Impairment of Cellular Functions

Rabbit Corneal Cell Cultures / Plasminogen Activator	(1985)
Bovine Cornea / Corneal Opacity	(1984)
Proposed Mouse Eye / Permeability Test	(1987)
Rabbit Corneal Epithelial Cells / Wound Healing	(1985)
Epidermal Slice / Electrical Conductivity	(1985)

Others

Enucleated Superfused Rabbit Eye System	(1981)
Rabbit Ileum / Contraction Inhibition	(1986)
EYTEX Assay	(1986)
Computer Based / Structure Activity Relationship (SAR)	(1982)
Tetrahymena / Motility	(1986)
Liposomes	(1988)

Note: Other recent developments in nonanimal methodologies are not included in this list.

From Frazier, J. M., *Scientific Criteria for Validation of In Vitro Toxicity Testing*, Organization for Economic Cooperation and Development, Paris, 1990.

- the nature and composition of the medium utilized;
- the procedures of preparation and maintenance of cellular cultures used in the test;
- cellular densities employed and their growth modalities, according to optimum temperatures;
- treatment time of chemical substances and relative solvents utilizable;
- the procedures to survey test results and their quantitative evaluation;

- the criteria to set maximum doses of the chemical substance employed in the test;
- the chemical substances utilizable as positive controls within the scope of that methodology, in relation to the experimental conditions employed;
- the systems of metabolic activation to employ for those substances subject to metabolism;
- the number of the test replicate, so that a valid and repeatable result may be obtained;
- result-confusing factors, such as pH, temperature, osmolality, antibiotic treatments, etc.

Once experimental limits are defined for each of the mentioned parameters within which the test may be considered acceptable (valid), a "standardized protocol" of test performance can be drafted for each methodology, so that it may be employed in any other laboratory, even one that has no specific experience in the use of this methodology.

The protocol developed during the 1970s on Ames' Test (genetic mutation) has allowed the diffusion of this methodology to thousands of biological laboratories all over the world, where a correct execution of the method has been carried out, is still in operation, and is submitted to continuous revaluation.

6.3 METHODOLOGY SPECIFICITY

Once a particular methodology is defined and the use standardization is fixed, it is necessary to verify its ability to identify chemical substances with different molecular structure that is toxic for the desired effects — for example, acute toxicity, skin irritation, eye irritation, skin sensitization, teratogenicity, etc.

In utilizing groups of chemical substances belonging to different chemical classes (e.g., aromatic amines, chlorinated solvents, naphthalenic compounds, polycyclic aromatic hydrocarbons, and secondary amines) it is necessary to determine whether that methodology can distinguish, within each chemical class, substances more or less toxic for a given endpoint, or if there are some chemical classes to which that methodology is not sensitive (all toxic or all nontoxic). In the latter case, that will necessitate a battery of methods fundamental in studying a chemical substance of new synthesis and structure.

6.4 METHODOLOGY PREDICTIVITY

This is a delicate subject, because it must include the current criteria of toxicological classification of chemical substances, based on results obtained from animal tests.

At present we cannot compile lists of chemical substances, ordered according to their toxic power, for particular toxic effects, as evaluated by a given alternative methodology.

It is most important that we establish the predictive value of each one of the new *in vitro* methodologies, relative to the entity of toxic effects found in animals. That is the reason why it is necessary to define for each methodology the degree of:

Sensitivity: represented by the percentage of toxic chemical substances, so stated by means of that methodology;

Specificity: represented by the percentage of nontoxic substances, so stated by means of that methodology;

Accuracy: represented by the percentage of correct results obtained by employing that methodology (identification of the greater percentage of toxic substances and of nontoxic substances as such);

Predictivity: represented by the percentage of toxic substances identified as such, among all the results indicating toxic substances.

It should be stressed that all these parameters never reach 100%, even in the case of the most highly developed animal models presently employed in toxicity testing to predict human toxic effects.

Obviously, those operations geared toward defining the effectiveness of a certain methodology need the cooperation of several other laboratories, so that it is possible for a certain methodology to be used in laboratories other than the one where it was originally developed.

We deem this work necessary and feel sure it is already in operation, even if results that can identify a methodology utilizable in a short time are not yet available. A further complication is caused by the wide heterogenicity of the biologic material utilized for the performance of the same type of test.

In our present studies focused on the constitution of databases, for example, we have noticed that for the Neutral Red Uptake, the following cellular lines can be used:

- Rabbit tracheal epithelium
- Rat hepatocytes
- Human epidermal keratinocytes
- SIRC cell line
- Balb/c 3T3-L1 cell line
- Keratinocytes, clonetics'
- Human fetal dermal fibroblast cell line

And for the Colony Formation Assay, the following cellular lines can be used:

- Rabbit cornea cells
- FRSK cell line
- ARLJ301-3 cell line
- Balb 3T3 cell line
- SIRC cell line

At the same time, different methodologies are utilized to measure the Total Protein Content; for example:

Lowry method	(SIRC cell line),
Bio-rad assay	(keratinocytes, clonetics'),
	(Human fetal dermal fibroblast cell line),
	(HEp-2 cell line),
	(Balb/c 3T3 cell line),
Kenacid blue method, KB	(3T3-L1 cell line)

Therefore, it is extremely necessary that future programs of validation of new and utilizable *in vitro* methodologies try to solve those problems of extreme heterogeneity that, if still present, do not allow the accurate assessment of the value of a certain methodology, and therefore of the reliability of the result obtained, or of its comparability with results relative to other substances studied by using a different cellular line.

6.5 ALTERNATIVE METHODS: PERSPECTIVES

If we consider the present knowledge in the scientific field and the state of development of alternative *in vitro* methodologies so far studied, it is possible to foresee a series of actions that may lead, if carried out with strict coordination, swiftness, and scientific strictness, to the availability of some methodologies utilizable by the administrative authorities of the European Community, as substitutes for the present types of toxicity studies based on the use of animals.

6.5.1 STANDARDIZATION OF SPECIFIC METHODOLOGIES FOR THE PREDICTIVE EVALUATION OF POTENTIAL TOXIC EFFECTS OF CHEMICAL SUBSTANCES

This is a task of primary importance and top priority for the Commission, if it wants to fully comply with the contents of 86/609/EEC Directive[10] and with the positions so far taken by the European Parliament, in connection with the modification of Directive 76/768/EEC[1] on cosmetic products, and, in the future, in connection with other sectors of chemical substances regulated by the EC.

The recent creation of the European Centre for Validation of Alternative Methodologies (ECVAM) will enable the achievement of European collaborative research aimed at the definition of alternative methodologies in the sector of acute toxicity, skin irritation, and eye irritation.[61]

6.5.2 IMPLEMENTATION OF A DATABASE FOR THE SECTOR OF COSMETIC INGREDIENTS

Information is needed on toxicity testing data of cosmetic ingredients derived from both *in vivo* and *in vitro* studies developed in the past, and those derived from *in vitro* alternative studies presently or to be developed in the near future, to be used for safety evaluation of cosmetic ingredients of concern for Directive 76/768/EEC,[1] as amended by Directive 93/35/EEC.[2] Literature examination or, preferably, data banks have been considered to be the first step of a toxicity testing.

According to Bawden,[62] an information system can help to reduce the number of animal experiments by contributing to:

- the removal of the necessity for experimentation, by showing that information already exists;
- the provision of adequate background information so that the extent of animal experimentation can be reduced;
- obtaining new perspectives on old data by applying statistical reduction and analysis to "wring out" information that may not be immediately obvious, or by correlating apparently disparate pieces of information;
- the provision of evidence as to the usefulness, or lack thereof, of experimental procedures, so that unproductive animal experiments can be eliminated;
- the support for systems for modeling, prediction, simulation, and risk assessment, which may in turn replace or reduce animal experimentation, or may increase the resolution power of validation studies.

The classical information resources available, such as MED-LINE, do not allow a set of information of reliable value, as the data present in the main on-line systems are not the result of a critical analysis of protocols, procedures, and data quality. However, no service can be so comprehensive to be reliable as a sole source.

Among EC organizations, the potential users of these types of data are the following:

1. small cosmetic industries not having access to research laboratories and which need information on the safety evaluation of cosmetic ingredients for their insertion in the dossier, as laid down by the Sixth Amendment (Directive 93/35/EEC);[2]

2. animal rights organizations, to develop their action as a follow-up of the use of alternatives in the cosmetic sector;
3. the TEC-Consumer Policy Service, for organizing a database system of the toxicological profiles of old and new cosmetic ingredients of concern for Directive 76/768/EEC;[1]
4. ECVAM, to organize validation studies and for their results' interpretation for future development;[61]
5. various groups of scientists intending to compare their data with a bigger database.

On the basis of considerations expressed hereafter, sources of information presently available to be used for the organization of a database for cosmetic ingredients are the following:

- *INVITTOX*: a data bank that provides detailed methodological protocols on *in vitro* methods of potential interest to toxicologists;[63]
- the Galileo Data Bank, which collects detailed information on results obtained from *in vitro* alternative toxicity testing of several thousand chemicals of different use, including information on protocols used, cell lines employed in toxicity studies, statistical analysis of data, etc.;[64,65]
- ZEBET (the Center for Documentation and Evaluation of Alternative Methods to Animal Experiments), at the German Federal Health Office, has established a data bank to facilitate the common use of all information available on *in vitro* methods. ZEBET collects and documents alternative methods to animal experiments from the international literature published;[66]
- cosmetic industries that have developed their own databases, by applying individual or batteries of alternative tests and comparing the results with *in vivo* data;
- different types of public organizations (health services, animal rights groups, individual scientific institutions, etc.).

As envisaged before, there is the need to collect and organize all these types of information so that they can be useful to interested groups. General principles for organizing such information are as follows:

- the definition of criteria for the selection of data to be included in a database;
- the way to process data to compare them between the same protocols or between various methodologies, including those *in vivo* as well;
- the organization of a network for the fastest acceptability of data from different users, including the capability to obtain documents in the electronic form;
- the identification of a reliable organization to be responsible for confidentiality of data, by limiting access to different levels of information.

We already have pointed out that in the future it will be necessary to create lists of comparison of "safety evaluation" results obtained from animal studies, in order to verify predictive values of alternative methodologies. Thus, we believe it appropriate to create a database containing all the results of toxicity animal studies, obtained for approximately 400 cosmetic ingredients that have been evaluated by the SCC since 1978.

Such a database should contain, for each toxic effect considered, the list of ingredients ranked according to the numeric value of the effect, for the following types of studies:

1. acute toxicity
2. dermal absorption
3. dermal irritation

4. mucous membrane irritation
5. skin sensitization
6. subchronic toxicity
7. toxicokinetics
8. mutagenicity
9. teratogenicity
10. cancerogenicity
11. human data

The creation of this database allows:

1. arrangement of all knowledge evaluated so far on cosmetic ingredients regulated by the Commission, which should enhance the safety evaluation of new cosmetic ingredients submitted to the Commission's attention in future years;
2. preparation of results for the comparison of data that will be obtained in the near future with alternative methodologies;
3. identification of reference substances for the validation of alternative methodologies.

6.5.3 ORGANIZATION OF A DATABASE OF CURRENTLY AVAILABLE RESULTS FOR THE EVALUATION OF SAFETY OF COSMETIC INGREDIENTS OBTAINED OR BEING DEVELOPED WITH ALTERNATIVE METHODOLOGIES

At present, in scientific literature we find several results of toxicity tests performed on cosmetic ingredients, or different formulations of cosmetic ingredients, obtained with *in vitro* alternative methodologies of different kinds (biotic and abiotic). Moreover, European cosmetic industries are deeply involved in the development of toxicity studies, using alternative methodologies, of cosmetic ingredients already on the market.

It would be appropriate to arrange a database containing all this information, which may define the following material:

*   the list of the chemical substances of cosmetic interest tested with alternative methodologies;
*   the list of alternative methodologies employed in the toxicological study of cosmetic ingredients;
*   the list of the different kinds of toxic effects (within the general frame of the studies requested) tested;
*   the comparison of toxicity between data obtained by using alternative methodologies, and those obtained by using animals;
*   the identification of the more specific and predictive methodologies utilized in the sector of toxicological research applied to cosmetic ingredients;
*   the elaboration of programs of control and validation of alternative methodologies in some sectors of safety evaluation.

Within the ambit of the Commission and ECVAM, the organization of a general database for results obtained *in vitro* has been achieved by the Galileo Data Bank.[64,65]

6.5.4 VALIDATION STUDIES ON ALTERNATIVE METHODOLOGIES

During 1993 several validation studies were concluded, mainly at the industrial level with the participation of academic groups. However, although these studies show that alternative methods could be used in toxicity testing, conclusions cannot yet be drawn from these validation studies to influence immediate implementation of the Sixth Amendment (Directive 93/35/EEC[2] or decisions by other administrative institutions).

As stated earlier, within the scope of Council Directive 76/768/EEC[1] there are some specific types of cosmetic ingredients for which the Commission receives from cosmetic industries extensive toxicological information according to the safety evaluation recommendations laid down in the SCC's Guidelines.[3] As already mentioned, these groups of chemicals are represented by preservatives, coloring agents, sunscreens, hair dyes, and a few other different chemical classes. All of these are biologically active chemicals whose use in cosmetic products is to be restricted within specific limitations, as they may represent various kinds of toxic risk to consumers.

The range of chemicals so far tested by alternative methodologies in validation studies carried out or in progress represents a series of chemical classes of various uses, such as industrial chemicals (mainly solvents), pharmaceutical drugs, mineral salts, and organic compounds of different types. Cosmetic ingredients also have been included in these programs; they mainly represent formulants of a general type employed in finished products, surfactants, and ingredients employed for the formulation of body lotions, creams, and detergent products. In addition, finished cosmetic products of unknown composition also have been tested. The scientific literature may include reports dealing with toxicity testing of cosmetic ingredients of some concern for Council Directive 76/768/EEC[1] (see Table 6.2).

In such validation studies, those chemicals for which animal data are already available, such as LD_{50} or eye irritant potential, have been considered in order to compare results obtained by alternative toxicity testing assays with those from the animal studies. In particular, cosmetic ingredients belonging to the groups of preservatives, hair dyes, coloring agents, sunscreens, etc., apart from a few exceptions, have to date scarcely been considered in validation studies carried out by alternative methods. Because there is presently no conclusive evidence that one or more specific alternative methods could be used for testing different classes of chemicals, it is not possible to extrapolate validation results obtained so far to all types of organic chemicals, including those of particular concern for Council Directive 76/768/EEC.[1]

The absence of scientifically defined validation studies applied to chemicals of different classes among preservatives, coloring agents, sunscreens, and hair dyes of the type included in the positive lists of Directive 76/768/EEC,[1] or considered by the SCC, is not to be ascribed to the lack of animal data for these chemicals. On the contrary, these are the best known, but existing toxicological data are the property of individual cosmetic industries even though they are known to the Commission, to whom they have presented all the toxicological dossiers.

Before developing appropriate validation studies of alternative methodologies for evaluating the safety of cosmetic ingredients subject to Directive 76/768/EEC,[1] it is crucial to develop an extensive computerized database system containing information on the results of the many toxicological studies applied to the safety evaluation of all such cosmetic ingredients evaluated by the SCC since its creation in 1978. These include all relevant ingredients in use to date for which human data are also available. These data represent the basis for further development of new safety evaluation methods.

The COLIPA is strongly involved in ongoing validation programs — for instance, the EC-UK Home Office Validation Program — on alternatives to the Draize eye irritation test, although this program is not strictly related to the safety evaluation of cosmetic ingredients; L'Oreal (France), Unilever (U.K.), and Henkel (Germany) are among the most active participants in the program.[67]

Moreover, in January 1994 COLIPA launched a new program on a further eye irritation validation study, involving the use of nine different alternative methodologies. The program intends to apply these methodologies to the safety evaluation of generic product formulations

TABLE 6.2
List of Chemicals and Products Tested on Validation Studies[94-148]

Name	CAS No.	Use	76/768/EEC Directive
1,3-diisoproprylbenzene	99-62-7		
1,5-dimethylcycloctadiene	3760-14-3		
1,5-hexadiene	592-42-7		
1,9-decadiene	1647-16-1		
1-butanol	71-36-3	Cosmetic denaturant (DIIC)	
1-methylpropylbenzene	135-98-8	Solvent	
1-nitropropane	108-03-2	Solvent	
1-pentanol	71-41-0	Industrial chemicals, Laboratory chemicals	
2,2-dimethylbutanoic acid	595-37-9		
2,4-dinitrofluoronitrobenzene	446-35-5		
2,6-dichlorobenzyl chloride	4659-45-4		
2-butoxyethyl acetate	112-07-2	Solvent	
2-ethyl-1-hexanol	104-76-7		
2-methoxyethanol	109-86-4	Cosmetic solvents (DIIC)	
2-methylpentane	107-83-5		
2-nitropropane	79-46-9	Solvent	
2-propanol	67-63-0	Cosmetic foaming agent (DIIC)	
3-butenyl-triethoxysilane			
3-butyl-4-hydroxyanisole		Food additives, Industrial & Natural chem.	
3-chloro-4-fluorintrobenzene	350-30-3		
3-ethyltoluene	620-14-4		
3-methylhexane	589-34-4		
3-nitrobenzoic acid	121-92-6	Industrial chemicals	
4,4-methylene-*bis*-(2,6-diterbutyl phenol)	118-82-3		
4-aminophenol	123-30-8	Cosmetic hair dyes (DIIC)	
4-bromophenetole	589-10-6		
4-carboxybenzaldehyde	619-66-9		
6-methyl coumarine	92-48-8	Cosmetic oral care agent	
8-MOP	298-81-7	Photo drugs	
acetaldehyde	75-07-0	Cosmetic (use not specified, CTFA)	
acetic acid	64-19-7	Cosmetic buffering agents (DIIC)	
acetone	67-64-1	Cosmetic solvent (DIIC)	
acetonitrile	75-05-8	Industrial chemicals	Annex II; No. 393
acrylamide	79-06-1	Not reported	
adult shampoos		Cosmetic formulation	
aftershave		Cosmetic formulation	
all-purpose cleaner		Formulation	

TABLE 6.2 (Continued)
List of Chemicals and Products Tested on Validation Studies[94-148]

Name	CAS No.	Use	76/768/EEC Directive
allantoin	97-59-6	Cosmetic oral care agents (DIIC)	
allyl alcohol	107-18-6	Industrial chemicals	
aluminium chlorohydrate			
aluminium hydroxide	21645-51-2	Industrial chemicals	
aluminium zirconium glycinate			
aminodarone	1951-25-3	Pharmaceutical Drug	
ammonium alkyl (C12)		Detergent	
ammonium alkyl (C6.5)		Detergent	
ammonium lauryl sulfate	2235-54-3	Cosmetic surfactants (DIIC)	
ammonium nitrate	6484-52-2	Cosmetic various uses (DIIC)	
amphoteric surfactants		Detergent	
aniline	62-53-3	Dyes, general	Annex II; No. 22
anionic surfactants		Detergent	
anthraquinone	84-65-1	Industrial chemicals	
anti-acne cream		Cosmetic formulation	
anti-dandruff products		Cosmetic formulation	
antiperspirant salts		Cosmetic formulation	
antiperspirant/deodorants		Cosmetic formulation	
avocado extract	977018-62-4	Cosmetic various uses (DIIC)	
baby shampoos		Cosmetic formulation	
bar soap		Cosmetic formulation	
bath preparations		Cosmetic formulation	
behemic alcohol			
behenic acid	112-85-6	Cosmetic Emulsifying Agents	
benzaldehyde	100-52-7	Cosmetic flavoring agents (DIIC)	
benzalkonium chloride	63449-41-2	Cosmetic Preservative	Annex VI; Part 2; No. 16
benzene sulfonate			
benzethonium chloride	121-54-0	Cosmetic preservatives (DIIC)	Annex VI; Part 2; No. 15
benzoic acid	65-85-0	Cosmetic preservatives (DIIC)	
benzophenone-3	131-57-7	Cosmetic UV agents (DIIC)	
benzyl alcohol	100-51-6	Cosmetic preservatives (DIIC)	
bithionol	97-18-7	Surfactant	Annex II; No. 275
Brij 35	9002-92-0	Cosmetic emulsifying agent	
bubble baths		Cosmetic formulation	
butyl cellosolve	111-76-2	Cosmetic solvent (DIIC)	
butyl methoxydibenzoyl-methane	70356-09-1	Cosmetic UV adsorber (DIIC)	

TABLE 6.2 (Continued)
List of Chemicals and Products Tested on Validation Studies[94-148]

Name	CAS No.	Use	76/768/EEC Directive
butyl methoxydibenzoyl-methane	70356-09-1	Cosmetic UV adsorber (DIIC)	
cadmium chloride	10108-64-2	Industrial chemicals	Annex II; No. 68
calcium pyrophosphate	7790-76-3	Cosmetic abrasives (DIIC)	
caprylic/capric triglyceride	73398-61-5	Cosmetic emollients (DIIC)	
cationic surfactants		Detergent	
cellosolve acetate	111-15-9	Cosmetic solvent (DIIC)	
cetearyl alcohol	67762-27-0		
cetyl piridimium chloride	123-03-5	Cosmetic anti-microbials	
chlorhexidine	55-56-1	Cosmetic preservatives (DIIC)	
chloroform	67-66-3	Industrial chemicals	Annex II; No. 366
chloropromazine	50-53-3	Pharmaceutical drug	
cinnamic aldehyde	104-55-2	Food and food additives	
cis-oclooctene	931-88-4		
Clayton Yellow	1829-00-1	Dyes, general	
cleansing cream		Cosmetic formulation	
cleansing lotion		Cosmetic formulation	
cleansing milks		Cosmetic formulation	
cloisorine red-ED		Cosmetic coloring additives (DIIC)	
cloisorine red-GI		Cosmetic coloring additives (DIIC)	
cocamidopropylhydroxysultaine	68139-30-0	Cosmetic surfactants (DIIC)	
cocoamphocarboxylglycinate	68650-39-5	Cosmetic surfactants (DIIC)	
coconut oil	8001-31-8	Cosmetic emollients (DIIC)	
cold-water detergent		Detergent	
colognes		Cosmetic formulation	
copper II sulfate	7758-98-7	Cosmetic various use (DIIC)	
coramide DEA			
corn oil	8001-30-7	Cosmetic emollients (DIIC)	
cosmetic cleanser		Cosmetic formulation	
cosmetic cleanser gel		Cosmetic formulation	
cream		Cosmetic formulation	
cuticle remover cream		Cosmetic formulation	
cyanuric acid chloride	108-77-0		
cyclohexanol	108-93-0	Industrial chemicals	
deodorant		Cosmetic formulation	
di-(2-ethylhexyl) phthalate	117-81-7	Cosmetic film former (DIIC)	
diazolinyl-urea	78491-02-8	Cosmetic preservative (DIIC)	
dibenzoyl peroxide	94-36-0	Industrial chemical	
dibutylethane dichloride		Industrial chemical	

TABLE 6.2 (Continued)
List of Chemicals and Products Tested on Validation Studies[94-148]

Name	CAS No.	Use	76/768/EEC Directive
dibutyltin chloride	683-18-1	Industrial chemical	
dimethylsulfoxide (DMSO)	67-68-5	Solvent	Annex II; No. 338
dishwashing liquid		Detergent	
disinfectant		Disinfectant	
distearyldimonium chloride	107-64-2	Cosmetic antistatic agents (DIIC)	
dodecane	112-40-3		
dodecyl dimethylamine oxide	1643-20-5		
doxycycline	564-25-0		
Ecsin Yellow			
EDTA	60-00-4	Cosmetic chelating agent (DIIC)	
Emcol E607	6272-74-8	Cosmetic unspecified use (CTFA)	
emollient cream		Cosmetic formulation	
ethanol	64-17-5	Cosmetic solvents (DIIC)	
ethoxylate sulfate			
ethyl acetate	141-78-6	Cosmetic solvent (DIIC)	
ethyl trimethyl acetate	3938-95-2		
ethyl-2-methylacetoacetate	609-14-3		
ethylacetate	141-78-6	Cosmetic solvents (DIIC)	
ethylene glycol	107-21-1	Cosmetic solvents (DIIC)	
eucalyptus oil	8000-48-4	Cosmetic various uses (DIIC)	
eyeliners		Cosmetic formulation	
fabric softener		Detergent	
face mask		Cosmetic formulation	
face powders		Cosmetic formulation	
fatty acids		Cosmetic formulant	
fluorescein	2321-07-5	Cosmetic hair dyes (DIIC)	
foot cream		Cosmetic formulation	
formaldehyde	50-00-0	Cosmetic preservatives (DIIC)	Annex III; Part 1; No. 13
foundations		Cosmetic formulation	
fragrance oils		Cosmetic formulation	
fragranced powder		Cosmetic formulation	
freshener		Cosmetic formulation	
Geropon AC-78			
glutaric acid	110-94-1		
glycerol	56-81-5	Cosmetic denaturants (DIIC)	
granular laundry detergent		Detergent	
hair conditioners		Cosmetic formulation	
hair masque		Cosmetic formulation	

TABLE 6.2 (Continued)
List of Chemicals and Products Tested on Validation Studies[94-148]

Name	CAS No.	Use	76/768/EEC Directive
hair spray		Cosmetic formulation	
hair tonics		Cosmetic formulation	
hair/body lotion		Cosmetic formulation	
hand cleaner		Detergent	
hand cream		Cosmetic formulation	
hand/nail lotion		Cosmetic formulation	
heavy duty washing-up liquid		Detergent	
hydrochloric acid	7647-01-0	Cosmetic buffering agents (DIIC)	
hydrogen peroxide	7722-84-1	Cosmetic antimicrobials (DIIC)	
hydrolyzed animal protein		Cosmetic formulant	
hydrophilic ointment		Cosmetic formulant	
Igepon AC-78	61789-32-0	Cosmetic use not specified (CTFA)	
imidazolidinyl urea	39236-46-9	Cosmetic preservatives (DIIC)	
isobutanol	78-83-1		
isopropanol	67-63-0	Cosmetic foaming agents (DIIC)	
isopropyl myristate	110-27-0	Cosmetic emollients (DIIC)	
isopropyl palmitate	142-91-6	Cosmetic emollients (DIIC)	
L-histidine	7006-35-1	Food additives, Industrial & Natural chem.	
lactic acid (D)	10326-41-7	Industrial chemicals	
lactic acid (DL)	598-82-3	Industrial chemicals	
lactic acid (L)	79-33-4	Industrial chemicals	
lanoline	8006-54-0	Cosmetic antistatic agents (DIIC)	
laundry detergent		Detergent	
lauramide DEA	120-40-1	Cosmetic controlling agents (DIIC)	
lauramidopropylbetaine	4292-10-8	Cosmetic antistatic agents (DIIC)	
lauroamphodiacetate		Cosmetic surfactant	
lauroamphoglycinate	68647-44-9	Cosmetic surfactant	
laurylmonophosphate	12751-23-4	Cosmetic (use not specified, CTFA)	
light duty liquid cleaner		Detergent	
light duty liquid detergent		Detergent	
light duty washing-up liquid		Detergent	
linear alkyl (C11.8)		Detergent formulant	
linear alkyl (C12.3)		Detergent formulant	
liquid hand soap		Detergent	
liquid laundry additive		Detergent	
liquid laundry detergent		Detergent	
liquid soaps		Detergent	
lotions		Cosmetic formulation	
lysin (L)	56-87-1	Cosmetic antistatic agents (DIIC)	

TABLE 6.2 (Continued)
List of Chemicals and Products Tested on Validation Studies[94-148]

Name	CAS No.	Use	76/768/EEC Directive
lysine (DL)	70-54-2	Food additives, Industrial & Natural chem.	
magnesium chloride	7786-30-3	Industrial chemical, laboratory	
make-up powders		Cosmetic formulation	
manganese violet	10101-66-3	Cosmetic coloring additives (DIIC)	
mascaras		Cosmetic formulation	
mercury II chloride	7487-94-7	Laboratory chemicals	Annex II; No. 221
methanol	67-56-1	Cosmetic solvents (DIIC)	Annex III; Part 1; No. 52
methyl acetate	79-20-9	Cosmetic solvent (DIIC)	
methyl amyl ketone	110-43-0		
methyl ethyl ketone	78-93-3	Cosmetic solvent (DIIC)	
methyl isobutyl ketone	108-10-1	Cosmetic denaturants (DIIC)	
methyl trimethyl acetate	598-98-1		
methyl/methylchloroisothiazo-linone	55965-84-9	Cosmetic preservatives (DIIC)	
methylcyclopentane	96-37-7		
methylparaben	99-76-3	Cosmetic preservatives (DIIC)	
mineral oil	8012-95-1	Cosmetic emollients (DIIC)	
moisturizing cream		Cosmetic formulation	
mouthwash		Detergent	
Myris 49			
n-butyl acetate	123-86-4	Cosmetic solvent (DIIC)	
n-hexane	110-54-3	Cosmetic (use not specified, CTFA)	
n-hexanol	111-27-3	Cosmetic foaming agents (DIIC)	
N-N-dimethyl guanidine sulfate	598-65-2		
natural extracts		Cosmetic formulant	
neutral red	553-24-2	Dyes general	
night creams		Cosmetic formulation	
nickel chloride	7718-54-9	Industrial chemicals	
nitrobenzene	99-95-3	Industrial chemicals	Annex II; No. 249
non-ionic surfactants		Detergent	
non-tear shampoos		Detergent	
nonoxynol-12	9016-45-9	Cosmetic surfactants (DIIC)	
octyl methoxycinnamate	5466-76-3	Cosmetic UV adsorber (DIIC)	
octyl palmitate	29806-73-3	Cosmetic emollients (DIIC)	
octyldimethyl PABA	21245-02-3	Cosmetic UV adsorber (DIIC)	
PABA	1501-31-0	Cosmetic UV adsorber (DIIC)	
palm oil	8002-75-3	Cosmetic emollients (DIIC)	

TABLE 6.2 (Continued)
List of Chemicals and Products Tested on Validation Studies[94-148]

Name	CAS No.	Use	76/768/EEC Directive
parafluoroaniline	371-40-4		
pareth-12 (C12-15)	68131-39-5	Cosmetic surfactants (DIIC)	
PEG-40 hydrogenated castor oil	61788-85-0	Cosmetic emulsifying agents (DIIC)	
penicillin G	61-33-6	Antibiotics	
perfumed skin lotion		Cosmetic formulation	
perfumes		Cosmetic formulation	
phenol	108-95-2	Cosmetic antimicrobials (DIIC)	Annex III; Part 1; No. 19
phenoxyethanol	122-99-6	Cosmetic preservatives (DIIC)	
phthalic anhydride	85-44-9	Industrial chemicals	
phthalic acid	88-99-3		
plant extracts		Cosmetic formulant	
polyethylene glycol 400	25322-68-3		
polyethylene glycol 600	25322-68-3	Cosmetic binders (DIIC)	
polysorbate 40 (TWEEN 40)	9005-66-7	Cosmetic surfactants (DIIC)	
polysorbate 60 (TWEEN 60)	9005-67-8	Cosmetic emulsifying agents (DIIC)	
preservatives		Cosmetic formulant	
prioxicam		Drugs	
promethazine	60-87-7	Pharmaceutical drugs	
propylbetaine			
propylene glycol	57-55-6	Cosmetic solvents (DIIC)	
psoralens		Drugs	
pyridine	110-86-1	Cosmetic solvents (DIIC)	
quaternium 15			
roll-on antiperspirant		Cosmetic formulation	
rose bengal	11121-48-5	Food additives, Industrial & Natural chem.	
salicocylamide			
salicylamide	65-45-2	Pharmaceutical drug	
salicylic acid	69-72-7	Cosmetic preservatives (DIIC)	
SD alcohol		Cosmetic formulant	
shampoos		Cosmetic formulation	
shaving cream		Cosmetic formulation	
shower gel		Cosmetic formulation	
silver nitrate	7761-88-8	Cosmetic antimicrobials (DIIC)	
skin moisturizers		Cosmetic formulation	
sodium benzoate	532-32-1	Cosmetic preservatives (DIIC)	
sodium C14-16 olefin sulfonate	68439-57-6	Cosmetic surfactants (DIIC)	
sodium cetearyl sulfate	59186-41-3	Cosmetic surfactants (DIIC)	

TABLE 6.2 (Continued)
List of Chemicals and Products Tested on Validation Studies[94-148]

Name	CAS No.	Use	76/768/EEC Directive
sodium chloride	7647-14-5	Cosmetic controlling agents (DIIC)	
sodium hydroxide	1310-73-2	Cosmetic buffering agents (DIIC)	
sodium laureth sulfate	9004-82-4	Cosmetic buffering agents (DIIC)	
sodium lauryl sarcosinate	137-16-6	Cosmetic surfactants (DIIC)	
sodium lauryl sulfate	151-21-3	Cosmetic surfactants (DIIC)	
sodium methyl cocoyl taurate	61791-42-2	Cosmetic surfactants (DIIC)	
sodium perborate tetrahydrate	10486-00-7		
sodium sesquicarbonate	533-96-0	Cosmetic buffering agents (DIIC)	
stain remover		Cosmetic formulation	
stearalkonium chloride	122-19-0	Cosmetic preservatives (DIIC)	
styrene	100-42-5	Industrial chemical	
sun lotion		Cosmetic formulation	
sunblock		Cosmetic formulation	
sunscreen cream		Cosmetic formulation	
sunscreens		Cosmetic formulation	
surface cleanser		Cosmetic formulation	
surfactant containing formulations		Cosmetic formulation	
TCSA	1154-59-2	Antimicrobial agents	
TEA-laurylsulfate	139-96-8	Cosmetic surfactants (DIIC)	
tetrachloroethylene	127-18-4	Solvent	Annex II; No. 314
tetracycline	60-54-8	Antibiotics	
tetrahydrofurfuryl alcohol	97-99-4	Cosmetic solvents (DIIC)	
thiourea	62-56-6	Industrial chemicals	Annex II; No. 321
thiourea lauryl sulfate			
tin II chloride	7772-99-8	Cosmetic various uses (DIIC)	
titanium dioxide coated mica		Cosmetic color additive	Annex IV; Part 1
toluene	108-88-3	Cosmetic solvents (DIIC)	
treatment cream		Cosmetic formulation	
triacetin	102-76-1	Cosmetic antimicrobials (DIIC)	
tributylethane chloride			
tributyltin chloride	1461-22-9	Industrial chemical	
trichloroacetic acid	76-03-9	Laboratory chemicals	
triethanolamine	102-71-6	Cosmetic buffering agents (DIIC)	
triethanolamine cocoyl glutamate	68187-29-1	Cosmetic surfactants (DIIC)	
Triton X-100	9002-93-1	Cosmetic emulsifying agents (DIIC)	
Tween 20	9005-64-5	Cosmetic surfactants (DIIC)	
Tween 80	9005-65-6	Cosmetic surfactants (DIIC)	
uvinul MS40	4065-45-6	Cosmetic UV adsorber (DIIC)	
xylene	1330-20-7	Cosmetic solvent (DIIC)	
zinc pyrithione	13473-41-7	Cosmetic preservatives (DIIC)	

and cosmetic ingredients for a total of 50 samples; the cosmetic ingredients considered in this program overlap with samples tested in the EC-UK Home Office program.

Attempts have been presented, based on results from scientific research developed by some cosmetic industries.

The *In Vitro* Ocular Toxicology Laboratory of the Procter & Gamble Company has presented the results of a study aiming to evaluate seven *in vitro* alternatives for ocular safety testing, to be used as screening procedures in ocular safety assessment.[61] The test material used for this study consisted of 17 materials of different uses, listed together with their "alternatives" in Table 6.3.[68]

The results of the *in vitro* test assay were compared with the maximum average eye irritation scores obtained in the low volume eye test: the relationship between *in vivo* and *in vitro* data was analyzed by calculating the rank correlation coefficient using Spearman's rank correlation test.

According to the authors, the study indicates that five of the seven *in vitro* assays evaluated may be useful in ocular safety assessment. They are (1) the silicon microphysiometer; (2) the luminescent bacteria test; (3) the neutral red assay; (4) the total protein assay; (5) the *T. thermophila* motility assay.

Therefore, the authors suggest that after thorough historical data analysis and evaluation of physical and chemical characteristics of a test substance, the materials should be assayed in an *in vitro* test battery that could make it possible to classify test materials into broad irritation categories. When possible, safety assessment should be performed without testing on animals.[68]

A different approach has been presented by the Basic Research Centre of L'Oreal.[69] Forty-one test materials have been studied using six to eight *in vitro* methods, each exploring one or two endpoints that could be linked to ocular irritation phenomena, and then comparing *in vitro* results with *in vivo* ocular irritation data obtained for these materials in previous studies. Test materials were compared for 20 individual chemicals and 21 cosmetic preparations (Tables 6.4 and 6.5).

TABLE 6.3
Test Materials and Alternative Methodologies Employed in the Procter & Gamble Study[68]

Test Substance	Alternative Methodologies
Tween 20	Silicon microphysiometer[72]
Triethanolamine	Luminescent bacteria toxicity test[78]
Bar soap A	Neutral red assay[73,74]
Bar soap B	Total protein content[75]
Fabric softener	*Tetrahymena thermophila* motility assay[149]
Hard surface cleaner A	Bovine/eye chorioallantoic membrane assay[150]
Hard surface cleaner B	EYTEX® system[151]
Light duty dishwashing liquid	
Liquid hand soap	
Shampoo A	
Shampoo B	
Shampoo C	
Shampoo D	
Heavy duty dishwashing liquid	
Benzalkonium chloride (10%)	
Sodium lauryl sulfate (40%)	
Heavy duty laundry detergent	

From Bruner et al., *Fundamental and Applied Toxicology,* 17, 136, 1991.

TABLE 6.4
Surfactants and Their *In Vivo* Draize Data Tested by L'OREAL

No.	Chemical Name	Category[a]	Draize Data MAS[b]	D7 Score[c]
1	Polyoxyethylene sorbitane monooleate	NI	3.8	0
2	Polyoxyethylene sorbitane monolaurate	NI	5.7	0
3	Pentadecanol (etherified)	NI	5.7	0
4	Industrial Tween 20	NI	10.1	0
5	Dodecanol (etherified)	NI	24.2	0
6	1,2 dodecanediol (etherified)	NI	31.7	1.2
7	Blend of decanol and dodecanol (both etherified)	NI	37.7	6.3
8	Octyl phenoxypolyethoxy ethanol (= Triton X 100)	NI	40.3	9.3
9	Blend of sodium and magnesium laurylethersulfate	AN	31.7	0
10	Acylamine polyglycol ethersulfate	AN	20.3	0
11	Sodium dodecyl sulfate (SDS)	AN	37.3	9.8
12	Sodium dodecylethersulfate	AN	42.3	15.5
13	Ammonium dodecylsulfate	AN	45.0	5.5
14	Triethanolamine dodecacylsulfate	AN	46.0	9.0
15	Sodium lauryl N methylglycinate	AN	63.7	3.7
16	Coprah amphoteric alkylimidazolium dicarboxylate	AM	32.7	2.7
17	Cocobetain derivative	AM	42.7	26.3
18	Tetradecyltrimethylammonium bromide (= MTAB)	CT	42.7	25.8
19	Hexadecyltrimethylammonium bromide (= CTAB)	CT	44.0	33.8
20	Pyridinium cotylbromide	CT	52.7	36.3

[a] NI: nonionic; AN: anionic; AM: amphoteric; CT: cationic.
[b] Maximum Average Scores (on a scale of 110).
[c] Mean scores 7 days after instillation of the product.

From Rougier et al., *Lens and Eye Toxicity Research,* 9, 229, 1992. With permission.

The *in vitro* test assays employed in this study were: the EYTEX® System,[70] the Silicon Microphysiometer,[71,72] the Neutral Red Assay,[73,74] the Total Protein Content Assay,[75] the Agar Diffusion Method,[76,77] the Luminescent Bacteria Toxicity Test,[78] the Isolated Cornea Opacity and Permeability Test,[79,80] and the Hen's Egg Test — Choriallantoic Membrane Assay (HETC-CAM).[81,82] All *in vitro* and *in vivo* comparative plotted data were submitted to Spearman's (rank) correlation computer analysis.

An extensive program aimed at developing toxicity testing experiments on a series of cosmetic formulations in order to assess their ocular irritation potential by means of a series of alternative methods has been developed by the U.S. Cosmetic, Toiletry and Fragrance Association (CTFA) and recently concluded.[83-91]

In Phase I, 10 representative hydroalcoholic personal care formulations (e.g., colognes, mouthwashes, deodorants, etc.) were subjected to the Draize primary irritation test and to 25 *in vitro* assay protocols (12 types of *in vitro* endpoints). Six of the assays evaluated were shown to have a high correlation with the *in vivo* eye irritation test: EYTEX®, Microphysiometer, HET-CAM I assay, Neutral Red Release assay, HET-CAM II assay, CAM-Vascular assay, Pollen Tube test).[91]

In Phase II, 18 oil/water emulsion formulations (representing products such as sunscreens, hair conditioners, and cleansing creams) were tested in an extensive variety of test assays: 16

TABLE 6.5
Cosmetic Preparations and Their *In Vivo* Draize Data[69]
Tested by L'OREAL

Sample	Idenity	*In Vivo* Draize Data	
		MAS[a]	D7 Score[b]
A	Eye make-up remover	2.7	0
B	Eye make-up remover	2.7	0
C	Eye make-up remover	3.0	0
D	Eye make-up remover	1.7	0
E	Eye make-up remover	2.3	0
F	Make-up remover	8.0	0
G	Make-up remover	8.7	0
H	Make-up remover	10.0	0
I	Make-up remover	16.0	0
J	Make-up remover	18.0	0
K	Make-up remover	23.3	0
L	Make-up remover	24.0	0.3
M	Make-up remover	32.7	8
N	Make-up remover	36.0	0
O	Mild shampoo	39.0	10.0
P	Shampoo	43.7	12.7
Q	Shampoo	47.0	10.0
R	Shampoo	42.7	12.0
S	Shampoo	42.3	25.0
T	Shampoo	45.3	21.8
U	Shower gel	50.3	23.2

[a] Maximum Average Scores (out of 110).
[b] Average Scores at day 7.

From Rougier et al., *Lens and Eye Toxicity Research*, 9, 229, 1992. With permission.

assays (including five already employed in Phase I) were found to be correlated with the *in vivo* eye irritation test.[88,90,91]

In Phase III, 25 representative surfactant-based personal care formulations (e.g., shampoos, facial cleansers, shower gels, etc.) were subjected to the Draize test and to 23 *in vitro* assays (41 endpoints). Of 41 *in vitro* endpoints, 21 were shown to have the highest correlation with the *in vivo* eye irritation test.[89,91]

These approaches could be well adapted for evaluation of the ocular safety potential of different types of materials and of the photoirritation and/or photoallergenic potential of individual test substances, provided that statistical analysis of data developed to date by these industrial research centers considers the intralaboratory variability of the various experiments performed by the same methodologies and test materials.

There are other examples in the literature supporting the hypothesis that a series of possible models soon will be available for different combinations of alternative methodologies. These would be applied to evaluation of the ocular safety of different types of materials, such as cosmetic formulations or cosmetic ingredients widely used in finished cosmetic products.

The establishment of ECVAM[61] at the EC's Joint Research Center located in Ispra, Italy, represents an important action undertaken by the Commission. This should allow further development of alternative methodologies to the use of animals in toxicity testing programs. The aim is to reach a stage that will include both validation of several alternative testing assays or of a battery of alternative methods and their acceptance by the regulatory authorities of the EC and of other supranational organizations, such as the OECD, or nations, such as the U.S. and Japan.

By virtue of its role, ECVAM has already embarked on coordination of a program, supported by the Commission in conjunction with the UK-Home Office, on the validation of a group of methods alternative to the Draize eye irritation test currently employed in the classification and labeling scheme of dangerous industrial chemicals. Several industries are taking part in this program, including European and U.S. chemical and cosmetic industries. Although the chemicals selected for this validation project belong to classical industrial chemicals rather than cosmetic ingredients, the experiments this group of chemicals requires could lay the groundwork for a similar future validation study, dealing specifically with cosmetic ingredients that could fall within Council Directive 76/768/EEC.[1]

A photoirritation *in vivo* assay system has never been defined at the OECD level because of the difficulty in predicting human chemically induced phototoxic effects by means of animal models. A broad spectrum of potential alternative methodologies is available to be defined and validated. This includes physical and chemical analysis, photobinding, absorption spectroscopy, light-induced oxidation of histidine, etc. In this case, the selection of adequate test methods to be analyzed has a fundamental motivation and it is one of ECVAM's top responsibilities.

Extensive human data also are available concerning phototoxicity of many chemical substances, which could be used to evaluate currently existing alternative methods. Moreover, the mechanisms of phototoxic and photoallergic effects known to occur in humans and to be caused by the action of visible or ultraviolet radiation on photosensitizing chemicals vary according to the initial reaction in human tissues. Such mechanisms include energy transfer, electron transfer, covalent binding to different cellular molecules, formation of photoproducts, formation of hapten as photoproduct, and binding of hapten to skin protein.

To facilitate legal acceptance of alternative methodologies in the safety testing of cosmetics and other components of the modern human lifestyle (drugs, food additives, detergents, etc.), development of basic research should be organized and promoted by the EC. A critical aspect of the advancement of alternative procedures to be used in toxicity testing procedures is the establishment of mechanistic data on a variety of methodologies that have been developed and applied to the toxicity testing of chemicals. Many of these methodologies have been developed on account of their simplicity and reproducibility, but there is still little understanding of the mechanism by which the biological system is affected by a given chemical. More research should be devoted to the mechanistic basis of these methodologies. For example, there are numerous *in vitro* biochemical assays that have multiple uses in toxicology, yet many of these test systems have not been applied as extensively to toxicology as they could be. Such applications include the use of the assays on enzymes or catalytic functions critical for cell communication, translocation of the external signals to internal apparatus of cell machinery, control of the process of cell proliferation or cell death, and inhibition of essential and specific cell division-controlling proteins.[92] An additional field of research is represented by the use of transgenic cell lines, which could present a tremendous improvement in development of new and specialized biological material of great use in applied toxicology.

Evaluation of photoirritation and photosensitization potential for chemicals absorbing UV light is a specific toxicological requirement for a group of chemicals well represented among cosmetic ingredients, such as UV filters, that represent a component of a variety of finished cosmetic products used not only as suntanning products, but also in a wider group of body and facial creams.

The results of this program could directly influence 1998 implementation of the Sixth Amendment to Directive 76/768/EEC.[1]

Another important issue facing those in charge of alternative methodologies for validation programs during the remaining time before January 1998 is represented by assessment of percutaneous absorption of chemicals in general, and of cosmetic ingredients in particular.

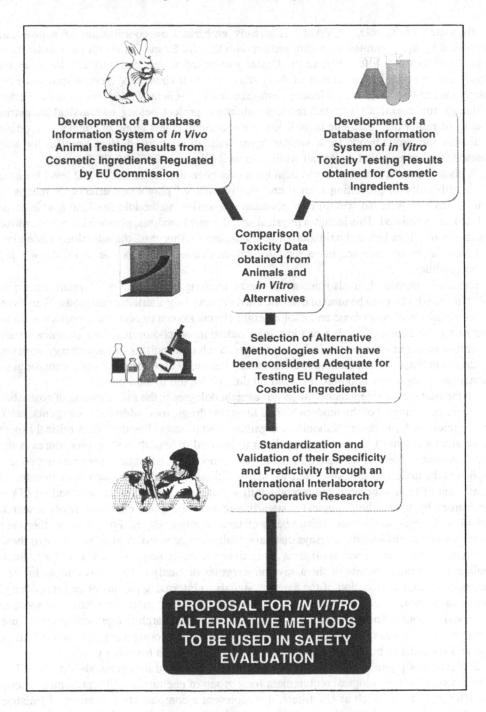

Figure 6.1 Development of *in vitro* methods in safety evaluation of cosmetic ingredients.

This sector has crucial priority and needs to be immediately coordinated and stimulated by ECVAM.

By recognizing the important role percutaneous absorption represents for cosmetic ingredients, the SCC already has been discussing currently available test methods for evaluation of such a property. Information on the amount of a cosmetic ingredient that penetrates the skin is a very important factor influencing the overall spectrum of toxicological information necessary for the final safety evaluation of cosmetic ingredients. Cutaneous penetration assessment is made possible by the presence of robust *in vitro* methods with high predictivity vs. the human *in vivo* process.

The cosmetic industry has devoted considerable scientific and technical resources to the study of the percutaneous absorption process for different cosmetic ingredients; again, in this case a series of extensive *in vivo* human data are available that have proved to be well predicted by means of *in vitro* methods.

The development of such basic research will permit identification of specific applications of individual methodologies, thus determining their reliability and acceptance.

One specific line of research potentially fruitful in promoting application and acceptance of alternative methodologies for safety evaluation of cosmetic ingredients could consist in retrospective *in vitro* analysis of key compounds identified among those cosmetic ingredients in use for which a variety of historical toxicological data are available. Such analysis would provide information on the real predictive value of proposed test systems regarding compounds for which there exists a great deal of data on *in vivo* target organ effects.

On the basis of knowledge and experience gained from development of other sectors of toxicity testing, the procedure outlined in Figure 6.1 represents the future course for *in vitro* alternative testing of cosmetic ingredients.

Chapter 7

IN VITRO TOXICITY DATABASE

7.1 INTRODUCTION

During the last ten years, hundreds of "Alternative Methodologies" to the use of animals in the toxicity testing of chemicals have been developed and applied to chemical safety evaluation or hazard identification. These methodologies make use of organs, tissues, or *in vitro*-grown animal/plant cells, mixtures or structures of synthetic and artificial chemicals, mathematical equation (QSARs) studies, etc.

One problem with the application of alternative methodologies to the evaluation and the regulation of toxicity testing of chemicals is the interpretation of results available to date; that is, the comparative evaluation of different methodologies and the extrapolation of their results to the prediction of human toxicity (*risk assessment*). All sectors of *in vitro* alternative methodologies applied to the toxicity testing of chemicals may increase their information value, if access to results of performed tests is improved through the organization of a data bank.[62]

Besides the validation programs already concluded[68,69] or currently being set up, the organization of a test data bank could contribute to the assessment of the reliability of a given alternative method by means of its evaluation based on a comparison of test results obtained by using the same test method in different laboratories. The existence of a factual data bank with *in vitro* toxicity data allows the development of analogy models based on mathematical patterns constructed with *in vitro* toxicity data and chemicophysical data related to different classes of chemical molecules (QSARs studies).

7.2 THE STRUCTURE OF THE GALILEO DATA BANK

The structure of the Galileo Data Bank (GDB) is composed of four archives: (1) Chemicals and Formulations; (2) Methods; (3) Biosystems; (4) Results.[64,65,152]

7.2.1 CHEMICALS AND FORMULATIONS

The number of individual materials described in the GDB is 2199 chemical compounds and 310 formulations represented by different combinations of ingredients. For each chemical or formulation, its principal use is reported; 24% are used as cosmetic materials, and 46% as other chemicals and formulations such as drugs, pesticides, food additives, industrial chemicals, etc. For each chemical, the IUPAC name and, when possible, CAS and EINECS reference numbers, as well as a series of physicochemical properties, are identified and reported. The formulations are treated in a way to include as much information as possible; the individual ingredients and their concentrations in the formulations are reported, up to a total of 15 different materials. For each ingredient, the GDB code is inserted in order to have the possibility to track both the single ingredient and the compound itself, when reported in another study as a compound alone, thus permitting in the future a comparison between the biological response of the same ingredient when tested alone, or in a formulation (Figure 1).

In cooperation with the Center for Alternatives to Animal Testing (CAAT) of Johns Hopkins University (Baltimore, MD, USA; Professors A.M. Goldberg and J.M. Frazier) and with the financial support of several public (EC Commission, Directorate Generale DGXI.A2; Consumer Policy Service; ECVAM; Italian National Research Council) and private (L'Oreal, General Direction of Research and Development, Paris, France; UNIPRO, Unione Italiana

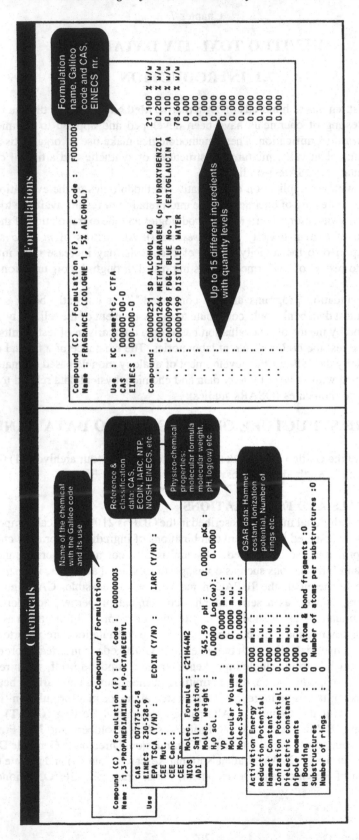

Figure 1. The Galileo Data Bank main screens: Chemicals and formulations.

Profumieri, Milan, Italy) the GDB was created 4 years ago in Pisa, specifically dealing with the organization of a database system of toxicity testing results by means of alternative methodologies.

The present composition of the group of experts includes university graduates in genetic toxicology, general toxicology, and foreign languages, and a Ph.D. in toxicology.

7.2.2 METHODS IN GDB

The structure of the archive of the methods is divided in two sections, one dealing with the *in vitro* methods, the other dealing with the *in vivo* methods. Each section is divided in subsections, for example, (*in vitro*): Cytotoxic, Genotoxic, Hepatotoxic, Neurotoxic methods, etc.; (*in vivo*): Acute toxic, Chronic toxic, Carcinogenic, Teratogenic, Genotoxic methods, etc. The archive of the methods includes a complete description of the experimental procedure employed in the test considered, according to the format of EEC[7,8] and OECD's Guidelines[9] (as the examples reported in Chapter 5) as well as *INVITTOX* protocols[63] (Figure 2).

A series of different toxic endpoints already has been considered and put into relation with different methodologies to test chemicals. Each archive is open: this allows the introduction of newly improved aspects, giving the chance to upgrade the methodologies already existing.

7.2.3 BIOSYSTEMS IN GDB

For each biosystem employed for the toxicity testing, the archive includes (Figure 1): the GDB code; the name; its biologic nature; its source; culture conditions, etc. In the GDB approximately 100 different biosystems, represented mainly by animal cell lines (55%), human cell lines (22%), and others, including plant materials, are reported.

7.2.4 RESULTS IN GDB

Each result or test is defined as a chemical or a formulation employed for the treatment of a biosystem, according to a specific experimental method that gives a result, such as:

different concentrations of Benzalkonium chloride (CAS No. 63449-41-2; EINECS No. 264-151-6; GDB code C0000054), employed on m3T3L-1 cell line, in a Neutral Red Uptake assay, for a treatment time of 24 h, have produced a series of results, represented by an average value, namely NRU50 of 8.4 µg/ml.

The test results are organized in the GDB through different steps (Figure 3): in the main data set, compounds or formulations, methods and biosystems are listed, as well as general test conditions, such as the treatment time and doses applied.

In the complementary data screens, results of tested compounds or formulations are reported as results of the negative and positive compounds, when reported. In addition, the GDB offers a complete description of the testing procedure, in a text file linked to the record, along with all other details that the literature can report.

The number of test data referring to different assay methods is approximately 21,000; the Neutral Red Uptake is the most represented with 1921 independent results. This method has been applied, on the basis of the data in the GDB, on 23 different biosystems tested in different laboratories, employing a treatment time ranging from 2 to 72 h.

7.3 USE OF GDB

Interrogating the GDB allows us to investigate problems of relevance to scientists, industries, and regulators. Some examples of the possibilities for evaluating the data present in the literature and included in the GDB are the following:

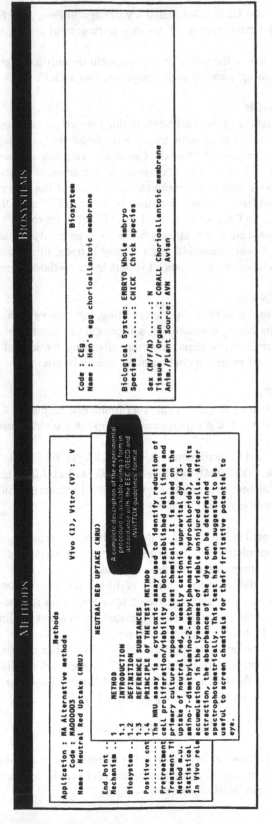

Figure 2. The Galileo Data Bank main screens: Methods and biosystems.

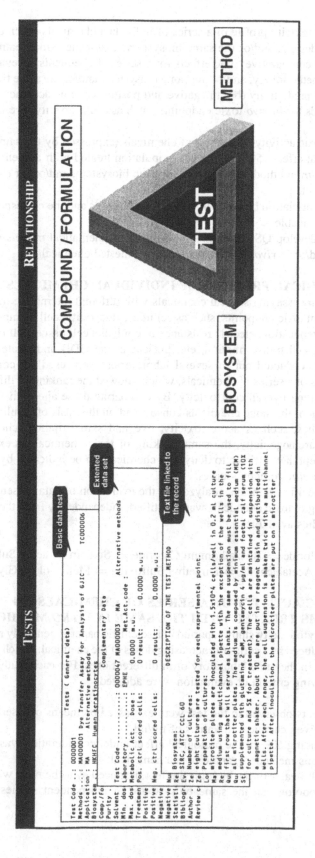

Figure 3. The Galileo Data Bank main screens: Tests and relationship design.

1. elaborating the toxicity profile of a series of individual chemicals ordered by the same *in vitro* methodology, and/or the same biosystem, and/or the same treatment time;
2. elaborating the comparative toxic effects for a series of chemicals, as evaluated by the same *in vitro* methodology, and/or the same biosystem, and/or the same treatment time;
3. elaborating the predictivity (both negative and positive) and its accuracy of a series of *in vitro* methods for *in vivo* toxic endpoints, such as acute toxicity, eye irritation, skin irritation, etc.;
4. ordering the toxic activity of a series of chemicals (expressed by the same value, such as the level that affects 50% of the cell population treated with a chemical) for each individual *in vitro* methodology, and/or for each biosystem, and/or for each individual treatment time etc.;
5. analyzing the correlation between *in vitro* toxicity results and the corresponding *in vivo* toxicity data available;
6. attempting to develop QSAR studies for defining mathematical models for predicting the *in vitro* and/or *in vivo* toxicity potential of untested chemicals.

7.3.1 TOXICOLOGICAL PROFILES OF INDIVIDUAL CHEMICALS

Results obtained by assaying several chemicals with different alternative methodologies, by analyzing different toxic endpoints, such as cellular cytotoxicity, cell membrane integrity, DNA synthesis/cell replication, electric resistance of epithelial cell tissue, cell-cell communication, genotoxicity, cell transformation, etc. present in the GDB and related to different independent studies conducted out in several laboratories, were used for constructing the toxicological profiles of a series of chemicals, which allowed the ranking of different chemicals on the basis of their overall cell toxicity. By comparing those alternative profiles with toxicological profiles of the same chemicals constructed on the basis of results from *in vivo* animal toxicity studies, such as acute toxicity, eye and skin irritation, chronic toxicity, teratogenicity and carcinogenicity, the same ranking of toxic chemicals is expressed, thus confirming the concept that intrinsic toxicity of a chemical can be indicated by means of the *in vivo* and/or the *in vitro* toxicity studies.

For a group of specific chemicals analyzed by the evaluation of data present in the GDB, the following ranking of toxic chemicals was identified, independently from the *in vivo* or the *in vitro* toxicity studies available:

Dibutyltin Chloride $\Rightarrow$ Benzalkonium Chloride $\Rightarrow$ Sodium Dodecyl Sulfate $\Rightarrow$
Toluene $\Rightarrow$ Acetaldehyde $\Rightarrow$ Dimethyl Sulfoxide $\Rightarrow$ Methanol $\Rightarrow$ Glycerol

7.3.2 CYTOTOXIC ACTIVITY OF A SERIES OF CHEMICALS ON DIFFERENT BIOSYSTEMS TREATED WITH THE SAME *IN VITRO* METHODS

Each individual cytotoxicity study reported in a scientific paper is generally represented by biological effects induced by a series of increasing doses of the chemical, which are confirmed by a reported assay, in the same laboratory of in different ones. For each study evaluated by the GDB, the following criteria of evaluation were adopted:

1. biological effects observed in the test were expressed by means of a series of concentrations of a given chemical in values of μg/ml;
2. the dose producing 50% of the biological effect under consideration was calculated by applying various methods, graphic or mathematical;
3. the average 50% value of the biological effect produced by a chemical when applied by a given methodology on the same biosystems, in independent studies for the same

treatment time was calculated: this represents the "quantitative" biological effect considered in the GDB;

4. whenever all these evaluations were not possible because of the inadequacy of the experimental report considered, the result of the biological effect reported in the GDB was expressed as "Positive" or "Negative".

By following these criteria, information relating to the cytotoxicity of 1500 chemicals evaluated by means of different methodologies — such as Neutral Red Uptake, Total Protein Content, Neutral Red Release, LDH Release, and MTT — is already available through the GDB. This information is being analyzed and will be illustrated in a series of outcoming scientific papers. Furthermore, it already allows the definition of the toxicological profiles of chemicals of different classes. A paper on Neutral Red Uptake already has been submitted for publication.

7.3.3 COMPARISON BETWEEN *IN VITRO* AND *IN VIVO* RESULTS

The most important prospect for alternative methods in the toxicity testing of chemicals is, of course, their use as a replacement for using animals in this type of study. Therefore, it is crucial to develop comparative analysis of the results obtained by applying *in vitro* or *in vivo* methods.

By using the GDB data, we constructed a list of chemicals or formulations tested by the *in vitro* Neutral Red Uptake (cytotoxic effect) and by the *in vivo* eye irritation method. In the first case, the cytotoxic effect is represented by the NRU_{50} value, while in the second the ocular irritation activity is represented by the MAS (Maximum Average Score).

Figure 4 shows the correlation between the two values for a series of 39 chemicals and/or formulations. In this comparison the value of R (= –0.51) is highly significant.

7.3.4 PREDICTIVITY OF *IN VITRO* METHODS VS. *IN VIVO* TOXIC ENDPOINTS

As for other *in vitro* toxicity methodologies, such as the genotoxicity testing employed for predicting the carcinogenic potential of chemicals, alternative cytotoxicity methods could be used for predicting *in vivo* toxic endpoints of different concern, such as the eye irritation potential.

In all cases it should be necessary to define a threshold dose of chemicals discriminating between cytotoxic and noncytotoxic chemicals; this assumption, in terms of mechanistic toxicology, would represent the number of molecules of a toxic chemical capable of inhibiting a biological process.

In order to test this hypothesis, and to make possible an evaluation of the predictive value of an Alternative, we have used the data present in the GDB of Neutral Red Uptake in the prediction of the eye irritation potential of a series of 85 test materials (64 individual chemicals, and 21 formulations), by assuming the dose of an $NRU_{50} = 1,000$ µg/ml as the threshold value between cytotoxic and noncytotoxic material. The complete analysis presented in our paper (6) has allowed the calculation of the following parameters concerning the predictivity:

Sensitivity: correct identification of eye irritant materials as cytotoxic = 62.9%
Specificity: correct identification of noneye irritant materials as noncytotoxic = 74.2%
Accuracy: the ability of a group of results to predict the results observed by another
  methodology = 67.0%

As recognized in many publications, the value of accuracy of the Neutral Red Uptake assay in the prediction of the ocular irritation potential of chemicals is not different from the value ascertained for other examples of animal toxicity prediction by means of *in vitro* methods.

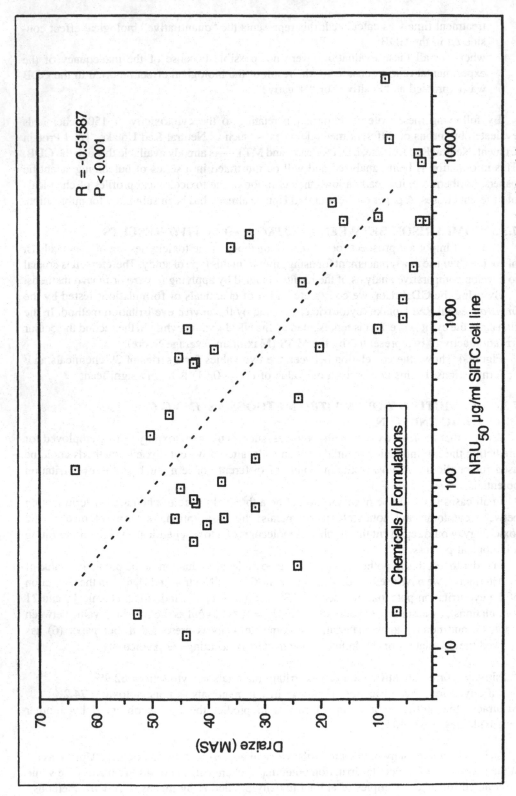

Figure 4. Linear regression analysis of NRU$_{50}$ on SIRC cell line vs. Draize MAS score for 39 chemicals and formulations.

7.4 COSMETIC INGREDIENTS

Cosmetic ingredients as defined in Council Directive 76/768/EEC[1] are chemical substances or preparations of both synthetic and natural origin used in the composition of cosmetic finished products. The core inventory requested by the Sixth Amendment (Council Directive 93/35/EEC[2]) and prepared for the European Inventory includes approximately 7000 individual substances, whereas Council Directive 76/768/EEC[1] includes 412 substances that must not be used in finished products and 303 substances that are used in finished products under some restrictions (reduced concentration, used by a selected group of consumers, or to be applied only to certain parts of the body). Animal data already exist for the majority of the 303 substances, especially for those submitted for SCC's opinion.

Results from alternative methodologies are available for a certain number of cosmetic ingredients of general use, and for some representatives of those regulated by Council Directive 76/768/EEC.[1]

The development of a database of toxicity testing results obtained from studies based on alternative methodologies could be useful in providing information to be used in the preparation of the dossier of finished products, especially for the section dealing with safety evaluation.

The development of a database of toxicity testing results obtained from animal studies applied to cosmetic ingredients regulated by Council Directive 76/768/EEC[1] and analyzed by the SCC could be useful in defining reference chemicals to be used as comparative information for evaluating results obtained by applying alternative methodologies.

Moreover, similar animal toxicity data should be collected for cosmetic ingredients not regulated by Council Directive 76/768/EEC,[1] to be used in the same way as specified above.

Table 7.1 reports cosmetic ingredients and formulations for which results from alternative testings are present in the Galileo Data Bank. Table 7.2 reports the alternative methods that have been applied to the safety evaluation of this group of cosmetic ingredients. Table 7.3 reports examples of results present in the Galileo Data Bank for the same group of chemicals and formulations, namely the Neutral Red Uptake, the Agar Overlay Test, and the Total Protein Content (Lowry Method and Bio-Rad).

TABLE 7.1

List of Cosmetic Compounds and Formulations Tested on Alternative *In Vitro* Methodologies
(the Galileo Data Bank, 1994)

Cas No.	EINECS	GAL Code	Name Compound / Formulation	Cosmetic Use	No.Test
71-55-6	200-756-3	C00001485	1,1,1-TRICHLOROETHANE (METHYLCHLOROFORM)	Cosmetic solvents (DIIC)	3
107-06-2	203-458-1	C00000393	1,2-DICHLOROETHANE	Cosmetic (use not specified, CTFA)	9
		C00000373	1,2-DODECANEDIOL (ETHERIFIED)	Cosmetic surfactant	4
		C00001633	1-(2'-HYDROXYETHYL)-AMINO-3,4-METHYLENEDIOXYBENZENE-HYDROCHLORIDE	Cosmetic hair dye	7
112-00-5	203-927-0	C00000005	1-DODECANAMINIUM, N,N,N-TRIMETHYL-, CHLORIDE	Cosmetic preservatives (DIIC)	1
124-30-1	204-695-3	C00000007	1-OCTADECANAMINE	Cosmetic antistatic agents (DIIC)	1
111-87-5	203-917-6	C00001508	1-OCTANOL (CAPRYLIC ALCOHOL)	Cosmetic controlling agents (DIIC)	18
3332-27-2	222-059-3	C00000008	1-TETRADECANAMINE, N,N-DIMETHYL-, N-OXIDE	Cosmetic surfactants (DIIC)	1
6219-67-6	228-290-6	C00000785	2,4-DIAMINOANISOLE SULFATE (CI 76051)	Cosmetic CTFA (use: hair dye)	4
56216-28-5		C00001646	2,6-DIMETHOXY-3,5-PYRIDINEDIAMINE HYDROCHLORIDE	Cosmetic CTFA (use: hair dye)	3
121-88-0	204-503-8	C00001502	2-AMINO-5-NITROPHENOL	Cosmetic hair dyes (DIIC)	13
78886-51-8		C00001647	2-AMINO-6-METHYLFENOL-HYDROCHLORIDE	Cosmetic hair dye	1
79352-72-0		C00001644	2-AMINOMETHYL-p-AMINOPHENOL HCl	Cosmetic CTFA (use: hair dye)	1
111-76-2	203-905-0	C00000077	2-BUTOXYETHANOL (BUTYL CELLOSOLVE)	Cosmetic solvents (DIIC)	3
		F00000215	2-CHLOROACETAMIDE & SODIUM BENZOATE (70/30) MIXTURE	Cosmetic preparation	1
110-80-5	203-804-1	C00001618	2-ETHOXYETHANOL	Cosmetic solvents (DIIC)	15
109-86-4	203-713-7	C00000014	2-METHOXYETHANOL (ETHYLENE GLYCOL METHYL ETHER)	Cosmetic solvents (DIIC)	45
5307-14-2	226-164-5	C00001401	2-NITRO-p-PHENYLENEDIAMINE	Cosmetic hair dyes (DIIC)	14
61566-66-3		C00001642	3,4-DIAMINOBENZOIC ACID DIHYDROCHLORIDE	Cosmetic hair dye	2

CAS	ID	Name	Use	Count
109-55-7	C00000447	3-(DIMETHYLAMINO)PROPYLAMINE	Cosmetic buffering agents (DIIC)	2
100418-33-5	C00001635	4-(2-HYDROXYETHYL)AMINO-3-NITROTOLUENE	Cosmetic CTFA (use: hair dye)	1
	C00001634	4-AMINO-2-HYDROXYMETHYLPHENOL-HYDROCHLORIDE	Cosmetic hair dye	6
119-34-6	C00001390	4-AMINO-2-NITROPHENOL	Cosmetic hair dyes (DIIC)	3
95-88-5	C00001643	4-CHLORORESORCINOL	Cosmetic hair dyes (DIIC)	1
104226-19-9	C00001637	4-DI(2-HYDROXYETHYL)AMINO-1-(3-HYDROXYPROPYL)-AMINO-2-NITROBENZENE-	Cosmetic hair dye	1
136-77-6	C00001532	4-HEXYLRESORCINOL	Cosmetic various uses (DIIC)	5
99-56-9	C00001415	4-NITRO-o-PHENYLENEDIAMINE (CI 76020)	Cosmetic hair dyes (DIIC)	11
27080-42-8	C00001641	4-NITROPHENYL AMINOETHYLUREA	Cosmetic CTFA (use: hair dye)	1
92-48-8	C00001500	6-METHYLCOUMARIN	Cosmetic oral care agents (DIIC)	8
7747-35-5	C00001751	7-ETHYLBICYCLOOXAZOLIDINE (OXABAN E)	Cosmetic preservatives (DIIC)	2
148-24-3	C00000338	8-QUINOLINOL (8-HYDROXYQUINOLINE)	Cosmetic antimicrobials (DIIC)	7
75-07-0	C00000022	ACETALDEHYDE	Cosmetic (use not specified, CTFA)	29
64-19-7	C00000023	ACETIC ACID	Cosmetic buffering agents (DIIC)	30
67-64-1	C00000083	ACETONE (2-PROPANONE)	Cosmetic solvents (DIIC)	19
	C00000374	ACYLAMINE POLYGLYCOL ETHERSULPHATE (GENAPOL)	Cosmetic surfactant	8
	F00000098	AFTERSHAVE (20% ALCOHOL) (Noxell)	Cosmetics, CTFA	58
97-59-6	C00000547	ALLANTOIN	Cosmetic oral care agents (DIIC)	56
7446-70-0	C00000581	ALUMINIUM CHLORIDE	Cosmetic antiperspirants agents (DIIC)	76
21645-51-2	C00002103	ALUMINUM HYDROXIDE	Cosmetic various uses (DIIC)	13
61788-94-1	C00000032	AMINES, (HYDROGENATED TALLOW ALKYL) DIMETHYL, N-OXIDE	Cosmetic surfactants (DIIC)	1
61788-90-7	C00000038	AMINES, COCO ALKYLDIMETHYL, N-OXIDE	Cosmetic surfactants (DIIC)	3
68439-73-6	C00000045	AMINES, N-TALLOW ALKYLTRIMETHYLENEDI-	Cosmetic emulsifying agents (DIIC)	1
61790-18-9	C00000047	AMINES, SOYA ALKYL	Cosmetic antistatic agents (DIIC)	1
61790-33-8	C00000050	AMINES, TALLOW ALKYL	Cosmetic emulsifying agents (DIIC)	1

TABLE 7.1 (Continued)

List of Cosmetic Compounds and Formulations Tested on Alternative *In Vitro* Methodologies (the Galileo Data Bank, 1994)

Cas No.	EINECS	GAL Code	Name Compound / Formulation	Cosmetic Use	No.Test
124-68-5	204-709-8	C00000257	AMINOMETHYL PROPANOL (1-PROPANOL, 2-AMINO-2-METHYL-)	Cosmetic buffering agents (DIIC)	69
7664-41-7	231-635-3	C00000597	AMMONIA (AMMONIUM HYDROXIDE)	Cosmetic buffering agents (DIIC)	1
12125-02-9	235-186-4	C00000598	AMMONIUM CHLORIDE	Cosmetic controlling agents (DIIC)	8
2235-54-3	218-793-9	C00001366	AMMONIUM LAURYL SULFATE	Cosmetic surfactants (DIIC)	7
977018-62-4		C00001765	AVOCADO EXTRACT	Cosmetic various uses (DIIC)	1
		F00000048	BABY SHAMPOO	Cosmetic preparation	5
		F00000245	BASE-IRIDESCENT COLOGNE	Cosmetic preparation	1
		F00000033	BATH FOAM	Cosmetic preparation	5
		F00000047	BATH GEL/BATH FOAM	Cosmetic preparation	5
112-85-6	204-010-8	C00001766	BEHENIC ACID	Cosmetic emulsifying agents (DIIC)	1
661-19-8	211-546-6	C00001767	BEHENYL ALCOHOL (1-DOCOSANOL)	Cosmetic emollients (DIIC)	1
100-52-7	202-866-7	C00000637	BENZALDEHYDE	Cosmetic flavoring agents (DIIC)	4
63449-41-2	264-151-6	C00000054	BENZALKONIUM CHLORIDE (QUATERNARY AMMONIUM COMPOUNDS, BENZYL-C8-18-)	Cosmetic preservatives (DIIC)	40
121-54-0	204-479-9	C00001302	BENZETHONIUM CHLORIDE	Cosmetic preservatives (DIIC)	93
65-85-0	200-618-2	C00000087	BENZOIC ACID	Cosmetic preservatives (DIIC)	8
131-55-5	205-028-9	C00000566	BENZOPHENONE-2	Cosmetic U.V. absorbers for products (DIIC)	70
131-57-7	205-031-5	C00001739	BENZOPHENONE-3 (OXYBENZONE)	Cosmetic U.V. absorbers (DIIC)	12
4065-45-6	223-772-2	C00000559	BENZOPHENONE-4	Cosmetic U.V. absorbers (DIIC)	127
		F00000301	BENZOYL PEROXIDE CREAM (2.5%) (ESTEE LAUDER)	Cosmetics, CTFA	69

100-51-6	202-859-9	C00000649	BENZYL ALCOHOL (BENZENEMETHANOL)	Cosmetic preservatives (DIIC)	10
80-05-7	201-245-8	C00001520	BISPHENOL A	Cosmetic antimicrobials (DIIC)	9
43143-11-9		C00001749	BISPYRITHIONE (AND) MAGNESIUM SULFATE (OMADINE MDS)	Cosmetic other ingredients (Blaue List)	3
		F00000025	BLEND OF DODECANOL AND DECANOL (BOTH ETHERIFIED)	Cosmetic surfactant	6
		F00000026	BLEND OF SODIUM AND MAGNESIUM ALKYL ETHER SULFATE	Cosmetic surfactant	6
10043-35-3	233-139-2	C00000458	BORIC ACID	Cosmetic antimicrobials (DIIC)	1
		C00001803	BRANCHED 12 CARBON DISULFONATE	Cosmetic surfactant	1
9002-92-0		C00000059	BRIJ 35 (LAURETH-23)	Cosmetic surfactants (DIIC)	43
9004-95-9		C00001498	BRIJ 58 (CETETH-20)	Cosmetic emulsifying agents (DIIC)	8
9005-00-9		C00000555	BRIJ 72 (STEARETH-2)	Cosmetic emulsifying agents (DIIC)	126
9005-00-9		C00000088	BRIJ 78 (STEARETH-20)	Cosmetic surfactants (DIIC)	16
9004-98-2		C00000556	BRIJ 97 (BRIJ 96; OLETH-10)	Cosmetic emulsifying agents (DIIC)	127
9004-98-2		C00000089	BRIJ 99 (BRIJ 98; OLETH-20)	Cosmetic surfactants (DIIC)	12
60-11-7	200-455-7	C00000696	BRILLIANT YELLOW (CI 11020)	Cosmetic hair dyes (DIIC)	3
70356-09-1	274-581-6	C00001732	BUTYL METHOXYDIBENZOYLMETHANE	Cosmetic U.V. absorbers (DIIC)	3
25013-16-5	246-563-8	C00000063	BUTYLATED HYDROXYANISOLE (BHA)	Cosmetic antioxidants (DIIC)	101
96-48-0	202-509-5	C00002104	BUTYROLACTONE	Cosmetic solvents (DIIC)	13
6373-74-6	228-921-5	C00000096	C.I. ACID ORANGE 3	Cosmetic (use not specified, CTFA)	6
3567-69-9	222-657-4	C00001524	C.I. ACID RED 14 (C.I. 14720)	Cosmetic color additives (DIIC)	6
2475-45-8	219-603-7	C00000304	C.I. DISPERSE BLUE 1	Cosmetic hair dyes (DIIC)	9
2832-40-8	220-600-8	C00000305	C.I. DISPERSE YELLOW 3	Cosmetic hair dyes (DIIC)	4
842-07-9	212-668-2	C00000312	C.I. SOLVENT YELLOW 14	Cosmetic hair dyes (DIIC)	9
		C00001785	C12-15 ALCOHOLS BENZOATE (FINSOLV TN)	Cosmetic emollients (DIIC)	1
68131-39-5		C00001793	C12-15 PARETH-12	Cosmetic surfactants (DIIC)	1
58-08-2	200-362-1	C00000065	CAFFEINE	Cosmetic various uses (DIIC)	10
62-54-4	200-540-9	C00000472	CALCIUM ACETATE	Cosmetic controlling agents (DIIC)	1

TABLE 7.1 (Continued)

List of Cosmetic Compounds and Formulations Tested on Alternative *In Vitro* Methodologies (the Galileo Data Bank, 1994)

Cas No.	EINECS	GAL Code	Name Compound / Formulation	Cosmetic Use	No.Test
1305-62-0	215-137-3	C00000720	CALCIUM HYDROXIDE	Cosmetic buffering agents (DIIC)	3
7790-76-3	232-221-5	C00001786	CALCIUM PYROPHOSPHATE	Cosmetic abrasives (DIIC)	1
73398-61-5	277-452-2	C00001768	CAPRYLIC/CAPRIC TRIGLYCERIDE	Cosmetic emollients (DIIC)	1
8023-77-6	232-424-9	C00000680	CAPSICUM OIL	Cosmetic various uses (DIIC)	4
8028-89-5	232-435-9	C00000726	CARAMEL (A)	Cosmetic abrasives (DIIC)	4
8028-89-5	232-435-9	C00000728	CARAMEL (B)	Cosmetic abrasives (DIIC)	3
8028-89-5	232-435-9	C00000729	CARAMEL (C)	Cosmetic abrasives (DIIC)	4
8028-89-5	232-435-9	C00000730	CARAMEL (D)	Cosmetic abrasives (DIIC)	4
8028-89-5	232-435-9	C00000731	CARAMEL (E)	Cosmetic abrasives (DIIC)	4
9007-20-9		C00000557	CARBOMER	Cosmetic controlling agents (DIIC)	127
8001-79-4	232-293-8	C00002027	CASTOR OIL	Cosmetic emollients (DIIC)	12
120-80-9	204-427-5	C00000739	CATECHOL (CI 76500)	Cosmetic (use not specified, CTFA)	2
111-15-9	203-839-2	C00000743	CELLOSOLVE ACETATE (ETHYLENEGLYCOL MONOETHYLETHER ACETATE; ETHANOL	Cosmetic solvents (DIIC)	2
67762-27-0	267-008-6	C00001769	CETEARYL ALCOHOL (ALCOHOLS, C16-18)	Cosmetic emollients (DIIC)	1
36653-82-4	253-149-0	C00000554	CETYL ALCOHOL	Cosmetic controlling agents (DIIC)	127
		C00001801	CETYLDIMETHYL AMMONIUM BROMIDE	Cosmetic surfactant	1
123-03-5	204-593-9	C00001303	CETYLPYRIDINIUM CHLORIDE (CEEPRYN)	Cosmetic antimicrobials (DIIC)	1
55-56-1	200-238-7	C00001701	CHLORHEXIDINE	Cosmetic preservatives (DIIC)	2
18472-51-0	242-354-0	C00000753	CHLORHEXIDINE DIGLUCONATE	Cosmetic preservatives (DIIC)	1
104-29-0	203-192-6	C00001660	CHLORPHENESIN	Cosmetic preservatives (DIIC)	3
72-80-0	200-789-3	C00001703	CHLORQUINALDOL	Cosmetic preservative	6

CAS	ID	Name	Category	N
3468-63-1	C00001752	CI 12075 (PIGMENT ORANGE 5; D&C ORANGE 17)	Cosmetic (use not specified, CTFA)	2
587-98-4	C00001067	CI 13065 (METANIL YELLOW; ACID YELLOW 36)	Cosmetic colorant, dye (Blaue List)	1
5160-02-1	C00000271	CI 15585:1 (D&C RED No. 9/ PIGMENT RED 53:1)	Cosmetic color additives (DIIC)	10
129-17-9	C00001734	CI 42045 (ACID BLUE 1)	Cosmetic color additives (DIIC)	1
8004-87-3	C00001078	CI 42535 (METHYL VIOLET)	Cosmetic (use not specified, CTFA)	1
548-62-9	C00001048	CI 42555 (GENTIAN VIOLET)	Cosmetic (use not specified, CTFA)	1
2580-56-5	C00001705	CI 44045 (CI BASIC BLUE 26; VICTORIA BLUE B)	Cosmetic color additives (DIIC)	3
27870-92-4	C00001735	CI 56238 (SOLVENT YELLOW 98)	Cosmetic color additives (DIIC)	2
1330-38-7	C00001750	CI 74180	Cosmetic color additives (DIIC)	4
1309-37-1	C00000963	CI 77491 (IRON OXIDES; IRON SESQUIOXIDE)	Cosmetic color additives (DIIC)	4
10101-66-3	C00001762	CI 77742 (MANGANESE VIOLET)	Cosmetic color additives (DIIC)	2
13463-67-7	C00000297	CI 77891 (TITANIUM DIOXIDE)	Cosmetic color additives (DIIC)	4
12220-24-5	C00001700	CI ACID RED 195	Cosmetic color additives (DIIC)	2
8007-80-5	C00000254	CINNAMON OIL	Cosmetic flavoring agents (DIIC)	74
5392-40-5	C00000782	CITRAL	Cosmetic flavoring agents (DIIC)	3
77-92-9	C00000783	CITRIC ACID	Cosmetic buffering agents (DIIC)	84
	F00000300	CLEANSING CREAM III (REVLON)	Cosmetics, CTFA	202
	F00000247	CLEANSING GEL	Cosmetic preparation	1
	F00000250	CLEANSING GEL LR25	Cosmetic preparation	3
	F00000246	CLEANSING MILK	Cosmetic preparation	1
	C00001760	CLOISONNE RED-EO (ETHYLENE OXIDE TREATED)	Cosmetic color additive	1
	C00001761	CLOISONNE RED-GI (ETHYLENE OXIDE GAMMA IRRADIATED)	Cosmetic color additive	1
68603-42-9	C00001778	COCAMIDE DEA	Cosmetic controlling agents (DIIC)	1
61789-40-0	C00000132	COCAMIDOPROPYL BETAINE (DEHYTON K)	Cosmetic surfactants (DIIC)	8
68155-09-9	C00001759	COCAMIDOPROPYLAMINE OXIDE	Cosmetic surfactants (DIIC)	1
1390-65-4	C00000765	COCHINEAL	Cosmetic color additives (DIIC)	2
	C00000368	COCOAMPHODIACETATE	Cosmetic surfactant	3
	C00000375	COCOBETAINE DERIVATIVE	Cosmetic surfactant	6

TABLE 7.1 (Continued)

List of Cosmetic Compounds and Formulations Tested on Alternative *In Vitro* Methodologies
(the Galileo Data Bank, 1994)

Cas No.	EINECS	GAL Code	Name Compound / Formulation	Cosmetic Use	No. Test
8001-31-8	232-282-8	C00001770	COCONUT OIL	Cosmetic emollients (DIIC)	1
		F00000095	COLOGNE 1 (5% ALCOHOL) (Johnson & Johnson)	Cosmetics, CTFA	70
		F00000099	COLOGNE 2 (83% ALCOHOL) (Revlon)	Cosmetics, CTFA	70
7758-98-7	231-847-6	C00000126	COPPER (II) SULFATE	Cosmetic various uses (DIIC)	1
11006-34-1	234-242-5	C00000768	COPPER CHLOROPHYLL	Cosmetic color additives (DIIC)	4
8001-30-7	232-281-2	C00001209	CORN OIL	Cosmetic emollients (DIIC)	1
56-72-4	200-285-3	C00000317	COUMAPHOS	Cosmetic colorant, dye (Blaue List)	6
91-64-5	202-086-7	C00001444	COUMARIN	Cosmetic flavoring agents (DIIC)	1
		F00000255	CREAM 1	Cosmetic preparation	1
		F00000256	CREAM 2	Cosmetic preparation	1
57-09-0	200-311-3	C00000127	CTAB (CETYLTRIMETHYL AMMONIUM BROMIDE)	Cosmetic preservatives (DIIC)	43
112-02-7	203-928-6	C00001379	CTAC (CETYL TRIMETHYL AMMONIUM CHLORIDE)	Cosmetic preservatives (DIIC)	10
		F00000292	CUTICLE REMOVER CREAM (AVON)	Cosmetics, CTFA	56
633-96-5	211-199-0	C00000567	D&C ORANGE No. 4 (CI 15510)	Cosmetic color additives (DIIC)	70
57-48-7	200-333-3	C00000387	D-FRUCTOSE	Cosmetic flavoring agents (DIIC)	5
50-99-7	200-075-1	C00001496	D-GLUCOSE	Cosmetic flavoring agents (DIIC)	11
69-65-8	200-711-8	C00001210	D-MANNITOL	Cosmetic flavoring agents (DIIC)	11
60812-23-9		C00001746	DECOMINOL (3-DECYLOXY-2-HYDROXY-1-AMINOPROPANE HYDROCHLORIDE)	Cosmetic preservative (Blaue List)	3
7732-18-5	231-791-2	C00001198	DEIONIZED WATER	Cosmetic solvents (DIIC)	3
		F00000102	DEODORANT (40% ALCOHOL) (Dial)	Cosmetics, CTFA	76
103-23-1	203-090-1	C00000852	DI(2-ETHYLHEXYL)ADIPATE	Cosmetic emollients (DIIC)	3

CAS	ID	Name	Category	Count
117-81-7	C00001365	DI-(2-ETHYLHEXYL) PHTHALATE (DEHP)	Cosmetic film former (DIIC)	7
123-42-2	C00002106	DIACETONE ALCOHOL	Cosmetic solvents (DIIC)	12
78491-02-8	C00001704	DIAZOLIDINYL UREA (GERMALL II)	Cosmetic preservatives (DIIC)	2
111-42-2	C00000248	DIETHANOLAMINE (ETHANOL, 2,2'-IMINOBIS-)	Cosmetic buffering agents (DIIC)	10
84-66-2	C00000425	DIETHYL PHTHALATE	Cosmetic denaturants (DIIC)	3
109-89-7	C00000494	DIETHYLAMINE	Cosmetic buffering agents (DIIC)	1
111-46-6	C00000916	DIETHYLENE GLYCOL (CARBITOL; PEG-2)	Cosmetic solvents (DIIC)	8
108-18-9	C00001828	DIISOPROPYLAMINE	Cosmetic buffering agents (DIIC)	2
64365-23-7	C00000253	DIMETHICONE COPOLYOL	Cosmetic antistatic agents (DIIC)	135
2867-47-2	C00001875	DIMETHYLAMINOETHYL METHACRYLATE	Cosmetic controlling agents (DIIC)	2
110-98-5	C00000241	DIPROPYLENE GLYCOL (2-PROPANOL, 1,1'-OXIBIS-)	Cosmetic solvents (DIIC)	1
	F00000237	DISODIUM COCOAMPHODIACETATE 19% & SDS 11% & HEXYLENE GLYCOL 8%	Cosmetic surfactant	18
139-33-3	C00000558	DISODIUM EDTA	Cosmetic controlling agents (DIIC)	128
107-64-2	C00001781	DISTEARYLDIMONIUM CHLORIDE	Cosmetic antistatic agents (DIIC)	1
54-12-6	C00001375	DL-TRYPTOPHAN	Cosmetic antistatic agents (DIIC)	4
	C00000372	DODECANOL (ETHERIFIED)	Cosmetic surfactant	4
	C00002101	DODECYL MERCAPTANS (ETHERIFIED 20 R)	Cosmetic surfactant	2
25155-30-0	C00000420	DODECYLBENZENE SULFONIC ACID, SODIUM SALT	Cosmetic surfactants (DIIC)	1
514-78-3	C00000851	DRY CANTHAXANTHIN	Cosmetic color additives (DIIC)	4
60-00-4	C00001482	EDTA (ETHYLENEDIAMINETETRAACETIC ACID)	Cosmetic chelating agents (DIIC)	3
64-02-8	C00000142	EDTA-Na SALT (TETRASODIUM EDTA; GLYCINE, N,N'-1,2-ETHANEDIYLBIS[N-	Cosmetic chelating agents (DIIC)	1
	F00000289	EMOLLIENT CREAM (MARY KAY)	Cosmetics, CTFA	68
89-65-6	C00000858	ERYTHORBIC ACID (ISOASCORBIC ACID)	Cosmetic antioxidants (DIIC)	4
16423-68-0	C00001000	ERYTHROSIN (ERYTHROSIN BLUISH; CI 45430)	Cosmetic color additives (DIIC)	4
64-17-5	C00000144	ETHANOL	Cosmetic solvents (DIIC)	67
141-43-5	C00001003	ETHANOLAMINE (2-AMINO-ETHANOL, MONOETHANOLAMINE)	Cosmetic buffering agents (DIIC)	1

TABLE 7.1 (Continued)

List of Cosmetic Compounds and Formulations Tested on Alternative *In Vitro* Methodologies
(the Galileo Data Bank, 1994)

Cas No.	EINECS	GAL Code	Name Compound / Formulation	Cosmetic Use	No.Test
111-90-0	203-919-7	C00000922	ETHOXYDIGLYCOL (CARBITOL CELLOSOLVE; CARBITOL)	Cosmetic solvents (DIIC)	1
141-78-6	205-500-4	C00001008	ETHYL ACETATE	Cosmetic solvents (DIIC)	10
		F00000031	ETHYL ACETATE, 10% IN TWEEN 80	Cosmetic solvents (DIIC)	5
58882-17-0	261-482-8	C00000561	ETHYL DIHYDROXYPROPYL PABA	Cosmetic U.V. absorbers (DIIC)	138
25087-06-3		C00000256	ETHYL ESTER PVM/MA COPOLYMER (2-BUTANEDIOIC, ACID (Z-) MONOETHYL	Cosmetic film former (DIIC)	69
107-21-1	203-473-3	C00000145	ETHYLENE GLYCOL (1,2-ETHANEDIOL)	Cosmetic solvents (DIIC)	25
120-47-8	204-399-4	C00000884	ETHYLPARABEN	Cosmetic preservatives (DIIC)	3
8000-48-4		C00001771	EUCALYPTUS OIL	Cosmetic various uses (DIIC)	1
97-53-0	202-589-1	C00001529	EUGENOL	Cosmetic various uses (DIIC)	7
		F00000070	EYE MAKE UP REMOVER 4	Cosmetic preparation	9
2353-45-9	219-091-5	C00001032	FAST GREEN FCF(CI 42053)	Cosmetic color additives (DIIC)	7
3844-45-9	223-339-8	C00000998	FD&C BLUE No. 1 (ERIOGLAUCIN A; CI 42090 - SODIUM SALT)	Cosmetic color additives (DIIC)	129
		C00000550	FD&C COLOR(S)	Cosmetic color additives (DIIC)	54
81-88-9	201-383-9	C00001156	FD&C RED No. 19 (RHODAMINE B; RHODAMINE S; CI 45170(:3))	Cosmetic colorant, dye (Blaue List)	4
915-67-3	213-022-2	C00000587	FD&C RED No. 2 (AMARANTH; CI 16185; ACID RED 27)	Cosmetic color additives (DIIC)	81
2321-07-5	219-031-8	C00000147	FLUORESCEIN	Cosmetic hair dyes (DIIC)	15
		F00000044	FOAMING BATH	Cosmetic preparation	5
2650-18-2	220-168-0	C00000903	FOOD BLUE NO. 1	Cosmetic hair dyes (DIIC)	4
860-22-0	212-728-8	C00000904	FOOD BLUE NO. 2	Cosmetic hair dyes (DIIC)	8

CAS	EINECS	ID	Name	Category	No.
2611-82-7	220-036-2	C00000905	FOOD RED NO. 102	Cosmetic color additives (DIIC)	2
3520-42-1	222-529-8	C00000906	FOOD RED NO. 106	Cosmetic color additives (DIIC)	3
		F00000294	FOOT CARE CREAM (AVON)	Cosmetics, CTFA	65
50-00-0	200-001-8	C00001040	FORMALDEHYDE (FORMALIN)	Cosmetic preservatives (DIIC)	5
75-12-7	200-842-0	C00000475	FORMAMIDE	Cosmetic solvents (DIIC)	1
64-18-6	200-579-1	C00000483	FORMIC ACID	Cosmetic preservatives (DIIC)	1
		F00000087	FRAGRANCE (COLOGNE 1, 5% ALCOHOL)	Cosmetics, CTFA	70
		F00000088	FRAGRANCE (FRESHENER)	Cosmetics, CTFA	55
		F00000090	FRAGRANCE (HAIR STYLING LOTION)	Cosmetics, CTFA	66
		F00000089	FRAGRANCE (PERFUMED SKIN LOTION)	Cosmetics, CTFA	127
		F00000093	FRAGRANCE (PUMP HAIR SPRAY)	Cosmetics, CTFA	69
		F00000091	FRAGRANCE 1 (COLOGNE 2, 83% ALCOHOL)	Cosmetics, CTFA	71
		F00000092	FRAGRANCE 2 (COLOGNE 2, 83% ALCOHOL)	Cosmetics, CTFA	69
		F00000097	FRESHENER (15% ALCOHOL) (Mary Kay)	Cosmetics, CTFA	55
111-30-8	203-856-5	C00001222	GLUTARALDEHYDE	Cosmetic preservatives (DIIC)	7
70-18-8	200-725-4	C00000489	GLUTATHIONE (REDUCED)	Cosmetic various uses (DIIC)	1
56-81-5	200-289-5	C00000150	GLYCEROL (GLYCERINE; 1,2,3-PROPANETRIOL)	Cosmetic denaturants (DIIC)	229
		F00000293	HAIR CONDITIONER (Mary Kay)	Cosmetics, CTFA	75
		F00000043	HAIR GEL	Cosmetic preparation	5
		F00000049	HAIR GEL 2	Cosmetic preparation	5
		F00000288	HAIR MASQUE (Chesebrough-Ponds)	Cosmetics, CTFA	62
		F00000101	HAIR STYLING LOTION (65% ALCOHOL) (Procter & Gamble)	Cosmetics, CTFA	66
		F00000290	HAND AND BODY LOTION (Chesebrough-Ponds)	Cosmetics, CTFA	68
		F00000303	HAND AND NAIL LOTION (Chesebrough-Ponds)	Cosmetics, CTFA	68
2784-94-3	220-495-9	C00000335	HC BLUE 1	Cosmetic hair dyes (DIIC)	5
102767-27-1		C00001639	HC BLUE NO. 10	Cosmetic CTFA (use: hair dye)	1
23920-15-2		C00001636	HC BLUE NO. 11	Cosmetic CTFA (use: hair dye)	1

TABLE 7.1 (Continued)

List of Cosmetic Compounds and Formulations Tested on Alternative *In Vitro* Methodologies
(the Galileo Data Bank, 1994)

Cas No.	EINECS	GAL Code	Name Compound / Formulation	Cosmetic Use	No.Test
33229-34-4	251-410-3	C00000306	HC BLUE NO. 2	Cosmetic hair dyes (DIIC)	4
114087-41-1		C00001640	HC BLUE NO. 9	Cosmetic CTFA (use: hair dye)	1
2871-01-4	220-701-7	C00000307	HC RED NO. 3	Cosmetic hair dyes (DIIC)	12
59320-13-7		C00001638	HC YELLOW NO. 12	Cosmetic CTFA (use: hair dye)	1
70-30-4	200-733-8	C00001274	HEXACHLOROPHENE	Cosmetic (use not specified, CTFA)	1
3811-75-4		C00001740	HEXAMIDINE	Cosmetic preservatives (DIIC)	4
141-94-6	205-513-5	C00001706	HEXETIDINE	Cosmetic preservatives (DIIC)	1
7647-01-0	231-595-7	C00000154	HYDROCHLORIC ACID	Cosmetic buffering agents (DIIC)	8
7722-84-1	231-765-0	C00001235	HYDROGEN PEROXIDE	Cosmetic antimicrobials (DIIC)	7
92113-31-0	295-635-5	C00001782	HYDROLYZED ANIMAL PROTEIN	Cosmetic antistatic agents (DIIC)	1
123-31-9	204-617-8	C00000155	HYDROQUINONE (1,4-BENZENEDIOL)	Cosmetic bleaching agents (DIIC)	2
5470-11-1	226-798-2	C00000491	HYDROXYLAMINE HYDROCHLORIDE	Cosmetic (use not specified, CTFA)	1
9004-64-2		C00000563	HYDROXYPROPYLCELLULOSE	Cosmetic controlling agents (DIIC)	138
39236-46-9	254-372-6	C00000549	IMIDAZOLIDINYL UREA (GERMAL 115)	Cosmetic preservatives (DIIC)	56
67-63-0	200-661-7	C00001285	ISOPROPYL ALCOHOL (2-PROPANOL; ISOPROPANOL)	Cosmetic foaming agents (DIIC)	36
110-27-0	203-751-4	C00001772	ISOPROPYL MYRISTATE	Cosmetic emollients (DIIC)	1
142-91-6	205-571-1	C00000551	ISOPROPYL PALMITATE (DELTYL)	Cosmetic emollients (DIIC)	128
9000-07-1	232-524-2	C00000738	KAPPA-CARRAGEENAN (Na SALT)	Cosmetic emulsion stabilizers (DIIC)	3
55965-84-9		C00001370	KATHON CG (MIXTURE OF METHYLCHLOROISO THIAZOLINONE 26172-55-4	Cosmetic preservatives (DIIC)	75
50-81-7	200-066-2	C00000086	L-ASCORBIC ACID	Cosmetic buffering agents (DIIC)	39
25395-66-8	246-944-9	C00000630	L-ASCORBYL STEARATE	Cosmetic antioxidants (DIIC)	4

52-89-1	200-157-7	C00000442	L-CYSTEINE HYDROCHLORIDE (MONOHYDRATE)	Cosmetic antioxidants (DIIC)	5
56-86-0	200-293-7	C00000149	L-GLUTAMIC ACID	Cosmetic antistatic agents (DIIC)	4
63-91-2	200-568-1	C00001455	L-PHENYLALANINE	Cosmetic antistatic agents (DIIC)	5
87-69-4	201-766-0	C00000502	L-TARTARIC ACID	Cosmetic buffering agents (DIIC)	4
73-22-3	200-795-6	C00001382	L-TRYPTOPHAN	Cosmetic antistatic agents (DIIC)	4
50-21-5	200-018-0	C00000159	LACTIC ACID (PROPANOIC ACID, 2-HYDROXY-)	Cosmetic buffering agents (DIIC)	58
120-40-1	204-393-1	C00001780	LAURAMIDE DEA	Cosmetic controlling agents (DIIC)	1
4292-10-8	224-292-6	C00001788	LAURAMIDOPROPYL BETAINE	Cosmetic antistatic agents (DIIC)	1
		C00001789	LAUROAMPHODIACETATE	Cosmetic surfactant	1
12751-23-4	235-799-7	C00001791	LAURYL PHOSPHATE	Cosmetic (use not specified, CTFA)	1
14933-08-5	239-002-3	C00002107	LAURYL SULTAINE (LAURYLSULFOBETAINE)	Cosmetic various uses (DIIC)	12
301-04-2	206-104-4	C00001412	LEAD ACETATE	Cosmetic hair dyes (DIIC)	2
		C00001798	LINEAR 10 CARBON DISULFONATE	Cosmetic surfactant	1
60-33-3	200-470-9	C00001474	LINOLEIC ACID	Cosmetic antistatic agents (DIIC)	1
		F00000034	LIQUID SOAP	Cosmetic preparation	5
		C00001758	LITHIUM DODECYL SULFATE	Cosmetic surfactant	1
		F00000248	LOTION 1	Cosmetic preparation	1
		F00000249	LOTION 2	Cosmetic preparation	1
591-27-5	209-711-2	C00000503	m-AMINOPHENOL	Cosmetic hair dyes (DIIC)	1
108-45-2	203-584-7	C00001598	m-PHENYLENDIAMINE (CI76025)	Cosmetic hair dyes (DIIC)	3
		F00000272	m/p CRESOL MIXTURE	Cosmetic preparation	4
546-93-0	208-915-9	C00001464	MAGNESIUM CARBONATE	Cosmetic color additives (DIIC)	3
7487-88-9	231-298-2	C00001495	MAGNESIUM SULFATE	Cosmetic controlling agents (DIIC)	6
		F00000077	MAKE UP REMOVER 6	Cosmetic preparation	18
110-16-7	203-742-5	C00001242	MALEIC ACID	Cosmetic buffering agents (DIIC)	1
		F00000253	MASCARA 1	Cosmetic preparation	1
		F00000254	MASCARA 2	Cosmetic preparation	1
108-78-1	203-615-4	C00000277	MELAMINE	Cosmetic controlling agents (DIIC)	6

TABLE 7.1 (Continued)

List of Cosmetic Compounds and Formulations Tested on Alternative *In Vitro* Methodologies
(the Galileo Data Bank, 1994)

Cas No.	EINECS	GAL Code	Name Compound / Formulation	Cosmetic Use	No.Test
89-78-1	201-939-0	C00001243	MENTHOL	Cosmetic flavoring agents (DIIC)	1
67-56-1	200-659-6	C00000165	METHANOL	Cosmetic solvents (DIIC)	56
79-20-9	201-185-2	C00001206	METHYL ACETATE	Cosmetic solvents (DIIC)	2
78-93-3	201-159-0	C00001071	METHYL ETHYL KETONE (2-BUTANONE)	Cosmetic solvents (DIIC)	2
68239-42-9		C00000560	METHYL GLUCETH-20	Cosmetic humectants (DIIC)	138
108-10-1	203-550-1	C00001074	METHYL ISOBUTYL KETONE	Cosmetic denaturants (DIIC)	13
85-91-6	201-642-6	C00000992	METHYL N-METHYLANTHRANILATE	Cosmetic ingredient	4
9004-67-5		C00001545	METHYLCELLULOSE	Cosmetic controlling agents (DIIC)	4
75-09-2	200-838-9	C00001250	METHYLENE CHLORIDE (DICHLOROMETHANE)	Cosmetic solvents (DIIC)	7
99-76-3	202-785-7	C00001264	METHYLPARABEN (p-HYDROXYBENZOIC ACID METHYL ESTER; PARABEN)	Cosmetic preservatives (DIIC)	64
15087-24-8	239-139-9	C00001756	MEXORYL SD (3-BENZYLIDENE CAMPHOR)	Cosmetic U.V. absorbers (DIIC)	6
56039-58-9		C00000056	MEXORYL SL : BENZENESULFONIC ACID, 4- [(4,7,7-TRIMETHYL-3-OXO-BICYCLO	Cosmetic U.V. absorbers (DIIC)	1
90457-82-2		C00000015	MEXORYL SX : 3,3'-(1,4-PHENYLENEDIMETHYLIDYNE) BIS[7,7-DIMETHYL-2-OXO-	Cosmetic U.V. absorbers (DIIC)	2
		F00000081	MILD SHAMPOO	Cosmetic preparation	2
8012-95-1	232-384-2	F00000146	MINERAL OIL (PARAFFIN OIL; VASELINE OIL)	Cosmetic emollients (DIIC)	1
8032-32-4	232-453-7	F00000282	MINERAL SPIRITS (PETROLEUM SPIRITS; PETROLEUM ETHER)	Cosmetic solvents (DIIC)	12
		F00000257	MIXED C8 AMPHOCARBOXYLATES	Cosmetic surfactant	1
		F00000129	MIXTURE I (HAIR DYE)	Cosmetic hair dye	1
		F00000130	MIXTURE II (HAIR DYE)	Cosmetic hair dye	1

CAS	EINECS	ID	Name	Use	No.
		F00000128	MIXTURE III (HAIR DYE)	Cosmetic hair dye	1
		F00000298	MOISTURIZING LOTION (MARY KAY)	Cosmetics, CTFA	74
142-47-2	205-538-1	C00001483	MONOSODIUM GLUTAMATE	Cosmetic various uses (DIIC)	4
		F00000096	MOUTHWASH (10% ALCOHOL) (Lever Brothers)	Cosmetics, CTFA	74
1119-97-7	214-291-9	C00000172	MTAB (MYRISTYLTRIMETHYLAMMONIUM BROMIDE; 1-TETRADECANAMINIUM, N,N,N-	Cosmetic preservatives (DIIC)	25
9004-99-3		C00000062	MYRJ 45 (PEG-8 STEARATE)	Cosmetic emulsifying agents (DIIC)	9
9004-99-3		C00000258	MYRJ 52 (PEG-40 STEARATE)	Cosmetic emulsifying agents (DIIC)	127
134-62-3	205-149-7	C00001095	N,N-DIETHYL-m-TOLUAMIDE	Cosmetic various uses (DIIC)	9
99-98-9	202-807-5	C00001266	N,N-DIMETHYL-p-PHENYLENEDIAMINE (CI 76075)	Cosmetic (use not specified, CTFA)	8
94158-14-2		C00001648	N-(2-HYDROXYETHYL)-3,4-METHYLENDIOXY ANILINE-HYDROCHLORIDE	Cosmetic hair dye	2
123-86-4	204-658-1	C00000702	n-BUTYL ACETATE (ACETIC ACID, BUTYL ESTER)	Cosmetic solvents (DIIC)	6
71-36-3	200-751-6	C00000002	n-BUTYL ALCOHOL (1-BUTANOL)	Cosmetic denaturants (DIIC)	40
110-54-3	203-777-6	C00000174	n-HEXANE	Cosmetic (use not specified, CTFA)	47
111-27-3	203-852-3	C00001121	n-HEXYL ALCOHOL (1-HEXANOL)	Cosmetic foaming agents (DIIC)	5
71-23-8	200-746-9	C00001504	n-PROPYL ALCOHOL (1-PROPANOL)	Cosmetic foaming agents (DIIC)	5
98-92-0	202-713-4	C00000176	NICOTINAMIDE (3-PYRIDINECARBOXAMIDE)	Cosmetic various uses (DIIC)	5
7697-37-2	231-714-2	C00000470	NITRIC ACID	Cosmetic buffering agents (DIIC)	1
5064-31-3	225-768-6	C00001392	NITRILOTRIACETIC ACID TRISODIUM SALT	Cosmetic chelating agents (DIIC)	4
9016-45-9		C00001792	NONOXYNOL-12	Cosmetic surfactants (DIIC)	1
95-55-6	202-431-1	C00001729	o-AMINOPHENOL (CI 76520)	Cosmetic hair dyes (DIIC)	13
72674-05-6		C00001802	B-OLEFIN SULFONATE (B-ALKENESULFONIC ACID)	Cosmetic surfactant	1
95-54-5	202-430-6	C00001599	o-PHENYLEDIAMINE (CI76010)	Cosmetic hair dyes (DIIC)	2
		C00002102	OCTODECYLMERCAPTANS (ETHERIFIED)	Cosmetic surfactant	1
21245-02-3	244-289-3	C00001736	OCTYL DIMETHYL PABA	Cosmetic U.V. absorbers (DIIC)	1
5466-77-3	226-775-7	C00001731	OCTYL METHOXYCINNAMATE	Cosmetic U.V. absorbers (DIIC)	4
29806-73-3	249-862-1	C00001773	OCTYL PALMITATE	Cosmetic emollients (DIIC)	1
118-60-5	204-263-4	C00001737	OCTYL SALICYLATE	Cosmetic U.V. absorbers (DIIC)	1

TABLE 7.1 (Continued)

List of Cosmetic Compounds and Formulations Tested on Alternative *In Vitro* Methodologies
(the Galileo Data Bank, 1994)

Cas No.	EINECS	GAL Code	Name Compound / Formulation	Cosmetic Use	No.Test
88122-99-0		C00001745	OCTYL TRIAZONE	Cosmetic U.V. absorbers (DIIC)	2
1936-15-8	217-705-6	C00001131	ORANGE G (CI ACID ORANGE 10; CI 16230)	Cosmetic color additives (DIIC)	5
144-62-7	205-634-3	C00001262	OXALIC ACID	Cosmetic chelating agents (DIIC)	5
		F00000295	P&G OINTMENT 1 (HYDROPHILIC OINTMENT, 5% SLS - Procter & Gamble)	Cosmetics, CTFA	59
		F00000296	P&G OINTMENT 2 (HYDROPHILIC OINTMENT, 10% SLS - Procter & Gamble)	Cosmetics, CTFA	60
123-30-8	204-616-2	C00000180	p-AMINOPHENOL (PHENOL, 4-AMINO-)	Cosmetic hair dyes (DIIC)	20
624-18-0	210-834-9	C00001417	p-PHENYLENEDIAMINE DIHYDROCHLORIDE	Cosmetic hair dyes (DIIC)	11
8002-75-3	232-316-1	C00001774	PALM OIL	Cosmetic emollients (DIIC)	1
103-90-2	203-157-5	C00000182	PARACETAMOL (ACETAMINOPHEN)	Cosmetic various uses (DIIC)	49
61788-85-0		C00001775	PEG-40 HYDROGENATED CASTOR OIL	Cosmetic emulsifying agents (DIIC)	1
		C00000370	PENTADECANOL (ETHERIFIED)	Cosmetic surfactant	5
8006-90-4		C00000546	PEPPERMINT OIL	Cosmetic various uses (DIIC)	78
		F00000100	PERFUMED SKIN LOTION (33% ALCOHOL) (Avon)	Cosmetics, CTFA	127
62-44-2	200-533-0	C00001493	PHENACETIN	Cosmetic various uses (DIIC)	14
108-95-2	203-632-7	C00000186	PHENOL	Cosmetic antimicrobials (DIIC)	15
122-99-6	204-589-7	C00001757	PHENOXYETHANOL	Cosmetic preservatives (DIIC)	1
770-35-4	212-222-7	C00001712	PHENOXYISOPROPANOL	Cosmetic preservatives (DIIC)	2
6441-77-6	229-225-4	C00001144	PHLOXINE (CI 45405)	Cosmetic color additives (DIIC)	4
7664-38-2	231-633-2	C00000471	PHOSPHORIC ACID	Cosmetic buffering agents (DIIC)	1
25322-68-3		C00001380	POLYETHYLENE GLYCOL 400 (PEG 400)	Cosmetic binders (DIIC)	2

CAS	EINECS	ID	Name	Use	No.
53633-54-8		C00001783	POLYQUATERNIUM-11 (QUATERNARIUM-23)	Cosmetic antistatic agents (DIIC)	1
7758-02-3	231-830-3	C00000407	POTASSIUM BROMIDE	Cosmetic various uses (DIIC)	5
584-08-7	209-529-3	C00001041	POTASSIUM CARBONATE	Cosmetic buffering agents (DIIC)	3
7447-40-7	231-211-8	C00000408	POTASSIUM CHLORIDE	Cosmetic controlling agents (DIIC)	4
7789-23-3	232-151-5	C00000422	POTASSIUM FLUORIDE	Cosmetic oral care agents (DIIC)	1
1310-58-3	215-181-3	C00001432	POTASSIUM HYDROXIDE	Cosmetic buffering agents (DIIC)	3
7681-11-0	231-659-4	C00001497	POTASSIUM IODIDE	Cosmetic various uses (DIIC)	10
7757-79-1	231-818-8	C00001096	POTASSIUM NITRATE	Cosmetic various uses (DIIC)	2
7778-77-0	231-913-4	C00000469	POTASSIUM PHOSPHATE, MONOBASIC	Cosmetic buffering agents (DIIC)	1
24634-61-5	246-376-1	C00001097	POTASSIUM SORBATE	Cosmetic preservatives (DIIC)	4
7778-80-5	231-915-5	C00000405	POTASSIUM SULFATE	Cosmetic controlling agents (DIIC)	1
9087-53-0		C00000544	PPG-5 CETETH-20	Cosmetic emulsifying agents (DIIC)	70
79-09-4	201-176-3	C00000485	PROPIONIC ACID	Cosmetic preservatives (DIIC)	1
121-79-9	204-498-2	C00000261	PROPYL GALLATE	Cosmetic antioxidants (DIIC)	10
57-55-6	200-338-0	C00000192	PROPYLENE GLYCOL (1,2-PROPANEDIOL)	Cosmetic solvents (DIIC)	11
94-13-3	202-307-7	C00002036	PROPYLPARABEN	Cosmetic preservatives (DIIC)	12
		F00000094	PUMP HAIR SPRAY (90% ALCOHOL) (Amway)	Cosmetics, CTFA	69
25086-89-9		C00000252	PVP/VA COPOLIMER (50% ALCOHOL)	Cosmetic antistatic agents (DIIC)	66
110-86-1	203-809-9	C00000194	PYRIDINE	Cosmetic solvents (DIIC)	17
87-66-1	201-762-9	C00001428	PYROGALLOL	Cosmetic hair dyes (DIIC)	1
130-95-0	205-003-2	C00000506	QUININE	Cosmetic various uses (DIIC)	1
108-46-3	203-585-2	C00001290	RESORCINOL (A11; 1,3-BENZENEDIOL)	Cosmetic hair dyes (DIIC)	1
		C00000203	REWOQUAT RTM 50 (RICINOPROPYL AMIDO TRIMETHYL AMMONIUM METHOSULFATE)	Cosmetic (use not specified, CTFA)	9
		F00000304	ROLL-ON ANTIPERSPIRANT (DIAL)	Cosmetics, CTFA	64
81-07-2	201-321-0	C00001663	SACCHARIN	Cosmetic flavoring agents (DIIC)	3
6485-34-3	229-349-9	C00001111	SACCHARIN CALCIUM	Cosmetic flavoring agents (DIIC)	3
128-44-9	204-886-1	C00000111	SACCHARIN SODIUM SALT	Cosmetic flavoring agents (DIIC)	10

TABLE 7.1 (Continued)

List of Cosmetic Compounds and Formulations Tested on Alternative *In Vitro* Methodologies (the Galileo Data Bank, 1994)

Cas No.	EINECS	GAL Code	Name Compound / Formulation	Cosmetic Use	No.Test
69-72-7	200-712-3	C00000205	SALICYLIC ACID (BENZOIC ACID, 2-HYDROXY)	Cosmetic preservatives (DIIC)	8
		C00000251	SD ALCOHOL 40	Cosmetic (use not specified, CTFA)	800
		C00001797	SD ALCOHOL 40-B	Cosmetic (use not specified, CTFA)	1
		F00000013	SHAMPOO 1	Cosmetic preparation	1
		F00000086	SHAMPOO 10	Cosmetic preparation	2
		F00000039	SHAMPOO 2	Cosmetic preparation	5
		F00000040	SHAMPOO 3	Cosmetic preparation	5
		F00000046	SHAMPOO 4	Cosmetic preparation	5
		F00000042	SHAMPOO 5	Cosmetic preparation	5
		F00000082	SHAMPOO 6	Cosmetic preparation	2
		F00000083	SHAMPOO 7	Cosmetic preparation	2
		F00000084	SHAMPOO 8	Cosmetic preparation	2
		F00000085	SHAMPOO 9	Cosmetic preparation	2
9000-59-3	232-549-9	F00000117	SHELLAC	Cosmetic controlling agents (DIIC)	4
		F00000038	SHOWER GEL 1	Cosmetic preparation	10
		F00000050	SHOWER GEL 1 WITH BABY OIL	Cosmetic preparation	5
		F00000064	SHOWER GEL 2	Cosmetic preparation	2
		F00000242	SHOWER GEL 3	Cosmetic preparation	1
7761-88-8	231-853-9	C00000209	SILVER NITRATE [NITRIC ACID, SILVER(1+) SALT]	Cosmetic antimicrobials (DIIC)	21
		F00000035	SKIN CLEANSER	Cosmetic preparation	5
127-09-3	204-823-8	C00000112	SODIUM ACETATE	Cosmetic buffering agents (DIIC)	4
9005-38-3		C00001117	SODIUM ALGINATE	Cosmetic controlling agents (DIIC)	4

CAS	EINECS	Code	Name	Category	Count
532-32-1	208-534-8	C00001166	SODIUM BENZOATE	Cosmetic preservatives (DIIC)	5
144-55-8	205-633-8	C00000460	SODIUM BICARBONATE	Cosmetic buffering agents (DIIC)	5
1303-96-4		C00000462	SODIUM BORATE DECAHYDRATE	Cosmetic (use not specified, CTFA)	1
		F00000243	SODIUM C14-16 OLEFIN SULFONATE 45% & Na.SULFATE 3.5% & Na.CHLORIDE 1.5	Cosmetic surfactant	1
497-19-8	207-838-8	C00001296	SODIUM CARBONATE	Cosmetic buffering agents (DIIC)	5
59186-41-3		C00001776	SODIUM CETEARYL SULFATE	Cosmetic surfactants (DIIC)	1
7647-14-5	231-598-3	C00000212	SODIUM CHLORIDE	Cosmetic controlling agents (DIIC)	24
		C00001799	SODIUM DODECYL ETHER SULFATE	Cosmetic surfactant	1
518-47-8	208-253-0	C00001172	SODIUM FLUORESCEIN (CI ACID YELLOW 73; CI 45350)	Cosmetic color additives (DIIC)	4
7681-49-4	231-667-8	C00001173	SODIUM FLUORIDE	Cosmetic oral care agents (DIIC)	10
1310-73-2	215-185-5	C00000213	SODIUM HYDROXIDE	Cosmetic buffering agents (DIIC)	27
70161-44-3	274-357-8	C00001713	SODIUM HYDROXYMETHYLGLYCINATE (SUTTOCIDE A)	Cosmetic antistatic agents (DIIC)	1
7772-98-7	231-867-5	C00001145	SODIUM HYPOSULFITE	Cosmetic various uses (DIIC)	4
7681-82-5	231-679-3	C00000395	SODIUM IODIDE	Cosmetic various uses (DIIC)	1
72-17-3	200-772-0	C00000548	SODIUM LACTATE	Cosmetic buffering agents (DIIC)	58
		F00000239	SODIUM LAURETH SULFATE 30%/BA	Cosmetic surfactant	6
68647-44-9	271-949-8	C00001790	SODIUM LAUROAMPHOACETATE (LAUROAMPHOGLYCINATE)	Cosmetic surfactants (DIIC)	2
137-16-6	205-281-5	C00000347	SODIUM LAUROYL SARCOSINATE	Cosmetic surfactants (DIIC)	4
		F00000241	SODIUM LAURYL SULFATE 30%/F	Cosmetic surfactant	80
61791-42-2	263-174-9	C00001794	SODIUM METHYL COCOYL TAURATE	Cosmetic surfactants (DIIC)	1
7632-00-0	231-555-9	C00001162	SODIUM NITRITE	Cosmetic anticorrosive (DIIC)	3
62-76-0	200-550-3	C00002046	SODIUM OXALATE	Cosmetic chelating agents (DIIC)	13
7632-04-4	231-556-4	C00001891	SODIUM PERBORATE	Cosmetic oxidizing agents (DIIC)	1
7558-80-7	231-449-2	C00001167	SODIUM PHOSPHATE, MONOBASIC	Cosmetic buffering agents (DIIC)	4
9003-04-7		C00001168	SODIUM POLYACRYLATE	Cosmetic controlling agents (DIIC)	4
137-40-6	205-290-4	C00001170	SODIUM PROPIONATE	Cosmetic preservatives (DIIC)	4

TABLE 7.1 (Continued)

List of Cosmetic Compounds and Formulations Tested on Alternative *In Vitro* Methodologies (the Galileo Data Bank, 1994)

Cas No.	EINECS	GAL Code	Name Compound / Formulation	Cosmetic Use	No.Test
533-96-0	208-580-9	C00001796	SODIUM SESQUICARBONATE	Cosmetic buffering agents (DIIC)	1
1344-09-8	215-687-4	C00001431	SODIUM SILICATE	Cosmetic buffering agents (DIIC)	3
7757-82-6	231-820-9	C00000401	SODIUM SULFATE	Cosmetic various uses (DIIC)	2
515-74-2	208-208-5	C00000499	SODIUM SULFANILATE	Cosmetic (use not specified, CTFA)	1
7757-83-7	231-821-4	C00000473	SODIUM SULFITE	Cosmetic preservatives (DIIC)	1
3398-33-2	222-264-8	C00001804	SODIUM UNDECYLENATE	Cosmetic preservatives (DIIC)	2
50-70-4	200-061-5	C00000545	SORBITOL	Cosmetic flavoring agents (DIIC)	78
122-19-0	204-527-9	C00001784	STEARALKONIUM CHLORIDE	Cosmetic preservatives (DIIC)	1
110-15-6	203-740-4	C00000477	SUCCINIC ACID	Cosmetic buffering agents (DIIC)	4
57-50-1	200-334-9	C00001427	SUCROSE (SACCHAROSE)	Cosmetic flavoring agents (DIIC)	9
7664-93-9	231-639-5	C00000216	SULFURIC ACID	Cosmetic buffering agents (DIIC)	6
2783-94-0	220-491-7	C00001179	SUN YELLOW (FD & C YELLOW No. 6; CI 15985)	Cosmetic color additives (DIIC)	12
		F00000103	SUNBLOCK (55% ALCOHOL) (Chesebrough-Ponds)	Cosmetics, CTFA	138
		F00000302	SUNSCREEN LOTION (SCHERING-PLOUGH)	Cosmetics, CTFA	59
		F00000291	SUNSCREEN SPF 15 (ESTEE LAUDER)	Cosmetics, CTFA	72
1934-21-0	217-699-5	C00001183	TARTRAZINE (CI 19140; FD&C YELLOW No. 5)	Cosmetic color additives (DIIC)	3
68187-29-1	269-084-6	C00001777	TEA-COCOYL GLUTAMATE	Cosmetic surfactants (DIIC)	1
139-96-8	205-388-7	C00000219	TEA-LAURYL SULFATE (TEXAPON T-42)	Cosmetic surfactants (DIIC)	19
126-92-1	204-812-8	C00000294	TERGITOL 08 [SODIUM(2-ETHYLHEXYL) ALCOHOL SULFATE]	Cosmetic (use not specified, CTFA)	5
5392-28-9	226-393-0	C00002105	TETRAAMINOPYRIMIDINE SULFATE	Cosmetic various uses (DIIC)	11
97-99-4	202-625-6	C00001346	TETRAHYDROFURFURYL ALCOHOL	Cosmetic solvents (DIIC)	1

7722-88-5	231-767-1	C00001042	TETRASODIUM PYROPHOSPHATE	Cosmetic buffering agents (DIIC)	3
		F00000066	TEXAPON ASV	Cosmetic (use not specified, CTFA)	7
		C00000218	TEXAPON MG (MAGNESIUM LAURETH SULFATE)	Cosmetic surfactants (DIIC)	7
54-64-8	200-210-4	C00000222	THIMEROSAL (THIOMERSAL; MERCURATE(1-), ETHYL[2-MERCAPTOBENZOATO(2-)-	Cosmetic preservatives (DIIC)	4
68-11-1	200-677-4	C00001349	THIOGLYCOLIC ACID (MERCAPTOACETIC ACID)	Cosmetic depilating agents (DIIC)	1
7772-99-8	231-868-0	C00000224	TIN (II) CHLORIDE	Cosmetic various uses (DIIC)	7
		F00000236	TITANIUM DIOXIDE COATED MICA	Cosmetic color additive	1
108-88-3	203-625-9	C00000225	TOLUENE (BENZENE, METHYL-)	Cosmetic solvents (DIIC)	32
102-76-1	203-051-9	C00000226	TRIACETIN (TRIACETYL GLYCERIN)	Cosmetic antimicrobials (DIIC)	23
102-71-6	203-049-8	C00000230	TRIETHANOLAMINE (TEA)	Cosmetic buffering agents (DIIC)	168
68-04-2	200-675-3	C00000492	TRISODIUM CITRATE.DIHYDRATE	Cosmetic buffering agents (DIIC)	4
150-38-9	205-758-8	C00001527	TRISODIUM EDTA	Cosmetic chelating agents (DIIC)	7
9002-93-1		C00001196	TRITON X-100	Cosmetic emulsifying agents (DIIC)	33
9005-64-5		C00000215	TWEEN 20 (POLYSORBATE 20)	Cosmetic surfactants (DIIC)	25
9005-66-7		C00000234	TWEEN 40 (POLYSORBATE 40)	Cosmetic surfactants (DIIC)	12
9005-67-8		C00001334	TWEEN 60 (POLYSORBATE 60)	Cosmetic emulsifying agents (DIIC)	86
9005-65-6		C00000235	TWEEN 80 (POLYSORBATE 80)	Cosmetic surfactants (DIIC)	31
9005-70-3		C00000440	TWEEN 85 (POLYSORBATE 85)	Cosmetic emulsifying agents (DIIC)	1
57-13-6	200-315-5	C00000298	UREA	Cosmetic antistatic agents (DIIC)	84
121-33-5	204-465-2	C00001374	VANILLIN	Cosmetic flavoring agents (DIIC)	4
		F00000299	WATERLESS HAND CLEANSER (Dial)	Cosmetics, CTFA	68
1330-20-7	215-535-7	C00000259	XYLENE (BENZENE, DIMETHYL-)	Cosmetic solvents (DIIC)	7
557-34-6	209-170-2	C00000386	ZINC ACETATE	Cosmetic antimicrobials (DIIC)	1
7646-85-7	231-592-0	C00000239	ZINC CHLORIDE	Cosmetic oral care agents (DIIC)	4
127-82-2	204-867-8	C00001764	ZINC PHENOLSULFONATE	Cosmetic antimicrobials (DIIC)	1
			Total Compounds/Formulations 467	Total Number of Tests	9585

TABLE 7.2
List of Alternative *In Vitro* Methodologies with Relative Number of Test and Compounds/Formulations (C/F)
(the Galileo Data Bank, 1994)

Code	Name of Method	Nr.Test	C/F
AM000001	Salmonella typhimurium — Reverse Mutation Assay (92/69/EEC Dir.)	65	26
CV000001	In Vitro Mammalian Cytogenetic Test (92/69/EEC Dir.)	471	127
GT000001	Unscheduled DNA Synthesis (87/302/EEC Dir. modified)	2	2
GT000002	Micronucleus Test	6	3
GT000004	In Vitro Sister Chromatid Exchange Assay (87/302/EEC Dir.)	8	5
GT000005	In Vitro Mammalian Cell Gene Mutation Test (87/302/EEC Dir.)	6	6
GT000006	*Escherichia coli* — Reverse Mutation Assay (92/69/EEC Dir.)	1	1
MA000003	Neutral Red Uptake (NRU)	1874	172
MA000004	Tetrazolium Salt Assay (MTT)	353	83
MA000005	LDH Release	107	50
MA000006	Colony Formation Assay	424	117
MA000007	Agar Overlay Test (AOT)	308	88
MA000008	Total Protein Content (Lowry Method)	124	89
MA000009	Total Protein Content (Bio-Rad Assay)	622	119
MA000010	Total Protein Content (Kenacid Blue Method, KB)	772	131
MA000011	Tetrahymena Motility Assay	309	74
MA000012	Neutral Red Release (NRR)	369	84
MA000013	In Vitro Mammalian Cell Transformation Test (87/302/EEC Dir.)	72	37
MA000014	Epidermal Slice Technique for Skin Corrosive Potential	37	25
MA000022	HET-CAM Test	541	134
MA000023	CAM Test	626	96
MA000024	Cell Metabolic Cooperation Assay	1	1
MA000025	Cell Metabolic Cooperation Assay for Analysis of GJIC	11	7
MA000027	Inhibition of Tumor Cell Attachment	4	4
MA000029	Co-culture Clonal Survival Assay	94	42
MA000030	EYTEX® Assay	561	181
MA000031	Dual Dye Staining (Acute Cellular Lethality)	538	67
MA000032	Chromium-51 Release Assay	297	56
MA000033	The Pollen Tube Test	520	74
MA000034	In Vitro Percutaneous Absorption Assay	67	33
MA000035	QSAR Applied to the Draize Eye Test 1	25	15
MA000037	QSAR Applied to the Draize Eye Test 3	21	21
MA000038	Protein Synthesis Inhibition	24	12
MA000039	Microtox Acute Toxicity Test	67	18
MA000040	Bovine Corneal Opacity and Permeability (BCOP) Assay	258	22
Total number of tests		9585	

TABLE 7.3

List of Compounds/Formulations and the Results Obtained with Five Different Methodologies
(the Galileo Data Bank, 1994)

Name of Compounds and Formulations	Neutral Red Uptake (BALB/3T3 clone A31; µg/ml)	Colony Formation Assay (SIRC cell line; µg/ml)	Total Protein Content Kenacid Blue (3T3-L1 cell line; µg/ml)	HET-CAM (Hen's egg chorio-allantoic memb.; HET-CAM score)	EYETEX® (EYETEX protein matrix.; EYETEX score)
AFTERSHAVE (20% ALCOHOL) (Noxell)	56950.00	248140.67	65959.80	5.31	5.55
ALLANTOIN	51650.00	277175.67	23448.25	8.52	4.19
ALUMINIUM CHLORIDE	1824.09	1150.67	790.00	11.94	48.22
AMINOMETHYL PROPANOL (1-PROPANOL, 2-AMINO-2-METHYL-)	18054.55	58059.00	8129.00	13.62	35.57
BENZETHONIUM CHLORIDE	1824.09	1150.67	790.00	11.94	48.61
BENZOPHENONE-2	1597.27	387.67	4411.33	13.78	31.77
BENZOYL PEROXIDE CREAM (2.5%) (ESTEE LAUDER)	258.00	256.33	2328.33	2.55	22.14
BUTYLATED HYDROXYANISOLE (BHA)	1597.27	387.67	2764.60	13.78	31.77
CINNAMON OIL	3649.09	1239.00	489.80	4.96	28.65
CITRIC ACID	3649.09	1239.00	489.80	6.30	28.65
CLEANSING CREAM I (COLGATE-PALMOLIVE)	1480.00	24144.33	2290.75	0.25	12.88
CLEANSING CREAM II (JOHNSON & JOHNSON)	3655.33	3962.00	354.00	13.33	22.22
COLOGNE 2 (83% ALCOHOL) (Revlon)	1597.27	387.67	4411.33	13.78	31.77
CUTICLE REMOVER CREAM (AVON)	12956.67	23482.50	25775.00	20.42	21.80
D&C ORANGE No. 4 (CI 15510)	1597.27	387.67	4411.33	13.78	31.77
DEODORANT (40% ALCOHOL) (Dial)	1824.09	1150.67	790.00	11.94	48.22
DIMETHICONE COPOLYOL	30872.73	43826.17	7521.56	13.18	23.36
EMOLLIENT CREAM (MARY KAY)	385.00	2414.00	765.33	1.64	10.60
ETHYL DIHYDROXYPROPYL PABA	13177.27	17139.14	4794.70	12.30	38.00
ETHYL ESTER PVM/MA COPOLYMER	18054.55	58059.00	8129.00	13.62	35.57
FD&C BLUE No. 1 (ERIOGLAUCIN A; CI 42090 - SODIUM SALT)	26103.50	124264.17	42879.13	9.54	14.29
FD&C COLOR(S)	52042.86	277175.67	23448.25	8.52	3.07
FD&C RED No. 2 (AMARANTH; CI 16185; ACID RED 27)	3649.09	1239.00	489.80	4.96	28.65

TABLE 7.3 (Continued)

List of Compounds/Formulations and the Results Obtained with Five Different Methodologies (the Galileo Data Bank, 1994)

Name of Compounds and Formulations	Neutral Red Uptake (BALB/3T3 clone A31; µg/ml)	Colony Formation Assay (SIRC cell line; µg/ml)	Total Protein Content Kenacid Blue (3T3-L1 cell line; µg/ml)	HET-CAM (Hen's egg chorio-allantoic memb.; HET-CAM score)	EYETEX® (EYTEX protein matrix.; EYTEX score)
FOOT CARE CREAM (AVON)	1155.00	716.67	420.33	1.96	8.92
FRAGRANCE (FRESHENER)	51650.00	277175.67	23448.25	8.52	3.07
FRAGRANCE (HAIR STYLING LOTION)	43690.91	29593.33	7035.60	12.74	17.25
FRAGRANCE (PUMP HAIR SPRAY)	18054.55	58059.00	8129.00	13.62	35.57
FRAGRANCE 1 (COLOGNE 2, 83% ALCOHOL)	1597.27	387.67	4411.33	13.78	31.77
FRAGRANCE 2 (COLOGNE 2, 83% ALCOHOL)	1597.27	387.67	4411.33	13.78	31.77
FRESHENER (15% ALCOHOL) (Mary Kay)	51650.00	277175.67	23448.25	8.52	3.07
GLYCEROL (GLYCERINE; 1,2,3-PROPANETRIOL)	23436.67	95150.10	23149.44	7.33	19.77
HAIR CONDITIONER (MARY KAY)	334.50	12858.67	603.00	1.15	14.76
HAIR MASQUE (CHESEBROUGH-PONDS)	98.60	5682.33	138.33	0.50	3.28
HAIR STYLING LOTION (65% ALCOHOL) (Procter & Gamble)	43690.91	29593.33	7035.60	12.74	17.25
HAND AND BODY LOTION (CHESEBROUGH-PONDS)	1498.50	7635.33	1609.75	2.10	6.13
HAND AND NAIL LOTION (CHESEBROUGH-PONDS)	242.47	50744.67	1101.00	0.30	6.48
HYDROXYPROPYLCELLULOSE	13177.27	17139.14	4794.70	12.30	38.00
IMIDAZOLIDINYL UREA (GERMAL 115)	51650.00	277175.67	23448.25	8.52	2.64
KATHON CG	711.36	55.00	206.40	6.07	0.60
LACTIC ACID (PROPANOIC ACID, 2-HYDROXY-)	51650.00	277175.67	23448.25	8.52	3.07
METHYL GLUCETH-20	13177.27	17139.14	4794.70	12.30	38.00
METHYLPARABEN (p-HYDROXYBENZOIC ACID METHYL ESTER; PARABEN)	56950.00	248140.67	47172.14	5.31	8.60
MOISTURIZING LOTION (MARY KAY)	354.67	632.25	548.00	3.50	11.25
MOUTHWASH (10% ALCOHOL) (Lever Brothers)	3649.09	1239.00	489.80	4.92	28.65
P&G OINTMENT 1 (HYDROPHILIC OINTMENT, 5% SLS - PROCTER & GAMBLE)	681.50	2906.00	200.67	7.58	20.18
P&G OINTMENT 2 (HYDROPHILIC OINTMENT, 10% SLS - PROCTER & GAMBLE)	2296.00	1321.67	234.33	11.33	12.12
PEPPERMINT OIL	3649.09	1239.00	489.80	4.96	28.65
PUMP HAIR SPRAY (90% ALCOHOL) (Amway)	16581.82	58059.00	8129.00	13.62	35.57
PVP/VA COPOLIMER (50% ALCOHOL)	43690.91	29593.33	7035.60	12.74	17.25
SD ALCOHOL 40	15721.07	53507.92	10318.02	9.99	23.35

Name of Compounds and Formulations	Neutral Red Uptake (BALB/3T3 clone A31; µg/ml)	Colony Formation Assay (SIRC cell line; µg/ml)	Total Protein Content Kenacid Blue (3T3-L1 cell line; µg/ml)	HET-CAM (Hen's egg chorio-allantoic memb.; HET-CAM score)	EYETEX® (EYTEX protein matrix.; EYETEX score)
SODIUM LACTATE	51650.00	277175.67	23448.25	8.52	3.07
SORBITOL	3649.09	1239.00	489.80	4.96	28.65
SUNBLOCK (55% ALCOHOL) (Cheesebrough-Pond's)	13177.27	17139.14	4794.70	12.30	38.00
SUNSCREEN LOTION (SCHERING-PLOUGH)	929.00	2674.67	2172.25	0.50	4.87
SUNSCREEN SPF 15 (ESTEE LAUDER)	344.00	5893.33	570.00	5.50	6.07
TRIETHANOLAMINE (TEA)	1237.32	2069.33	1255.82	3.26	18.84
TWEEN 60 (POLYSORBATE 60)	3627.27	1239.00	448.83	4.96	22.74
UREA	1824.09	1150.67	790.00	11.94	48.22
WATERLESS HAND CLEANSER (DIAL)	582.50	23.69	301.67	7.88	23.32

REFERENCES

1. **Council Directive 76/768/EEC,** On the approximation of the laws of the member states relating to cosmetic products, *Official Journal of the European Communities,* No. l262, p. 169, 1976.
2. **Council Directive 93/35/EEC,** Amending for the sixth time Directive 76/768/EEC on the approximation of the laws of the Member States relating to cosmetic products, *Official Journal of the European Communities,* No. L151, p. 32, 1993.
3. **Loprieno, N.,** Guidelines for safety evaluation of cosmetic ingredients in the EC countries, *Food & Chemical Toxicology,* Vol. 30, p. 809, 1992.
4. **Commission Decision 78/45/EEC,** Establishing a Scientific Committee on Cosmetology, *Official Journal of the European Communities,* No. L13, p. 24, 1978.
5. **De Klerck, W.,** personal communication, 1993.
6. **Anon,** General Toxicological Requirements for Cosmetic Ingredients and Finished Products, Report EUR 8794/83, Brussels, Belgium, 1983.
7. **Commission Directive 87/302/EEC,** 18 November 1987, Adapting to technical progress for the ninth time Council Directive 67/548/EEC on the approximation of laws, regulations and administrative provisions relating to the classification, packaging and labelling of dangerous substances, *Official Journal of the European Communities,* No. L133, Vol. 31, p. 1, 1988.
8. **Annex to Commission Directive 92/69/EEC,** 31 July 1992, Adapting to technical progress for the seventeenth time Council Directive 67/548/EEC on the approximation of laws, regulations and administrative provisions relating to the classification, packaging and labelling of dangerous substances, *Official Journal of the European Communities,* No. L383A, Vol. 35, p. 1, 1992.
9. OECD Guidelines for the Toxicity Testing of Chemicals, Section 4: Health Effects, Organization for Economic Cooperation and Development, Paris, 1993.
10. **Council Directive 86/609/EEC,** On the approximation of laws, regulations and administrative provisions of the Member States regarding the protection of animals used for experimental and other purposes, *Official Journal of the European Communities,* No. L358, p. 1, 1986.
11. **Anon,** SCC: General Scheme for Determining the Safety Margin of Preservatives Used in Cosmetic Products, DOC SPC/1247/93 EN, rev. 02/94, approved 9 March 1994, SPC-EC, Brussels, Belgium.
12. **Siemer, E.,** Sunscreen preparation, in *Cosmetic and Toiletries: Development Production and Use,* Umbach, W., Ed., Ellis Horwod, New York, 1991, Chap. 5.
13. **Koh, H. K. and R. A. Lew,** Sunscreens and melanoma: Implications for prevention, *Journal of the National Cancer Institute,* Vol. 86, p. 78, 1994.
14. **Wright, B.,** Sunscreens and the protection racket, *New Scientist,* No. 1909, p. 21, 1994.
15. **IARC Monograph,** Occupational exposures of hairdressers and barbers, and personal use of hair colourants; Some hair dyes, cosmetic colourants, industrial dyestuff and aromatic amines, International Agency for Research on Cancer, World Health Organization, Lyon, France, 1993, Vol. 57.
16. **Frazier, J. M. and A. M. Goldberg,** Alternative to and reduction of animal use in biomedical research, education and testing, *The Cancer Bulletin,* Vol. 42, p. 238, 1980.
17. **Council Directive 79/831/EEC,** Amending for the sixth time Council Directive 67/548/EEC on the approximation of laws, regulations and administrative provisions relating to the classification, packaging and labelling of dangerous substances, *Official Journal of the European Communities,* No. L196, p. 1, 1967.
18. **Commission Directive 91/325/EEC,** Adapting to technical progress for the twelfth time Council Directive 67/548/EEC on the approximation of laws, regulations and administrative provisions relating to the classification, packaging and labelling of dangerous substances, *Official Journal of the European Communities,* No. L180, p. 1, 1991.
19. **Van Den Heuvel, M. J., D. G. Clark, R. T. Fielder, P. P. Koundakjian, G. J. A. Oliver, D. Pelling, N. J. Tomlinson and A. P. Walker,** The international validation of a fixed-dose procedure as an alternative to the classical LD_{50} test, *Food & Chemical Toxicology,* Vol. 28, No. 7, p. 469, 1990.
20. **Motoyoshi, K., Y. Toyoshima, M. Sato and M. Yoshimura,** Comparative studies on the irritancy of oils and synthetic perfumes to the skin of rabbit, guinea pig, rat, miniature swine, and man, *Cosmetic Toiletries,* No. 94, p. 41, 1979.
21. **Spielmann, H., W. W. Lovell, E. Höltze, B. E. Johnson, T. Maurer, M. Miranda, W. J. W. Pape, O. Sapora and D. Sladowski,** *In vitro* phototoxicity testing. The report and recommendations of the ECVAM Workshop 2, *ATLA,* Vol. 22, p. 314, 1994.
22. **Loprieno, N., G. Boncristiani, G. Loprieno and M. Tesoro,** Data Selection and Treatment of Chemicals Tested for Genotoxicity and Carcinogenicity, *Environmental Health Perspectives,* Vol. 96, p. 121, 1991.
23. **De Serres, F. J. and J. Ashby,** *Progress in Mutation Research,* Vol. 1: *Evaluation of Short-Term Tests for Carcinogens,* Elsevier/North-Holland, New York, 1981.

24. **Ashby, J., F. J. De Serres, M. D. Shelby, B. H. Margolin, M. Ishidate, Jr. and G. C. Becking,** Evaluation of short-term tests for carcinogens — Report of the international programme on chemical safety's collaborative study on *in vivo* assays, Vol. 1, WHO, Cambridge University Press, Cambridge, U. K., 1988.

25. **Anon,** *FRAME News,* G. Griffin, Ed., No. 25, p. 2, 1990.

26. Statistics of scientific procedures on living animals — Great Britain 1992, Home Office, HMSO, London, October 1993.

27. **Balls, M., R. J. Riddell and A. N. Worden, Eds.,** *Animals and Alternatives in Toxicity Testing,* Academic Press, London, 1983.

28. **U.S. Office of Technology Assessment,** Alternatives to Animal Use in Research, Testing and Education, U.S. Congress, Washington, D.C., 1986, p. 9.

29. **Mehlman, M. A., Ed.,** *Benchmarks: Alternative Methods in Toxicology,* Princeton Scientific Publishing, Princeton, NJ, 1989, p. 1.

30. **Goldberg, A. M. and J. M. Frazier,** Alternatives to animals in toxicity testing, *Scientific American,* No. 261, p. 16, 1989.

31. **Zurlo, J., D. Rudacille and A. M. Goldberg,** *Animals and Alternatives in Testing,* Mary Ann Libert, New York, 1994.

32. **National Research Council,** *Use of Laboratory Animals in Biomedical and Behavioral Research,* National Academy Press, Washington, D.C., 1988.

33. **Bourdeau, P., E. Somers, G. M. Richardson and J. R. Hickman, Eds.,** *Short-term Toxicity Tests for Non-Genotoxic Effects. Scope 41.* IPCS Joint Symposia 8, John Wiley & Sons, New York, 1990, p. 4.

34. **Balls, M., J. Bridges and J. Southee, Eds.,** *Animals and Alternatives in Toxicology. Present Status and Future Prospects,* Macmillan, London, 1991, p. 375.

35. **Frazier, J. M., Ed.,** *In Vitro Toxicity Testing. Applications to Safety Evaluation,* Marcel Dekker, New York, 1992.

36. **Zbinden, G.,** Acute toxicity testing, public responsibility and scientific challenges, in *Benchmarks: Alternative Methods in Toxicology,* M. A. Mehlman, Ed., Princeton Scientific, Princeton, 1989, p. 3.

37. **Blanquart, C., S. Romet, A. Baeza, C. Guennou and E. Marano,** Primary cultures of tracheal epithelial cells for the evaluation of respiratory toxicity, *Toxicology In Vitro,* Vol. 5. No. 5/6, p. 499, 1991.

38. **Fautrel, A., C. Chesné, A. Guillozo, G. De Sousa, M. Placidi, R. Rhamani, F. Braut, J. Pichon, H. Hoellinger, P. Vintezous, I. Diarte, C. Melcion, A. Cordier, G. Lorenzon, M. Benincourt, B. Vannier, R. Fournex, A. F. Peloux, N. Bichet, D. Gouy and J. P. Cano,** A multicentre study of acute *in vitro* cytotoxicity in rat liver cells, *In Vitro Toxicology,* Vol. 5, No. 5/6, p. 543, 1991.

39. **Commission of the European Communities,** Collaborative study on the relationship between *"in vivo"* primary irritation and *"in vitro"* experimental models, Doc. CEC/V/E/3/Lux/157/188 Rev. 1, Brussels, 1989.

40. **Gettings, S. D., J. J. Teal, D. M. Bagley, J. L Demetrulias, L. C. Di Pasquale, K. L Hintze, M. G. Rozen, S. L. Weise, M. Chudkowski, K. D. Marenus, W. J. W. Pape, M. Roddy, R. Schnetzeinger, P. M. Silber, S. M. Glaza and P. J. Kurtz,** The CTFA Evaluation of Alternatives Program: An evaluation of *In Vitro* alternatives to the Draize primary eye irritation test (Phase I) Hydroalcoholic formulations; (Part 2) Data analysis and biological significance, *In Vitro Toxicology,* Vol. 4, No. 4, p. 247, 1991.

41. **Sasaki, K., N. Tanaka, M. Watanabe and M. Yamada,** Comparison of cytotoxic effects of chemicals in four different cell types, *In Vitro Toxicology,* Vol. 5 No. 5/6, p. 403, 1991.

42. **Paganuzzi-Stammati, A., V. Silano and F. Zucco,** Toxicology investigations with cell culture systems, *Toxicology,* Vol. 20, p. 91, 1981.

43. **Deleo, V. A.,** Cutaneous irritancy, in *In Vitro Toxicity Testing. Applications to Safety Evaluation,* Frazier, J. M., Ed., Marcel Dekker, New York, 1992, Chap. 8.

44. **ECETOC,** Monograph No. 15, July 20, 1990 — Skin Irritation, ECETOC, Brussels, 1990, p. 1.

45. **Anon,** *Evaluation of the Alternatives to the Draize Eye Test,* PMA Drug Safety Subsection — *In vitro* Toxicology Task Force, Washington, D.C., 1991.

46. **Frazier, J. M., S. C. Gad, A. M. Goldberg and J. P. McCulley,** *Evaluation of Alternatives to Acute Ocular Irritation Testing — Alternative Methods in Toxicology 4,* Mary Ann Liebert, New York, 1987.

47. **Fielder, R. J., I. F. Gaunt, C. Rhodes, F. M. Sullivan and D. W. Swanson,** A hierarchical approach to the assessment of dermal and ocular irritancy: A Report by the British Toxicology Society Working Party on Irritancy, *Human Toxicology,* No. 6., p. 269, 1987.

48. **Turner, L., F. Choplin, P. Dugard, J. Hermens, R. Jaeckh, M. Marsmann and D. Roberts,** Structure-activity relationships in toxicology and ecotoxicology: An assessment, *Toxicology In Vitro,* Vol. 1, No. 3, p. 143, 1987.

49. **Klopman, G., D. Ptchelintsev, M. Frierson, S. Pennisi, K. Renskers and M. Dikens,** Multiple computer automated structure evaluation methodology as an alternative to *in vivo* eye irritation testing, *ATLA,* No. 21, p. 14, 1993.

50. **Enslein, K.,** An overview of structure-activity relationships an as alternative to testing in animals for carcinogenicity, mutagenicity, dermal and eye irritation, and acute oral toxicity, in *Benchmarks: Alternative Methods in Toxicology,* M. A. Mehlman, Ed., Princeton Scientific, Princeton, 1989, p. 59.

51. **Ashby, J.,** Two million rodent carcinogens? The role of SAR and QSAR in their detection, *Mutation Research,* No. 305, p. 3, 1994.

52. **Nadolney, C. H., N. Chernoff, R. L. Dixon, K. S. Khera, R. Krowke, B. V. Leonov, D. Neubert and S. Tabacova,** Potential short-term tests to detect chemicals capable of causing reproductive and developmental dysfunction, in *Short-term Toxicity Tests for Non-Genotoxic Effects. Scope 41*, Bourdeau, P., E. Somers, G. M. Richardson, and J. R. Hickman, Eds., IPCS Joint Symposia 8, John Wiley & Sons, New York, 1990, Chap. 16

53. **Daston, G. P. and R. A. D'Amato,** *In vitro* technique in teratology, in *Benchmarks: Alternative Methods in Toxicology*, M. A. Mehlman, Ed., Princeton Scientific, Princeton, 1989, p. 79.

54. **Loprieno, N.,** *In vitro* assay systems for testing photomutagenic chemicals, *Mutagenesis*, Vol. 6, No. 5, p. 331, 1991.

55. **Dean, S. W., M. Lane, R. H. Dunmore, S. P. Ruddock, C. N. Martin, D. J. Kirkland and N. Loprieno,** Development of assays for the detection of photomutagenicity of chemicals during exposure to UV light; 1. Assay development, *Mutagenesis*, Vol. 6, No. 5, p. 335, 1991.

56. **Dean, S. W., R. H. Dunmore, S. P. Ruddock, J. C. Dean, C. N. Martin and D. J. Kirkland,** Development of assays for the detection of photomutagenicity of chemicals during exposure to UV light. II. Results of testing three sunscreen ingredients, *Mutagenesis*, Vol. 7, No. 3, p. 179, 1992.

57. **Russel, W. M. S. and R. L. Burch,** *The Principles of Humane Experimental Technique*, Methen, London, 1959.

58. **Anderson, D., M. H. L. Green, I. E. Mattern and M. J. Godley,** An international collaborative study of "genetic drift" in *Salmonella typhimurium* strains used in the Ames test, *Mutation Research*, No. 130, p. 10, 1984.

59. **Margolin, B. H., K. J. Risko, M. D. Shelby and E. Zeiger,** Sources of variability in Ames *Salmonella typhimurium* tester strains: Analysis of the international collaborative study on "genetic drift", *Mutation Research*, No. 130, p. 11, 1984.

60. **Agnese, G., D. Risso and S. De Flora,** Statistical evaluation of the inter- and intra-laboratory variations of the Ames test, related to the genetic stability of *Salmonella* tester strains, *Mutation Research*, No. 130, p. 27, 1984.

61. **Anon,** *ECVAM News & Views*, ECVAM — JRC, Ispra, Italy, 1993.

62. **Bawden, D.,** Information systems and databases as alternatives, *ATLA*, Vol. 18, p. 83, 1990.

63. **Ungar, K.,** *INVITTOX* — Promoting *in vitro* methods for toxicity testing, *AATEX*, Vol. 2, p. 37, 1993.

64. **Loprieno, N., G. Boncristiani, E. Bosco, M. Nieri and G. Loprieno,** The Galileo Data Bank on toxicity testing with *in vitro* alternative methods, I. General structure, *ATLA*, 22, p. 20, 1994.

65. **Loprieno, N., G. Boncristiani, E. Bosco, M. Nieri and G. Loprieno,** The Galileo Data Bank on toxicity testing with *in vitro* alternative methods; II. Toxicology profiles of 20 chemicals, *ATLA*, 22, p. 82, 1994.

66. **Spielmann, H., B. Grune-Wolf, S. Ewe, S. Skolik, M. Liebsch, D. Traue and J. Heuer,** ZEBET's data bank and information service on alternatives to the use of experimental animals in Germany, *ATLA*, 20, p. 362, 1992.

67. **COLIPA,** *The Cosmetic Industry and Its Efforts to Develop and Validate Alternatives to Animal Testing*, European Association of Cosmetic Industries, Brussels, 1993.

68. **Bruner, L. H., D. J. Kain, D. A. Roberts and R. D. Parker,** Evaluation of seven *in vitro* alternatives for ocular safety testing, *Fundamental and Applied Toxicology*, Vol. 17, p. 136, 1991

69. **Rougier, A., M. Cottin, O. De Silva, R. Roguet, P. Catroux, A. Toufic and K. G. Dossou,** *In vitro* methods: Their relevance and complementarity in ocular safety assessment, *Lens and Eye Toxicity Research*, Vol. 9, No. 3–4, p. 229, 1992.

70. **Gordon, V. C. and C. P. Kelly,** An *in vitro* method for determining ocular irritation, *Cosmetics and Toiletries*, Vol. 14, p. 69, 1989.

71. **Bruner, L. H., R. Miller, J. C. Owicki, J. W. Parce and V. C. Muir,** Testing ocular irritancy *in vitro* with the silicon microphysiometer, *Toxicology In Vitro*, Vol. 5, p. 272, 1992.

72. **Parce, J. W., J. C. Owicki, K. M. Kercso, G. B. Sigal, H. G. Wada, V C. Muir, J. Muir, L. J. Bousse, K. L. Rosse, B. I. Sikic and H. M. McConnel,** Detection of cell-affecting agents with a silicon biosensor, *Science*, Vol. 246, p. 243, 1989.

73. **Borenfreund, E. and J. A. Puerner,** Toxicity determined *in vitro* by morphological alterations and neutral red absorption, *Toxicology Letters*, Vol. 24, p. 119, 1985.

74. **Rouget, R., K. G. Dossou and A. Rougier,** Prediction of eye irritation potential of surfactants using SIRC-NR cytotoxity test, *ATLA*, Vol. 20, p. 451, 1992.

75. **Tachon, P., J. Cotovio, J., K. G. Dossou and M. Prunerias,** Assessment of surfactant cytotoxicity: comparison with the Draize eye test, *International Journal of Cosmetic Science*, Vol. 11, p. 233, 1989.

76. **Rosenbluth, S. A., G. R. Weddington, W. L. Guess and J. Autian,** Tissue culture method for screening toxicity of plastic materials to be used in medical practice, *Journal of Pharmaceutical Sciences*, Vol 54, p. 156, 1965.

77. **O'Brien, K. A. F., P. A. Jones and J. Rockley,** Evaluation of an agarose overlay assay to determine the eye irritation potential of detergent-based products, *Toxicology in Vitro*, Vol. 4, p. 311, 1990.

78. **Bulich, A. A.,** Use of luminescent bacteria for determining toxicity in aquatic environments, in *Aquatic Toxicology ASTM 667*, Markings, F. and R. A. Kimerle, Eds., American Society for Testing Materials, Philadelphia, 1979, p. 98.

79. **Muir, C. K.,** Four simple methods to assess surfactant-induced bovine corneal opacity *in vitro:* Preliminary findings, *Toxicology Letters*, No. 22, p. 199, 1984.

80. **Gautheron, P., M. Dukic, D. Alix and J. F. Sina,** Bovine corneal opacity and permeability test: An *in vitro* assay of ocular irritancy, *Fundamental and Applied Toxicology*, Vol. 18, p. 442, 1992.

81. **Lüpke, N. P. and F. H. Kemper,** The HET-CAM test — An alternative to the Draize eye test, *Food and Chemical Toxicology,* Vol. 23, p. 287, 1985.
82. **De Silva, O., A. Rougier and K. G. Dossou,** The HET-CAM test: A study of the irritation potential of chemicals and formulations, *ATLA,* Vol. 20, p. 432, 1992.
83. **Gettings, S. D.,** The current status of *in vitro* test validation (evaluation) in the United States, *ATLA* Vol. 19, 432, 1991.
84. **Gettings, S. D.,** Pride and prejudice: Ten years of CAAT — An industry perspective, in *In Vitro Toxicology: Tenth Anniversary Symposium of CAAT,* Goldberg, A. M., Ed., Mary Ann Liebert, New York, 1993, p. 121.
85. **Gettings, S. D.,** The CTFA evaluation of alternatives program: Objectives and overview, in *Proceedings of the 2nd CTFA Ocular Safety Testing Workshop: Evaluation of In Vitro Alternatives, Summit,* Gettings, S. D. and G. N. McEwen, Jr., Eds., New York, Sept. 1990, CTFA, Washington, 1991.
86. **Gettings, S. D. and G. N. McEwen, Jr.,** Development of potential alternatives to the Draize Eye Test: The CTFA Evaluation of Alternatives Program, *ATLA,* Vol. 17, p. 317, 1990.
87. **Gettings, S. D., J. J. Teal, D. M. Bagley, J. L. Demetrulias, L. C. Di Pasquale, K. L. Hintze, M. G. Rozen, S. L. Weise, M. Chudkowski, K. D. Marenus, W. J. W. Pape, M. Roddy, R. Schnetzinger, P. M. Silber, S. M. Glaza and P. J. Kurtz,** The CTFA evaluation of alternatives program: An evaluation of *in vitro* alternatives to the Draize primary eye irritation test (phase 1) hydro-alcoholic formulations; (part 2) data analysis and biological significance, *In Vitro Toxicology,* Vol. 4, No. 4, p. 247, 1991.
88. **Gettings, S. D., D. M. Bagley, M. Chudkowski, J. L. Demetrulias, L. C. Di Pasquale, C. L. Galli, R. Gay, K. L. Hintze, I. Janus, K. D. Marenus, M. J. Muscatiello, W. J. W. Pape, K. J. Renskers, M. T. Roddy and R. Schnetzinger,** Development of potential alternatives to the Draize Eye Test: The CTFA Evaluation of Alternatives Program; Phase II: Review of materials and methods, *ATLA,* Vol. 20, p. 164, 1992.
89. **Gettings, S. D., K. L. Hintze, D. M. Bagley, P. L. Casterton, M. Chudkowski, R. D. Curren, J. L. Demetrulias, L. K. Earl, P. I. Feder, C. L. Galli, R. Gay, S. M. Glaza, V. C. Gordon, P. J. Kurtz, R. A. Lordo, K. D. Marenus, I. Moral, W. J. W. Pape, K. J. Renskels, L. A. Rheins, M. T. Roddy, M. G. Rozen, J. P. Tedeschi and J. Zyracki,** The CTFA Evaluation of Alternatives Program; Phase III (surfactant-based formulations), *World Congress on Alternatives and Animal Use in the Life Sciences,* Baltimore, November 1993.
90. **Gettings, S. D., L. C. Di Pasquale, D. M. Bagley, P. L. Casterton, M. Chudkowski, R. D. Curren, J. L. Demetrulias, P. I. Feder, C. L. Galli, R. Gay, S. M. Glaza, K. L. Hintze, J. Janus, P. J. Kurtz, R. A. Lordo, K. D. Marenus, J. Moral, M. J. Muscatiello, W. J. W. Pape, K. J. Renskers, M. T. Roddy and M. G. Rozen,** The CTFA Evaluation of Alternatives Program: An evaluation of potential *in vitro* alternatives to the Draize primary eye irritation test (Phase II) oil/water emulsions, *Food & Chemical Toxicology,* (in press), 1994.
91. **Gettings, S. D., K. L. Hintze, D. M. Bagley, P. L. Casterton, M. Chudkowski, R. D. Curren, J. L. Demetrulias, L. K. Earl, P. I. Feder, C. L. Galli, R. Gay, S. M. Glaza, V. C. Gordon, P. J. Kurtz, R. A. Lordo, K. D. Marenus, I. Moral, W. J. W. Pape, K. J. Renskels, L. A. Rheins, M. T. Roddy, M. G. Rozen, J. P. Tedeschi and J. Zyracki,** The CTFA Evaluation of Alternatives Program: An evaluation of potential *in vitro* alternatives to the Draize primary eye irritation test (Phase III) Surfactant-based formulations, in press.
92. **Loprieno, N. and A. M. Goldberg,** The importance of alternatives to animal testing, in *Handbook of Carcinogen Testing,* Milman, H. A. and E. K. Weisburger, Eds., Noyes Publishing, Park Ridge, New Jersey, 1994.
93. **Frazier, J. M.,** *Scientific Criteria for Validation of In Vitro Toxicity Testing,* Organization for Economic Cooperation and Development, Paris, 1990.
94. **Loprieno, N.,** Progress in development validation and legal acceptance of methods alternative to those involving experiments on animals, *Bio. Re. Pla. SAS,* Pisa, 1994. Report to European Commission.
95. **Advanced Tissue Sciences,** Skin2™ ZK1300 CEC validated — high correlation to *in vivo* scores, *The Lab Partner,* No. II, p. 7, 1992.
96. **Advanced Tissue Sciences,** Amway® moves toward *in vitro* testing as standard screening tool, *The Lab Partner,* No. II, p. 9, 1992.
97. **Api, A. M.,** Fragrances and the skin: Animal alternatives, in *Proceedings of the 6th International Information Exchange,* Research Institute for Fragrance Materials, Princeton, NJ, 1992.
98. **Bason, M. M., J. Harvell, B. Realica, V. Gordon and H. L. Maibach,** Comparison of *in vitro* and human *in vivo* dermal irritancy data for four primary irritants, *In Vitro Toxicology,* Vol. 6, p. 383, 1992.
99. **Batelle,** CTFA Evaluation of Alternatives Program, Phase II: Oil-water emulsions. Preliminary results of data analysis, Batelle Corporation, Columbus, OH, August 1991.
100. **Blein, O., M. Adolphe, B. Lakhdar, J. Cambar, G. Gubanski, D. Castelli, C. Contie, F. Hubert, F. Latrille, P. Masson, J. Clouzeau, J. F. Le Bigot, O. De Silva and K.-G. Dossou,** Correlation and validation of alternative methods to the Draize eye irritation test (OPAL project), *Toxicology In Vitro,* Vol. 5, p. 555, 1991.
101. **Booman, K. A., T. M. Cascieri, J. Demetrulias, A. Driedger, J. F. Griffith, G. T. Grochoski, B. Kong, W. C. McCormick III, North-H. Root, M. G. Rozen and R. L. Sedlak,** *In vitro* methods for estimating eye irritancy of cleaning products, Phase 1: Preliminary assessment, *J. Toxicol. Cutan. Ocular. Toxicol.,* Vol. 7, p. 173, 1988.
102. **Botham, P. A., T. L. Hall, R. Dennet, J. C. McCall, D. A. Basketter, E. Whittle, M. Cheeseman, D. J. Esdaile and J. Gardner,** The skin corrosivity test *in vitro.* Results of an inter-laboratory trial, *Toxicology In Vitro,* Vol. 6, p. 191, 1992.

103. **Cannon, C. L., P. J. Neal, J. A. Southee, I. Kubilus and M. Klausner,** New epidermal model for dermal irritancy testing, *Toxicology In Vitro,* Vol. 8, p. 889, 1994.

104. **Casterton, P. L., L. F. Potts and B. D. Klein,** Use of *in vitro* methods to rank surfactants for irritation potential in support of new product development, *Toxicology In Vitro,* Vol. 8, p. 835, 1994.

105. **Courtellemont, P., P. Hebert and G. Redziniak,** Evaluation of the EYTEX^{TM} system as a screening method for ocular tolerance: Application to raw materials and finished products, *ATLA,* Vol. 20, p. 466, 1992.

106. **Decker, D. and R. Harper,** Evaluation of the EYTEX system, for use as a predictor of ocular irritancy; I. Shampoos, *J. Toxicol. Cutan. Ocul. Toxicol.,* Vol. 12, p. 35, 1993.

107. **Decker, D. and R. Harper,** Evaluation of a 3-dimensional human dermal model as a predictor of ocular irritation of shampoos, paper presented at *First World Congress on Alternatives and Animal Use in the Life Sciences, In Vitro Toxicology,* Vol. 7, p. 190, 1994.

108. **Doyle, J. M., W. E. Dressler, E. T. Spence and S. Rachui,** Utility of two *in vitro* ocular irritation models (the bovine corneal opacity and permeability assay BCOP and the Skin2™ model ZK1200) in categorising and ranking the relative ocular irritancy potential of chemicals and personal care products, *In Vitro Toxicology,* Vol. 7, p. 191, 1994.

109. **Earl, L. K., P. A. Jones, M. B. Dixit and K. A. F. O'Brien,** Comparison of five potential methods for assessing ocular irritation *in vitro, In Vitro Toxicology,* Vol. 7, p. 165, 1994.

110. **Ekwall, B., C. Clemendson, F. Barile, M. C. Calleja, J. Castell, J. Chesne, R. Clothier, R. Curren, P. Dierickx, E. McFarlane-Abdullah, M. Ferro, G. Fiskejo, L. Garza-Ocanas, M. J. Gomez-Lechon, M. Gulden, J. D. Harvell, B. Isomaa, J. Vanus, G. Kerszman, U. Kristen, M. Kunimoto, S. Karenlampi, K. Lavrijsen, L. Lewan, T. Ohno, G. Persoone, R. Roguet, L. Romert, T. Sawyet, H. Seibert, R. Shrivastava, K. Stadtlander, A. Stammati, N. Tanaka, D. Triglia, M. Valentino, E. Walum, X. Wang, F. Zucco and H. Maibach,** Comparison between human skin irritancy and *in vitro* cytotoxicity from 77 systems for the first 12 MEIC chemicals, *In Vitro Toxicology,* Vol. 7, p. 156, 1994.

111. **Gettings, S. D., K. L. Hintze, D. M. Bagley, P. L. Casterton, M. Chudkowski, R. D. Curren, J. L. Demetrulias, L. K. Earl, P. L. Feder, C. L. Galli, R. Gay, S. M. Glaza, V. C. Gordon, Kurtz, P. J., R. A. Lordo, K. D. Marenus, J. Moral, W. J. W. Pape, K. J. Renskers, L. A. Rheins, M. T. Roddy, M. G. Rozen, L. P. Tedeschi and J. Zyracki, J.,** The CTFA Evaluation of Alternatives Program: Phase III, Surfactant-based formulations, *In Vitro Toxicology,* Vol. 7, p. 166, 1994.

112. **Gordon, V. C.,** Evaluation of EYTEX®, a target biomacromolecular *in vitro* method to predict ocular irritation, *In Vitro Toxicology,* Vol. 7, p. 126, 1994.

113. **Gordon, V. C. and S. Boone,** Photoreactivity of chemicals and formulations in the SOLATEX®-PI® system, *In Vitro Toxicology,* Vol. 7, p. 126, 1994.

114. **Harvell, J. D., V. Gordon and H. Maibach,** Use of the Skintex High Sensitivity Assay for predictive assessments of cutaneous fatty acid irritancy in man, *In Vitro Toxicology,* Vol. 6, p. 91, 1993.

115. **Heinze, J., E. T. Spence, S. R. Rachui, M. A. Duke and W. D. Robertson,** Predicting ocular irritation potential of surfactant *in vitro* using the Skin2™ model ZK1200, *In Vitro Toxicology,* Vol. 7, p. 192, 1994.

116. **Hincks, J. R., K. Dahmus and E. I. Fischer,** Additional evaluation and a proposed testing strategy using *in vitro* assays as prescreens for *in vivo* ocular irritation of pharmaceutical products, *In Vitro Toxicology,* Vol. 7, p. 190, 1994.

117. **Juneja, C. and C. W. Stott,** Evaluation of eighteen shampoo formulations using a dual dye cytotoxicity assay, *In Vitro Toxicology,* Vol. 7, p. 168, 1994.

118. **Kalweit, S., R. Besoke, I. Gerner and H. Spielmann,** A national validation project of alternative methods to the Draize rabbit eye test, *Toxicology In Vitro,* Vol. 4, p. 702, 1990.

119. **Koslo, R. J., A. Butler and V. Farina,** Use of Microtox as an *in vitro* adjunct to *in vivo* dermal irritation testing, *The Toxicologist,* Vol. 12, p. 296, 1992.

120. **Kristen, U., F. Barile, P. Dierickx, B. Ekwall and W. G. W. Pape,** Toxicity assessment by the pollen tube growth test (PTG-Test), *In Vitro Toxicology,* Vol. 7, p. 156, 1994.

121. **Kruszewski, F. H., L. J. Moore, K. J. Renskers, M. Balls and M. S. Dickens,** Evaluation of neutral red release assays as predictive tests for the ocular irritancy potential of alcohol and surfactant-based cosmetics formulations, paper presented at *First World Congress on Alternatives and Animal Use in the Life Sciences,* Baltimore, 1993.

122. **Kruszewski, F. H., L. H. Hearn, K. T. Smith, J. J. Teal, V. C. Gordon and M. S. Dickens,** Application of the EYTEX^{TM} system to the evaluation of cosmetic products and their ingredients, *ATLA,* Vol. 20, p. 146, 1992.

123. **Kurtz, P. J., P. I. Feder and R. A. Lordo,** Evaluation of *in vitro* alternatives to the Draize test: Alcohol-containing product. Final report. Battelle, Columbus, Ohio, p. 153, 1990.

124. **Lewis, R. W., J. C. McCall, P. A. Botham and R. Trebilcock,** A comparison of two cytotoxicity tests for predicting ocular irritancy of surfactants, *Toxicology In Vitro,* Vol. 8, p. 867, 1994.

125. **Lewis, R. W., J. C. McCall and P. A. Botham,** Development of an *in vitro* test battery for use within a stepwise approach to the assessment of ocular irritant *in vivo, Toxicology In Vitro,* Vol. 8, p. 865, 1994.

126. **McCormick III, W. C.,** The SDA approach to phase 3 and beyond, *J. Toxicol. Cutan. Ocular Toxicol.,* Vol. 8, p. 115, 1989.

127. **Moore, L. J., K. Rollin, A. W. Hubbard and R. Clothier,** The use of an *in vitro* methodology to predict the irritancy potential of surfactants, paper presented at Practical, *In vitro Toxicology III,* Nottingham, U.K., 1993.

128. **Ohno, Y., T. Kaneko, T. Kobayashi, T. Inoue, Y. Kuroiwa, T. Yoshida, J. Momma, M. Hayashi, J. Alciyarna, T. Atsumi, T. Chiba, T. Endo, A. Fuji, H. Hakishima, H. Kojima, K. Masarnoto, M. Masuda, S. Matsukawa, K. Ohkoshi, J. Okada, K. Sakamoto, K. Takano and A. Takanaka,** First phase validation of the *in vitro* eye irritation tests for cosmetic ingredients, *In Vitro Toxicology*, Vol. 7, p. 147, 1994.

129. **Osborne, R. and M. A. Perkins,** *In vitro* skin irritation testing with human skin cell cultures, *Toxicology In Vitro*, Vol. 5, p. 563, 1991.

130. **Paller, B., G. Ziets, E. T. Spence, S. R. Rachui, M. A. Duke and W. D. Robertson,** Predicting ocular irritation potential of cosmetics and personal care products using two *in vitro* models, *In Vitro Toxicology*, Vol. 7, p. 192, 1994.

131. **Pape, W. J. W., M. Brandt, U. Pfannenbecker and U. Hoppe,** Combined *in vitro* assay for photohaemolysis and haemoglobin oxidation as part of a phototoxicity test system assessed with various phototoxic substances, *Toxicology In Vitro*, Vol. 8, p. 755, 1994.

132. **Pirovano, R., P. Zaninelli, J. Noben, P. Logemann, J. Southee, P. Joller and A. Coquette,** A European interlaboratory evaluation study of an *in vitro* ocular irritation model (Skin2™ Model ZK1100) using 15 chemicals and 3 shampoos, *ATLA*, Vol. 21, p. 81, 1993.

133. **Potthast, J. M., G. Klecak, F. Klammers, W. Hering and J. Ciullo,** Validation study on *in vitro* photoirritation with the 3T3 neutral red assay, the SRBC hemolysis method, the Solatex® Pl kit and the yeast growth inhibition assay, *In Vitro Toxicology*, Vol. 7, p. 198, 1994.

134. **Reece, B., M. Rozen, D. Long and B. Bryan,** Assessment of the ocular irritancy potential of surfactants using several different *in vitro* systems, *In Vitro Toxicology*, Vol. 7, p. 163, 1994.

135. **Roberts, D. A., M. A. Perkins, K. Wallace, G. Mun and R. D. Curren,** Interlaboratory validation of a new *in vitro* tissue equivalent assay (TEA) for eye irritation assessments, *In Vitro Toxicology*, Vol. 7, p. 191, 1994.

136. **Roguet, R., C. Cohen, K. G. Dossou and A. Rougier,** Use of an *in vitro* human reconstituted epidermis to assess the irritative potential of topically applied products, *In Vitro Toxicology*, Vol. 7, p. 166, 1994.

137. **Rougier, A., M. Cottin, O. De Silva, P. Catroux, R. Roguet and K. G. Dossou,** The use of *in vitro* methods in the ocular irritation assessment of cosmetic products, *Toxicology In Vitro*, Vol. 8, p. 893, 1994.

138. **Sanders, C., T. D. Swedlung, R. J. Stephens and P. M. Silber,** Evaluation of six *in vitro* toxicity assays: Comparison with *in vivo* ocular and dermal irritation potential of prototype cosmetic formulations, *The Toxicologist*, Vol. 11, p. 181, 1991.

139. **Sivak, J. G. and K. L. Herbert,** An *in vitro* Draize alternative using the bovine lens: Preliminary validation, *In Vitro Toxicology*, Vol. 7, p. 167, 1994.

140. **Spielmann, H., M. Balls, M. Brandt, B. Döring, H. G. Holzhutter, S. Kalweit, G. Klecak, H. L. Eplattenier, M. Liebsch, W. W. Lovell, T. Maurer, F. Moldenhauer, F. Moore, W. J. W. Pape, U. Pfannenbecker, J. Potthast, O. De Silva, W. Steiling and A. Willshaw,** EEC/Colipa project on *in vitro* phototoxicity testing: First results obtained with a BALB/c 3T3 cell phototoxicity assay, *Toxicology In Vitro*, Vol. 8, p. 793, 1994.

141. **Spielmann, H., S. Kalweit, M. Liebsch, T. Wirnsberger, T. Gerner, E. Bertram-Neis, K. Krauser, R. Kreiling, H. G. Miltenburger, W. G. W. Pape and W. Steiling,** Validation study of alternatives to the Draize eye irritation test in Germany: Cytotoxicity testing and HET-CAM test with 136 industrial chemicals, *Toxicology In Vitro*, Vol. 7, p. 505, 1993.

142. **Steer, S., M. Balls, R. H. Clothier and V. Gordon,** The development and evaluation of *in vitro* tests for photoirritancy, *Toxicology In Vitro*, Vol. 8, p. 719, 1994.

143. **Stott, C. W. and C. Juneja,** A new protocol for the prediction of the ocular irritation potentials of surfactants and shampoos using primary human keratinocytes in culture, paper presented at *First World Congress on Alternatives and Animal Use in the Life Sciences*, Baltimore, 1993.

144. **Sugai, S. and K. Murata,** Investigation of the *in vitro* evaluation method of eye irritation potential using rat red blood cells, *Fragrance Journal*, Vol. 20, p. 47, 1992.

145. **Sussman, R., D. M. Galer, J. W. Harbell, K. A. Wallace and R. D. Curren,** Ability of the bovine corneal opacity and permeability (BCOP) assay and the CAMVA assay to identify potential ocular irritancy of pharmaceutical intermediates, *In Vitro Toxicology*, Vol. 7, p. 165, 1994.

146. **Waters, D. K., D. M. Bagley and B. M. Kong,** Evaluation of the 10-day chorioallantoic membrane vascular assay (10-day CAMVA) as an alternative to eye irritation testing, paper presented at *First World Congress on Alternatives and Animal Use in the Life Sciences*, Baltimore, 1993.

147. **Whittle, E., D. Basketter, M. York, L. Kelly, T. Hall, J. McCall, P. Botham, D. Esdaile and J. Gardner,** Findings of an inter-laboratory trial of the enucleated eye method as an alternative eye irritation test, *Toxicology In Vitro*, in press.

148. **Wilhelm, K. P., M. Samblebe and C. P. Siegers,** Toxicity screening of N-alkyl sulfates in human keratinocytes (HaCaT) in comparison with *in vivo* human irritation test, *The Toxicologist*, Vol. 12, p. 110, 1992.

149. **Silverman, J. and S. Pennisi,** Evaluation of *Tetrahymena thermophila* as an *in vitro* alternative to ocular irritation studies in rabbits, *J. Toxicol. Cutaneous Ocul. Toxicol.*, Vol. 6, p. 33, 1987.

150. **Weterings, P. J. and Y. H. M. Van Erp,** Validation of the BECAM assay — An eye irritancy screening test, in *In Vitro Toxicology Approaches to Validation*, Vol. 5, Goldberg, A. M., Ed., Mary Ann Liebert, New York, 1987, p. 515.

151. **Gordon, V. C. and H. C. Bergman,** EYTEX™: An *in vitro* method for evaluation of ocular irritancy, in *In Vitro Toxicology*, Vol. 5, Goldberg, A. M., Ed., Mary Ann Liebert, New York, 1987, p. 293.

152. **Loprieno, G., G. Boncristiani, E. Bosco, N. Loprieno and M. Nieri,** The Galileo Data Bank of Alternative Methodologies to the Use of Animals in the Toxicity Testing. In *Alternative Methods in Toxicology and the Life Sciences*, Vol. 11, Goldberg, A.M. and Van Zutphen, L.F.M., Eds., Mary Ann Liebert, New York, 1995, p. 463.

APPENDIX A: ACRONYMS

2-AAF = 2-acetylaminofluorene
4-NQO = 4-nitroquinoline-N-oxide
6TG = 6-thioguanine
7,12-DMBA = 7,12-dimethylbenzanthracene
AB = alcian blue
ACD = allergic contact dermatitis
ACP = acid phosphatase
AG = 8-azaguanine
ALP = alkaline phosphatase
ALT = alanine transaminase
AMA = EYTEX® alkaline membrane assay
AST = aspartate transaminase
ATCC = American Type Culture Collection
BrdU = bromodeoxyuridine
CAM = chorioallantoic membrane
CCD camera = coupled charged device camera
CCL = certified cell line
CFU-C = colony-forming unit culture
cpm = counts per minute
CR_{50} = concentration of test chemical resulting in 50% release of ^{51}Cr compared to controls
CTFA = Cosmetic, Toiletry and Fragrance Association
DDS = dual dye staining
DDS_{50} = concentration of test chemical required to damage 50% of the cell population
DIIC = Dictionary of Cosmetic Ingredients
DMEM = Dulbecco's modification of Eagle's medium
dmp = disintegrations per minute
DMSO = dimethylsulphoxide
EBS = Earle's balanced salt solution
EC = Commission of the European Union
EC_{50} = effective concentration fifty
EDE = EYTEX®/Draize equivalent
EDTA = ethylenediaminetetraacetic acid
EES = EYTEX® classification equivalent to the Draize classification
EET = enucleated eye test
EGTA = ethylenebis(oxyethylenenitrilo)tetraacetic acid
EIE = EYTEX® irritation equivalent
EIJ = eye irritation judgment
EU = European Union
FAV = fibronectin-albumin-collagen mixture
FBS = fetal bovine serum
FCS = fetal calf serum
FdU = fluorodeoxyuridine
FRAME = Fund for the Replacement of Animals in Medical Experiments
FRSK = fetal rat skin keratinocytes cell line
GDB = Galileo Data Bank
GGT = γ-glutamyl transpeptidase
GJIC = gap junction intercellular communication
GLC/HPLC = gas-liquid chromatography/high-performance liquid chromatography

HBSS = Hank's balanced salt solution

HCM = high calcium medium

HEPES, buffer = N-(2-hydroxyethyl)piperazine-N¢-(2-ethanesulfonic acid), buffer

HET = hen's egg test

HFC = hair follicle cell

his = histidine

HOMO = highest occupied molecular orbital

HPRT = hypoxanthine guanine phosphoribosyl transferase

HSA = EYTEX® high sensitivity assay

IC_{50} = inhibition concentration 50%

ID_{50} = inhibition dose 50%

$IL1\alpha$ = interleukin lα

IRMA = immunoradiometric assay

KB = kenacid blue

KGM = keratinocyte growth medium

KRH medium = Krebs ringer heps medium

LB = limb cells

LC_{50} = lethal concentration fifty

LCM = low calcium medium

LD_{50} = lethal dose fifty: the dose that kills 50% of treated animals

LDH = lactate dehydrogenase

$LDHR_{50}$ = concentration of test chemical at which 50% of the LDH is released into the medium

LSC = liquid scintillation counting

LUMO = lowest occupied molecular orbital

MEK = mouse skin epidermal keratinocyte

MEM = minimum essential medium Eagle

MES = 2-(N-morpholino)ethanesulfonic acid

MI = mitotic index

MPA = EYTEX® membrane partition assay

MT = microtubule

MTT= 3-(4,5-dimethylthiazol-2-yl)-2,5-diphenyltetrazolium bromide

NCTC = national cancer tissue culture

NEAA = non-essential amino acids

NR = neutral red

NRR = neutral red release

NRR_{50} = concentration of the test chemical that cause 50% loss of the neutral red dye

NRU = neutral red uptake

NRU_{50} = the concentration producing 50% inhibition of growth

NSE = neurone-specific enolase

OD = optical density

OECD = Organization of Economic Cooperation and Development

PBS = Dulbecco's phosphate buffered saline

PEG = polyethylene glycol

PGE_2 = prostaglandin E_2

PHA = phytohemagglutinin

PIPES = piperazine-N-N¢-bis(2-ethanesulfonic acid)

POL_{50} = the concentration of test substance that reduces pollen tube growth to 50% of the control

PSI_{50} = the concentration producing 50% protein synthesis inhibition

PVP= polyvinylpyrrolidone
QSAR = quantitative structure-activity relationship
RCE = relative cloning efficiency
RIA = radioimmunoassay
RMA = EYTEX® rapid membrane assay
SCC = Scientific Committee for Cosmetology of the EC
SCE = sister chromatid exchange
SEM = standard error of the medium
SLRL = sex-linked recessive lethal
SPC = Consumer Policy Service of the EC
STD = EYTEX® standard assay
T_3 = triiodothyronine
T_4 = thyroxine
TCDD = tetrachlorodibenzodioxine
TdR = tritium labeled thymidine
TFT = trifluorothymidine
TK = thymidine kinase
TPA = 12-O-tetradecanoyl-phorbol-13-acetate
tpr = tryptophan
TSH = thyroid stimulating hormone
UDS = unscheduled DNA synthesis
UMA = EYTEX® upright membrane assay
UV = ultraviolet

APPENDIX B: CELL LINES REPORTED IN THE METHODS

3T3-L1, ATCC (CCL 92.1)
3T3-Swiss albino, ATCC (CCL 92)
ARLJ 301-3
BALB/3T3 clone A31, ATCC (CCL 163)
BALB/3T3 clone A31
CH3/10T1/2
CHL
CHO
FaO
FRSK
HEL/30
Hep G-2
HEp-2, ATCC (CCL 23)
IMR-32
L5178Y
L929, ATCC (CCL 1), NCTC 929, clone of strain L
L929, ATCC (CCL 1)
LLC-PK1
P815
SHE
SIRC, ATCC (CCL 60)
V79

Cell Lines	Methods
3T3-L1, ATCC (CCL 92.1)	Neutral red release
	Neutral red uptake
	Total protein content (kenacid blue method, KB)
3T3-Swiss albino, ATCC (CCL 92)	Microtubule disassembly
ARLJ 301-3	Colony formation assay
BALB/3T3 clone A31, ATCC (CCL 163)	Co-culture clonal survival assay
	In vitro mammalian cell transformation test
	LDH release
	Neutral red uptake
	Tetrazolium salt assay (MTT)
	Total protein content (bio-rad assay)
	Total protein content (kenacid blue method, KB)
BALB/3T3 clone A31–1–1	Colony formation assay
	In vitro mammalian cell transformation test
CH3/10T1/2	*In vitro* mammalian cell transformation test
CHL	*In vitro* mammalian cytogenetic test

Cell Lines	Methods
CHO	*In vitro* mammalian cell gene mutation test *In vitro* mammalian cytogenetic test *In vitro* sister chromatid exchange assay
FaO	LDH release Neutral red uptake Tetrazolium salt assay (MTT) Total protein content (bio-rad assay)
FRSK	Colony formation assay
HEL/30	Protein synthesis inhibition
Hep G-2	LDH release
HEp-2, ATCC (CCL 23)	LDH release Total protein content (bio-rad assay)
Human diploid fibroblasts	Unscheduled DNA synthesis
Human fetal dermal fibroblasts, CCRL 1475	Tetrazolium salt assay (MTT) Total protein content (bio-rad assay)
IMR-32	Method for *in vitro* neurotoxicity test
Keratinocytes, Clonetics' Epipack®	Tetrazolium salt assay (MTT) Total protein content (bio-rad assay)
L5178Y	*In vitro* mammalian cell gene mutation test
L929, ATCC (CCL 1)	Agar overlay test Dual dye staining Neutral red uptake Tetrazolium salt assay Total protein content (bio-rad assay)
L929, ATCC (CCL 1), NCTC 929, clone of strain L	Agar overlay test
LLC-PK1	Method for *in vitro* cytotoxicity testing
P815	Chromium-51 release assay
SHE	*In vitro* mammalian cell transformation test
SIRC, ATCC (CCL 60)	Colony formation assay Neutral red uptake Total protein content (kenacid blue method, KB)
V79	Agar overlay test Cell metabolic cooperation assay for analysis of GJIC Cell metabolic cooperation assay Colony formation assay

INDEX

A

Accuracy, 19, 186
Acute cellular lethality, 69–71
Acute toxicity tests, 2, 13, 20–22, 27–29
    alternative methods to animal tests for, 27–29
    assessment of, 27
    eye irritation, 36
    hepatotoxicity, 92–94
Agar Overlay Test (AOT), 28, 48, 49–52, 236
Agrochemicals, 9, see also specific types
Alkaline Unwinding Genotoxicity Test, 48
Allium Test, 48
Alternative methods to animal tests, 25–43, 187–205
    for acute hepatotoxicity tests, 94
    for acute toxicity tests, 27–29
    Agar Overlay Test, 51
    Bio-Rad assay, 173
    Bovine Corneal Opacity and Permeability assay, 52–54
    for carcinogenicity tests, 42–43
    cell lines used in, 252–253
    Cell Metabolic Cooperation assay, 59, 61
    Cell Proliferation assay, 63
    Chorioallantoic Membrane test, 56, 91
    Chromium-51 Release assay, 65
    Co-Culture Clonal Survival assay, 66
    Colony Formation assay, 69
    for cytotoxicity tests, 119
    databases for, 190
    development of, 10
    Dual Dye Staining, 71
    Dye Transfer assay, 73
    Enucleated Eye Test, 77
    Epidermal Slice Technique, 78
    Escherichia coli test, 81
    for eye irritation tests, 31–37
    EYTEX® assay, 86
    future of, 183–184
    Gene Mutation Test, 89, 97
    for genotoxicity tests, 42–43
    Hen's Egg Test, 91
    for hepatotoxicity tests, 94
    for inflammatory mediator measurement, 104
    in vitro, 32–35, see also *In vitro* toxicity tests
    Kenacid Blue method, 175
    LDH release tests, 117
    Lowry method, 177
    for mammalian cell transformation tests, 100
    for mammalian cytogenetic tests, 102
    for micromass teratogenicity tests, 125
    Micronucleus Test, 127
    for microtubule disassembly, 129
    Mitotic Recombination Test, 132
    for mucous membrane irritation tests, 31–37
    for neurotoxicity tests, 121
    Neutral Red Release test, 134
    Neutral Red Uptake test, 140
    Photomutagenicity Bacterial assay, 143
    for photomutagenicity mammalian cytogenetic tests, 110
    Pollen Tube Test, 170
    problems with application of, 207
    Protein Synthesis Inhibition test, 146
    Reverse Mutation assay, 81, 158
    Saccharomyces cerevisiae test, 89, 132
    safety requirements and, 25
    Salmonella typhimurium tests, 158
    for sister chromatid exchange assays, 113
    for skin irritation tests, 29–31
    state of art of, 183–184
    for structure-activity relationship studies, 37–40
    for teratogenicity tests, 41–42
    Tetrahymena thermophyla Motility assay, 162
    Tetrazolium Salt Assay, 166
    for thyrotoxicity tests, 123
    Total Protein Content assay, 173, 175, 177
    for tumor cell attachment inhibition, 115
    Unscheduled DNA Synthesis, 182
    validation studies on, 10, 190–191, 192–199
Ames Test, 48, 186
Animal rights groups, 25
Animals needed for Toxicity tests, 19–20
Animal toxicity tests, 11, 13–23, see also specific types
    accuracy of, 19
    acute, 13, 20–22, 27–29
    alternative methods to, see Alternative methods to animal testing
    animals needed for, 19–20
    for carcinogenicity, 16, 21
    chronic, 15–16, 21, 23, 28
    cytogenetic, 23
    eye, 15, 22
    inhalation, 21, 22
    in vitro, see *In vitro* toxicity tests
    mucous membrane irritation, 20
    for mutagenicity, 17–19, 21
    oral, 21, 22, 23
    predictivity of, 19
    prevalence in, 19
    protocols for, 13
    purpose of, 13
    repeated dose, 21, 23
    reproduction, 16–17, 21, 23
    sensitivity of, 19
    short-term, 26
    skin, 21, 22, 23
    skin absorption, 17, 20
    skin irritation, 13–15, 20, 22, 29–31
    skin sensitization, 20, 21, 23
    specificity of, 19
    subacute, 15–16
    subchronic, 15–16, 20, 21, 23

for teratogenicity, 16–17, 21, 23
toxicokinetic, 17, 21, 23
types of, 10
wastefulness of, 25
Antioxidants, 1, see also specific types
AOT, see Agar Overlay Test; Agar overlay test
Authorized substances, 1, see also specific types

B

Bacteria, 27
BCOP, see Bovine Corneal Opacity and Permeability
Bio-Rad assay, 29, 49, 170–174, 236
Bone marrow cytogenetic tests, 23
Bovine Corneal Opacity and Permeability (BCOP)
    assay, 52–54, 236
Bovine Isolated Cornea Test, 48
Bovine Spermatozoa Cytotoxicity Test, 48

C

CAAT, see Center for Alternatives to Animal Testing
CAM, see Chorioallantoic Membrane
Carcinogenicity tests, 2, 16, 21, 40, 42–43
Cell culture tests, 27, 30, 41, 45
Cell gene mutation test, 95–97, 236
Cell lines, 252–253
Cell Metabolic Cooperation assay, 57–61, 236
Cell migration, 30
Cell proliferation assays, 28, 62–63
Cell surface activities, 29
Cell transformation tests, 18, 98–100, 236
Cellular lethality, 69–71
Cellular toxicity tests, see Cytotoxocity tests
Center for Alternatives to Animal Testing (CAAT),
    207
Chorioallantoic Membrane (CAM) test, 54–56,
    89–92, 236
Chromium-51 Release assay, 63–65, 236
Chronic toxicity tests, 15–16, 21, 23, 28
Cleaners, 9
Co-Culture Clonal Survival assay, 65–66, 236
COLIPA, see European Association of Cosmetic
    Industries
Colony Formation assay, 28, 66–69, 236
Coloring agents, 1, 6, see also specific types
Corneal Cup Model/Leukocyte Chemotactic Factors,
    31
Corneal Opacity Test, 31
Cosmetic, Toiletry and Fragrance Association
    (CTFA), 201
Cosmetic ingredients, see Ingredients
Council Directive 67/548/EEC, 9
Council Directive 76/768/EEC, 1, 2, 6, 20
    Annex III of, 1, 2, 5, 6
    Annex II of, 1, 5, 6, 7
    Annex IV of, 1, 2, 5, 6
    Annex VII of, 1, 2, 5, 6, 7
    Annex VI of, 1, 2, 5, 6, 7
    Article 2 of, 1

Article 4 of, 3
    databases and, 188
    future of, 183, 188
    ingredients defined in, 215
    Sixth Amendment to, 203
    validation studies and, 190, 191, 203
Council Directive 79/831/EEC, 9
Council Directive 86/609/EEC (Protection of
    Animals), 2, 3, 10, 21, 183, 188
Council Directive 87/18/EEC, 5
Council Directive 87/302/EEC, 9, 10, 18
    future of, 183
    in vitro mammalian cell gene mutation test and,
        95–97
    in vitro mammalian cell transformation test and,
        98–100
    in vivo toxicity tests and, 20, 21
    Mitotic Recombination Test and, 111–114
    Saccharomyces cerevisiae test and, 111–114
    Sex-Linked Recessive Lethal test and, 158–160
    sister chromatid exchange assay and, 111–114
    unscheduled DNA Synthesis and, 178–182
Council Directive 91/325/EEC, 10
Council Directive 92/69/EEC, 9, 10, 13, 18
    future of, 183
    in vitro mammalian cytogenetic tests and,
        100–103
    in vivo toxicity tests and, 20, 21
    reverse mutation assay and, 156–158
    Salmonella typhimurium test and, 156–158
    skin irritation tests and, 14
Council Directive 93/21/EEC, 13
Council Directive 93/35/EEC, 1, 3, 4, 188, 190
CTFA, see Cosmetic, Toiletry and Fragrance
    Association
Cultures, see also specific types
    cell, 27, 30, 41, 45
    organ, 41
    tissue, 27, 30–31
    whole embryo, 41–42
Cytogenetic tests, 18, 23, 100–103, 109–111, 236
Cytotoxicity tests, 28, 45
    Bovine Spermatozoa, 48
    flow cytometric, 48
    Galileo Data Bank and, 212–213
    human lymphocyte, 48
    in vitro, 118–119
    methods for, 118–119

D

Databases, see also specific types
    Galileo, see Galileo Data Bank (GDB)
    implementation of, 188–190
    In vitro Techniques in Toxicology (INVITTOX),
        45, 47–49, 189
    ZEBET, 189
DES, see Diethylstilbestrol
Descriptive toxicology, 10–11
Detergents, 9

Diethylstilbestrol (DES), 10
Diffusion cells, 105
Dioxins, 10
DNA damage, 18, 43
DNA fragmentation, 45
DNA repair, 18, 19
DNA synthesis tests, 23, 43, 48, 49, 178–182
  description of method in, 178–181
  Galileo Data Bank and, 236
  reporting of results of, 181–182
Dose
  lethal, 13, 25, 39
  lowest effective, 27
  repeated, 21, 23
Draize Eye Test 1, 49, 146–151, 236
Draize Eye Test 2, 49, 151–155
Draize Eye Test 3, 49, 155–156, 236
Drosophila melanogaster tests, 49, 158–160
Drugs, see also specific types
Dual Dye Staining, 69–71, 236
Dyes, 1, 7, 9, 69–71, 236, see also specific types
Dye Transfer assay, 71–73

E

ECVAM, see European Centre for Validation of
    Alternative Methodologies
EET, see Enucleated Eye Test
Enucleated Eye Test (EET), 73–77
Enucleated Superfused Rabbit Eye System, 31
Enzyme release, 29, 45
Epidermal Slice Technique, 77–78, 236
Escherichia coli test, 18, 79–81, 236
European Association of Cosmetic Industries
    (COLIPA), 2, 20, 191
European Centre for Validation of Alternative
    Methodologies (ECVAM), 188–190, 202,
    203, 207
Eye irritation tests, 31–37, 200, see also Eye toxicity
    tests
  acute, 36
  Tetrahymena thermophyla, 48
Eye toxicity tests, 15, 22, 200, see also Eye irritation
    tests; specific types
  Draize Eye Test 1, 146–151
  Draize Eye Test 2, 151–155
  Draize Eye Test 3, 155–156
EYTEX® assay, 81–87, 236

F

Filters, 1, see also specific types
Flow Cytometric Cytotoxicity Test, 48
Food additives, 5, see also specific types
FRAME, see Fund for the Replacement of Animals
    in Medical Experiments
Fund for the Replacement of Animals in Medical
    Experiments (FRAME), 29, 48
Future, 183–205
  of alternative methods, 183–184

of predictivity of methodology, 186–187
of specificity of methodology, 186
of standardization of methodology, 184–186, 188

G

Galileo Data Bank (GDB), 190, 207–239
  biosystems in, 209, 210
  Chemicals and Formulations archives of, 207–209,
      214, 236
  cytotoxicity tests and, 212–213
  ingredients and, 215
  list of compounds and formulations tested in, 216–
      235
  methods in, 209, 210
  results in, 209
  structure of, 207–209
  tests and relationship design in, 211
  toxicological profiles in, 212
  use of, 209–216
Gap junction intercellular communication (GJIC)
  Cell Metabolic Cooperation assay for analysis of,
      59–61, 236
  Dye Transfer assay for, 71–73
GDB, see Galileo Data Bank
Gene Mutation Test, 18, 87–89, 95–97, 236
General guidelines, 2
Genetic toxicology, 23
Genotoxicity tests, 2, 40, 42–43, 48
GJIC, see Gap junction intercellular communication
Good Laboratory Practice, 5

H

Hair dyes, 1, 7, 9
Hazard identification, 184
HEMP, see Human Embryonic Palatal Mesenchyme
Hen's Egg Test (HET), 48, 49, 89–92, 236
Hepatoma Cell Cultures, 48
Hepatotoxicity tests, 48, 92–94
HET, see Hen's Egg Test
Household products, 9, see also specific types
Human data, 2
Human Embryonic Palatal Mesenchyme (HEMP)
    cells, 42
Human Lymphocyte Cytotoxicity test, 48

I

ICSU, see International Council of Scientific Unions
ILO, see International Labor Organization
Industrial solvents, 9, see also specific types
Inflammatory mediator measurement, 103–104
Ingredients, 5–7, see also specific types
  defined, 4, 5, 215
  function of, 4
  Galileo Data Bank and, 215
  identity of, 4
  inventory of, 4
Inhalation toxicity tests, 13, 21, 22

International Council of Scientific Unions (ICSU), 27
International Labor Organization (ILO), 27
International Program on Chemical Safety (IPCS), 27
Inventory of ingredients, 4
In vitro Techniques in Toxicology (INVITTOX)
      database, 45, 47–49, 189
In vitro toxicity tests, 22, 26, 45–182, see also
      specific types
  acute hepatotoxicity, 92–94
  Agar Overlay Test, 28, 48, 49–52, 236
  Alkaline Unwinding Genotoxicity Test, 48
  Allium Test, 48
  alternative methods to animal tests for, 32–35
  Ames Test, 48
  Bio-Rad assay, 49, 170–174, 236
  Bovine Corneal Opacity and Permeability assay,
      52–54, 236
  Bovine Isolated Cornea Test, 48
  Bovine Spermatozoa Cytotoxicity Test, 48
  cell gene mutation, 95–97
  Cell Metabolic Cooperation assay, 57–61, 236
  Cell Proliferation assay, 28, 62–63
  cell transformation, 18, 98–100, 236
  Chorioallantoic Membrane test, 54–56, 89–92, 236
  Chromium-51 Release assay, 63–65, 236
  Co-Culture Clonal Survival assay, 65–66, 236
  Colony Formation assay, 28, 66–69, 236
  cytogenetic, 18, 100–103
  cytotoxicity, 118–119
  databases for, see Galileo Data Bank (GDB);
      In vitro Techniques in Toxicology
  development of, 204
  Draize Eye Test 1, 49, 146–151, 236
  Draize Eye Test 2, 49, 151–155
  Draize Eye Test 3, 49, 155–156, 236
  Drosophila melanogaster tests, 49, 158–160
  Dual Dye Staining, 69–71, 236
  Dye Transfer assay, 71–73
  Enucleated Eye Test (EET), 73–77
  Epidermal Slice Technique, 77–78, 236
  Escherichia coli test, 18, 79–81, 236
  EYTEX® assay, 81–87, 236
  future of, 184
  Gene Mutation Test, 18, 87–89, 95–97
  genotoxicity, 2, 40, 42–43
  Hen's Egg Test, 48, 49, 89–92, 236
  hepatotoxicity, 48, 92–94
  Human Lymphocyte Cytotoxicity test, 48
  inflammatory mediator measurement in, 103–104
  in vivo tests vs., 213–216
  Isolated Rat Glomeruli and Proximal Tubules, 48
  Kenacid Blue method, 29, 48, 49, 174–176, 236
  LDH release, 28, 49, 116–118, 236
  Lowry method, 29, 49, 176–178, 236
  mammalian cell gene mutation, 95–97
  mammalian cell transformation, 18, 98–100, 236
  mammalian cytogenetic, 100–103, 109–111
  micromass teratogenicity, 123–125
  Micronucleus Test, 125–127, 236
  Microtox Acute Toxicity Test, 236
  microtubule disassembly and, 127–129
  Mitotic Recombination Test, 18, 49, 129–132
  Model Cavity method, 48
  neurotoxicity, 23, 119–121
  Neutral Red Release test, 29, 48, 49, 132–134,
      236
  Neutral Red Uptake test, see Neutral Red Uptake
      (NRU) test
  percutaneous absorption tests, 105–108, 236
  Photomutagenicity Bacterial assay, 141–143
  photomutagenicity mammalian cytogenetic tests,
      109–111
  Pollen Tube Test, 49, 167–170, 236
  Polymorphonuclear Leukocyte Locomotion, 48
  predictivity of, 205, 213–216
  Protein Synthesis Inhibition test, 49, 143–146, 236
  protocols for, 46
  Rabbit Isolated Terminal Ileum test, 48
  Reverse Mutation assay, 18, 79–81, 156–158, 236
  Saccharomyces cerevisiae test, 49, 87–89,
      129–132
  Salmonella typhimurium tests, 49, 156–158, 236
  Sex-linked Recessive Lethal Test, 49, 158–160
  sister chromatid exchange assays, 18, 43, 111–114,
      236
  synthesis of, 184
  Tetrahymena thermophyla Motility assay, 29, 49,
      160–162, 236
  Tetrahymena thermophyla Ocular Irritancy Test,
      48
  Tetrazolium Salt Assay, 28, 48, 49, 162–167, 236
  thyrotoxicity, 121–123
  Total Protein Content assays, see Total Protein
      Content assays
  tumor cell attachment inhibition and, 114–116, 236
  Unscheduled DNA Synthesis, see Unscheduled
      DNA Synthesis (UDS)
  Whole Rat Brain Reaggregate Culture, 48
INVITTOX, see *In vitro* Techniques in Toxicology
In vivo toxicity tests, 20–23, 28, 201, 202
  in vitro tests vs., 213–216
  for mutagenicity, 19
  predictivity of, 213–216
IPCS, see International Program on Chemical Safety
Isolated Rat Glomeruli and Proximal Tubules, 48

K

KB, see Kenacid Blue
Kenacid Blue (KB) method, 29, 48, 49, 174–176, 236
Keratinization, 30

L

LD, see Lethal dose
LDH release tests, 28, 49, 116–118, 236
LED, see Lowest effective dose
Legislative basis, 1–5
Lethal dose (LD), 13, 25, 39
L'Oreal, 191, 200–202

Lowest effective dose (LED), 27
Lowry method, 29, 49, 176–178, 236

M

Mammalian cell gene mutation test, 95–97, 236
Mammalian cell transformation tests, 18, 98–100, 236
Mammalian cytogenetic tests, 100–103, 236
Manufacturing methods, 4
Mechanistic toxicology, 10
MED-LINE, 188
Metabolic pathways, 29
Methodology predictivity, 19, 186–187, 205, 213–216
Methodology specificity, 19, 186
Methodology standardization, 184–186, 188
Methylmercury poisoning, 10
Microbiological specifications, 4
Micromass teratogenicity tests, 123–125
Micronucleus Test, 125–127, 236
Microtox Acute Toxicity Test, 236
Microtubule disassembly, 127–129
Minamata disease, 10
Mitotic Recombination Test, 18, 49, 129–132
Model Cavity method, 48
MOT, see Mouse ovarian tumor
Mouse heritable assays, 21, 23
Mouse ovarian tumor (MOT) cells, 42
Mouse spot test, 21, 23
MTT, see Tetrazolium Salt Assay
Mucous membrane irritation tests, 2, 20, 31–37
Mutagenicity tests, 2, 21, 40, 42
    animal, 17–19
    in vivo, 19
    photo-, 2, 109–111, 141–143
Mutation tests, see also specific types
    gene, 18, 87–89, 95–97, 236
    mammalian cell gene, 95–97, 236
    reverse, 18, 79–81, 156–158, 236

N

National Toxicology Program (NTP), 42
Neurotoxicity tests, 23, 119–121
Neutral Red Release (NRR) test, 29, 48, 49, 132–134, 236
Neutral Red Uptake (NRU) test, 28, 48, 49, 134–141
    Galileo Data Bank and, 236
    method used in, 134–140
    reporting of results of, 140
NRR, see Neutral Red Release
NRU, see Neutral Red Uptake
NTP, see National Toxicology Program

O

Ocular, see Eye
OECD, see Organization for Economic Cooperation and Development
Oral toxicity tests, 13, 21, 22, 23
Organ cultures, 41

Organic compounds, 9, see also specific types
Organization for Economic Cooperation and Development (OECD), 3, 9, 22–23
Organophosphorus substances, 23, see also specific types

P

Paints, 9
Percutaneous absorption tests, 105–108, 236
Phagocytosis, 30
Photoallergic reactions, 14
Photomutagenicity, 2
Photomutagenicity Bacterial assay, 141–143
Photomutagenicity mammalian cytogenetic tests, 109–111
Phototoxicity tests, 2, 14–15, 48
Physicochemical specifications, 4, 30, 207
P.I., see Product information
Pollen Tube Test, 49, 167–170, 236
Polymorphonuclear Leukocyte Locomotion, 48
Precipitation test systems, 30
Predictivity, 19, 186–187, 205, 213–216
Preservatives, 1, 6, 7, see also specific types
Prevalence, 19
Procter & Gamble, 200
Product information, 4, 5
Protection of Animals (Council Directive 86/609/EEC), 2, 3, 10, 21, 183, 188
Protein content tests, 29, 45, 170–174
    total, see Total Protein Content
Protein Synthesis Inhibition test, 49, 143–146, 236
Protocols, 13, 46

Q

QSAR, see Quantitative structure-activity relationship
Qualitative composition, 4
Qualitative data, 9
Quantitative data, 4, 9
Quantitative structure-activity relationship (QSAR) studies, 37–40
    chemical descriptors for, 38, 40
    Draize Eye Test 1 and, 146–151, 236
    Draize Eye Test 2 and, 151–155
    Draize Eye Test 3 and, 155–156, 236
    Galileo Data Bank and, 207
    techniques in, 39–40
    toxicological data and, 38–39

R

Rabbit Isolated Terminal Ileum test, 48
Raw materials, 4
Receptor binding, 39
Receptor fluid, 106
Repeated dose toxicity tests, 21, 23
Reporting
    of acute hepatotoxicity test results, 94
    of Agar Overlay Test results, 51

of Bio-Rad assay results, 173
of Bovine Corneal Opacity and Permeability assay
    results, 52–54
of Cell Metabolic Cooperation assay results,
    59, 61
of Cell Proliferation assay results, 63
of Chorioallantoic Membrane test results, 56, 91
of Chromium-51 Release assay results, 64–65
of Co-Culture Clonal Survival assay results, 66
of Colony Formation assay results, 68–69
of cytotoxicity test results, 119
of *Drosophila melanogaster* test results, 160
of Dual Dye Staining results, 70–71
of Dye Transfer assay results, 73
of Enucleated Eye Test results, 76–77
of Epidermal Slice Technique results, 78
of *Escherichia coli* test results, 80–81
of EYTEX® assay results, 86
of Gene Mutation Test results, 89, 97
of Hen's Egg Test results, 91
of inflammatory mediator measurement results,
    104
of Kenacid Blue method results, 175
of LDH release test results, 117
of Lowry method results, 177
of mammalian cell transformation test results,
    99–100
of mammalian cytogenetic test results, 102
of micromass teratogenicity test results, 125
of Micronucleus Test results, 127
of microtubule disassembly results, 129
of Mitotic Recombination Test results, 131–132
of neurotoxicity test results, 121
of Neutral Red Release test results, 134
of Neutral Red Uptake test results, 140
of Photomutagenicity Bacterial assay results, 142–
    143
of photomutagenicity mammalian cytogenetic test
    results, 110
of Pollen Tube Test results, 169–170
of Protein Synthesis Inhibition test results, 146
of Reverse Mutation assay results, 80–81, 158
of *Saccharomyces cerevisiae* test results, 89,
    131–132
of *Salmonella typhimurium* test results, 158
of Sex-linked Recessive Lethal Test results, 160
of sister chromatid exchange assay results, 113
of *Tetrahymena thermophyla* Motility assay
    results, 161–162
of Tetrazolium Salt Assay results, 166
of thyrotoxicity test results, 122–123
of Total Protein Content assay results, 173, 175,
    177
of tumor cell attachment inhibition results, 115
of Unscheduled DNA Synthesis results, 181–182
Reproduction toxicity tests, 2, 16–17, 21, 23
Respiratory tract irritation, 39
Reverse Mutation assay, 18, 79–81, 156–158, 236
Risk assessment, 184, 207

S

Saccharomyces cerevisiae test, 18, 49, 87–89, 129–132
Safety evaluation, 4–5, 25, 184
Salmonella typhimurium tests, 18, 39, 49, 156–158,
    236
SAR, see Structure-activity relationship
SCC, see Scientific Committee on Cosmetology
SCE, see Sister chromatid exchange
Scientific Committee on Cosmetology (SCC), 1–2, 4,
    6, 7, 20
  databases and, 189
  validation studies and, 191
Scientific Committee on Problems of the
    Environment (SCOPE), 27
SCOPE, see Scientific Committee on Problems of the
    Environment
Sensitivity, 19, 186
Sex-linked Recessive Lethal Test in *Drosophila*
    melanogaster, 49, 158–160
Shampoo, 9
Sister chromatid exchange (SCE) assays, 18, 43, 111–
    114, 236
Skin absorption tests, 2, 17, 20, 39
Skin corrosive potential, 77–78
Skin explants, 30–31
Skin irritation tests, 2, 13–15, 20, 22, 29–31
Skin membranes, 106
Skin metabolism, 106
Skin sensitization tests, 2, 14, 20, 21, 23
Skin toxicity tests, 13, 21–23, 48, see also specific
    types
Solvents, 9, see also specific types
Specificity of methodology, 19, 186
Standardization of methodology, 184–186, 188
Structure-activity relationship (SAR) studies, 37–40
  quantitative, see Quantitative structure-activity
    relationship (QSAR)
Subacute toxicity tests, 15–16
Subchronic toxicity test, 2
Subchronic toxicity tests, 15–16, 20, 21, 23
Sunscreens, 7, 9
Surfactants, 201

T

Tanning agents, 7
Teratogenicity tests, 2, 21, 23, 39, 41–42
  animal, 16–17
  micromass, 123–125
Tetrahymena motility assays, 29, 236
Tetrahymena thermophyla Motility assay, 29, 49,
    160–162, 236
Tetrahymena thermophyla Ocular Irritancy Test, 48
Tetrazolium Salt Assay (MTT), 28, 48, 49, 162–167,
    236
Thalidomide, 10
"Three R" principle, 184
Thyrotoxicity tests, 121–123

Tissue culture methods, 27, 30–31
Total Protein Content assays, 29, see also specific
    types
  Bio-Rad assay, 49, 170–174, 236
  Kenacid Blue Method, 48, 49, 174–176, 236
  Lowry Method, 49, 176–178, 236
Toxicity tests, see also specific types
  accuracy of, 19
  acute, see Acute toxicity tests
  animal, see Animal toxicity tests
  for carcinogenicity, 2, 16, 21, 40, 42–43
  chronic, 15–16, 21, 23, 28
  cyto-, see Cytotoxicity tests
  cytogenetic, 18, 23, 100–103, 109–111, 236
  eye, see Eye toxicity tests
  hepato-, 92–94
  inhalation, 13, 21, 22
  in vitro, see *In vitro* toxicity tests
  in vivo, see *In vivo* toxicity tests
  for mutagenicity, see Mutagenicity tests
  for mutations, see Mutation tests
  neuro-, 23, 119–121
  ocular, see Eye toxicity tests
  oral, 13, 21–23
  photo-, 2, 14–15, 48
  predictivity of, 19
  prevalence in, 19
  purpose of, 9, 13
  repeated dose, 21, 23
  reproduction, 2, 16–17, 21, 23
  sensitivity of, 19
  short-term, 26
  skin, 13, 21–23
  skin absorption, 17
  skin irritation, 13–15, 22, 29–31
  skin sensitization, 21, 23
  specificity of, 19
  subacute, 15–16
  subchronic, 2, 15–16, 21, 23
  for teratogenicity, see Teratogenicity tests
  thyro-, 121–123

  toxicokinetic, 2, 17, 21, 23
Toxicokinetic tests, 2, 17, 21, 23
Toxicology
  data in, 38–39
  descriptive, 10–11
  genetic, 23
  mechanistic, 10
  role of, 9–11
Tumor cell attachment inhibition, 114–116, 236
Turbidity, 30

U

UDS, see Unscheduled DNA Synthesis
Ultraviolet filters, 1
Undesirable effects, 5
UNEP, see United Nations Environmental Program
United Nations Environmental Program (UNEP), 27
Unscheduled DNA Synthesis (UDS), 43, 48, 49,
    178–182
  description of method in, 178–181
  Galileo Data Bank and, 236
  reporting of results of, 181–182

V

Validation studies, 10, 190–191
  Galileo Data Bank and, 207
  list of chemicals and products tested on, 192–199
"Very toxic" classification, 13
Volatile organic compounds, 9, see also specific types

W

Whole embryo cultures, 41–42
Whole Rat Brain Reaggregate Culture, 48

Z

ZEBET database, 189